SAUNDERS' QUESTION-COMPENDS, NO. 7

ESSENTIALS OF MATERIA MEDICA, THERAPEUTICS AND PRESCRIPTION WRITING

ARRANGED IN THE FORM OF QUESTIONS AND ANSWERS

PREPARED ESPECIALLY FOR STUDENTS OF MEDICINE

SAUNDERS' QUESTION-COMPENDS, NO. 7

ESSENTIALS
OF
MATERIA MEDICA, THERAPEUTICS AND PRESCRIPTION WRITING

ARRANGED IN THE FORM OF QUESTIONS AND ANSWERS

PREPARED ESPECIALLY FOR STUDENTS OF MEDICINE

BY

HENRY MORRIS, M.D.

Fellow of the College of Physicians of Philadelphia; Associate Member of the Association of Military Surgeons of the United States.

SEVENTH EDITION, THOROUGHLY REVISED

And adapted to the Eighth Revision (1905) of the United States Pharmacopoeia.

By

W. A. Bastedo, Ph. G., M.D.

Instructor in Materia Medica and Pharmacology at Columbia University (College of Physicians and Surgeons), New York; Assistant Attending Physician to the Roosevelt Hospital Dispensary and to the Vanderbilt Clinic

GYAN

Published by

GYAN

Gyan Publishing House
5, Ansari Road
Daryaganj, New Delhi-110002
Phone: 011-47034999, 9811692060
E-mail: books@gyanbooks.com

Distribution Network
gyanbooks.com
India, USA, Canada, UK, Australia, France

ISBN : 978-81-212-2227-3 (HB)
First Published, 1906

2nd Impression 2021

Printed at: Gyan Press, Delhi.

Essentials
of
Materia Medica Therapeutics and Prescription Writing
Arranged in the Form of
Questions and Answers
Prepared Especially for Students of Medicine
Author: Henry Morris

SAUNDERS' QUESTION-COMPENDS, No. 7

ESSENTIALS

OF

MATERIA MEDICA, THERAPEUTICS

AND PRESCRIPTION WRITING

ARRANGED IN THE FORM OF

QUESTIONS AND ANSWERS

PREPARED ESPECIALLY FOR STUDENTS OF MEDICINE

BY

HENRY MORRIS, M.D.

Fellow of the College of Physicians of Philadelphia; Associate Member of the Association of Military Surgeons of the United States.

SEVENTH EDITION, THOROUGHLY REVISED

And adapted to the Eighth Revision (1905) of the United States Pharmacopoeia.

BY

W. A. BASTEDO, PH.G., M.D.

Instructor in Materia Medica and Pharmacology at Columbia University (College of Physicians and Surgeons), New York; Assistant Attending Physician to the Roosevelt Hospital Dispensary and to the Vanderbilt Clinic

PHILADELPHIA AND LONDON

W. B. SAUNDERS COMPANY

1906

To the Memory of

DR. THEODORE HORWITZ,

WHOSE EARLY DEATH

DEPRIVED THE MEDICAL PROFESSION OF AN EARNEST

AND TALENTED WORKER,

THIS BOOK IS AFFECTIONATELY INSCRIBED

BY HIS FRIEND,

THE AUTHOR.

PREFACE TO THE SEVENTH EDITION.

In the present revision, the definitions, nomenclature, and official preparations have been made to conform with those of the Eighth Decennial Revision of the United States Pharmacopœia, which became the official standard on Sept. 1, 1905. In addition articles have been inserted on Diphtheria Antitoxin, Thyroid Extract, and Organotherapy; and a few of the obsolete drugs have been dropped.

W. A. BASTEDO.

PREFACE TO THE FIRST EDITION.

The object of this little book is, not to replace or attempt to replace with the student the larger text-books on Materia Medica, but simply to give him, in condensed form, the principles of this branch of medicine, without a knowledge of which he can neither pass his final examinations, nor practice his profession intelligently.

The author hopes that, if properly used, this book will be of service to the student and young practitioner, but he is sure, from his experience as a teacher, that neither this nor any other "compend" will suffice to form the groundwork of what is really the study of a lifetime—the Science of Medicine.

In regard to the classification of drugs, he would say that this work was commenced before the excellent arrangement contained in the last edition of Prof. Wood's Therapeutics was published, and not being satisfied with any of the groupings which he had seen, he was induced to adopt a classification based on therapeutic rather than physiological grounds, which, however, he is pleased to think agrees very nearly with that of the latest edition of Wood. In conclusion he must acknowledge his indebtedness not only to the standard text-books, such as the admirable works of Wood, Bartholow, Ringer, Lauder Brunton and many others, but also to many writers in the medical journals, both of this and other countries, to whom want of space has prevented him from giving due credit in the appropriate place. He must also acknowledge the kindness of his friend, Dr. Henry D. Moore, to whom he is indebted for the preparation of the index.

Believing that the critic is the best friend of the medical author, he will thankfully receive any criticisms or hints from either public or private sources.

HENRY MORRIS.

313 South 16th St., Philadelphia.

CONTENTS

PAGES

DEFINITIONS.—(Materia Medica, Pharmacy, Pharmacology, Therapeutics, Remedies, Pharmacopeia, Dispensatory, Official Preparations) 17-24

WEIGHTS AND MEASURES.—(Troy or Apothecaries' weights, Wine or Apothecaries' measures, Metric or decimal system of weights, Tables showing the value of Apothecaries' weight in the metric system, Tables showing the value of Apothecaries' measure in the metric system, Approximate measures) 24-26

PRESCRIPTION WRITING.—(Purposes for which medicines are combined, Precautions to be observed in prescription writing, Component parts of a prescription, Method of writing a prescription, Calculation of dose, General rules for dosage) 26-31

INFLUENCES THAT MODIFY EFFECTS OF MEDICINES.—(Age, Sex, Idiosyncrasy, Constitution, Habitual Use, Condition of digestive and absorbent systems, Diseases, Mode of administration) 31, 32

ADMINISTRATION OF MEDICINES.—(Enepidermic, Epidermic, Endermic, and Hypodermic methods, By the mucous membranes, By intravenous injection) 32

CLASSIFICATION OF MEDICINES 33, 34

SYSTEMIC MEDICINES 34-247

MEDICINES ACTING ON THE BODY AT LARGE BY THEIR INFLUENCE ON DIGESTION, NUTRITION (tissue waste and repair), AND CALORIFICATION 34-88

Digestants—(Pepsin, Ingluvin, Pancreatin, Papain) . 34-36

Tonics—(Quassia, Gentian, Calumba, Chirata, Berberis Serpentaria, Eucalyptus, Prunus Virginiana, Anthemis, Matricaria, Eupatorium, Cascarilla, Absinthium, Cinchona and its alkaloids, Hydrastis, Preparations of Iron and of Manganese, Phosphorus, Mineral acids, Lactic acid) . . . 36-59

PAGES

Alteratives—(Preparations of Mercury and of Gold, Iodin, the Iodids, Arsenical preparations, Cod-liver oil, the Phosphates and Hypophosphites, Calcium chlorid. Ammonium chlorid, Colchicum, Sarsaparilla, Guaiac, Mezereum, Calendula, Sassafras, Stillingia, Lappa) . . . 59–77

Antipyretics—(Antipyrin, Acetanilid, Phenacetin, Phenocoll, Quinin, Salicin, the Salicylates, Salol, Salophen, Guaiacol, Resorcin, Hydroquinon, Pyrocatechin, Chinolin, Thallin, Kairin) 77–88

MEDICINES ACTING ON THE BODY BY THEIR EFFECTS ON THE VARIOUS ORGANS 89–204

ON THE NERVOUS SYSTEM 89–146

Hypnotics—(Opium and its alkaloids, Chloral, Chloralamid, the Bromids, Scopolamin hydrobromid, Hyoscin, Paraldehyd, Sulphonal, Trional, Tetronal, Urethran, Cannabis indica, Humulus, Lactucarium) 89–106

Mydriatic Anodyns — (Belladonna, Homatropin hydrobromid, Stramonium, Hyoscyamus, Scopola, Coca, and their alkaloids) 106–116

Anesthetics—(Ether, Chloroform, Nitrous oxid, Bromoform, Methylene bichlorid, Ethyl bromid.) *Local Anesthetics*—(Cold, Rhigolene, Ether, Ethyl chlorid, Cocain, Eucain, Menthol, Guaiacol, Tincture of aconite) 116–126

Antispasmodics—(Musk, Sumbul, Valerian, the Valerianates, Asafetida, Camphor, Ethereal oil, Hoffmann's anodyn, Cypripedium, Scutellaria) 126–131

Excitomotors—(Nux vomica and its alkaloids) 132–135

Depressomotors—(Physostigma, Chloral, the Bromids, the Nitrites, Gelsemium, Prussic acid, the Cyanids, Oil of bitter almond, Lobelia, Conium, Woorara, Tobacco) . 135–146

ON THE ORGANS OF CIRCULATION 146–169

Stimulants—(Alcohol, Ether, Ammonium, Atropin, Digitalis, Suprarenal extract, Caffein, Adonidin, Strophanthus, Spartein, Cimicifuga, Convallaria) 146–160

Sedatives—(Antimonial preparations, Aconite and its alkaloids, Veratrum, Veratrin, Gelsemium, Arnica, the Vegetable acids) 161–167

ON THE SEXUAL ORGANS 169–178

Aphrodisiacs—(The Tonics generally, especially Phosphorus, Zinc phosphid, and Iron. The Phosphates and Hypophosphites, Gold, Arsenic, Cod-liver oil, Opium, Alcohol, Cannabis indica, Musk, Camphor, Nux vomica, Stimulants, Hamamelis, Ergot, Cantharides, Myrrh) . . 169

PAGES

Anaphrodisiacs—(Nauseants, Purgatives, Opium (full doses), the Bromids, Monobromated camphor, Iodin and the Iodids, Potassium nitrate, Ammonium chlorid, Belladonna, Tobacco, Conium, Cardiac sedatives, Digitalis, Cocain, Sabal) 170

Oxytocics—(Ergot, Hydrastis, Hydrastinin hydrochlorid, Stypticin, Cotton-root bark, Quinin) 170–175

Uterine Sedatives—(Opium, Cannabis indica, the Bromids, Chloral, Tartar emetic, Ether, Viburnum prunifolium, Viburnum opulus) 175, 176

Emmenagogues—(Preparations of Iron, of Arsenic, and of Manganese, Myrrh, Aloes, the Salines, Potassium permanganate, Savin, Tansy, Apiol, Cantharides, Guaiac) . 176–178

ON THE ALIMENTARY CANAL 178–204

Emetics—(Ipecac, Apomorphin, Mustard, Zinc sulphate, Copper sulphate, Alum, Turpeth mineral, Tartar emetic) 178–182

Gastric Sedatives—(Calomel, Ice, Lime-water, Brandy, Champagne, Morphin, Diluted hydrocyanic acid, Creasote, Resorcin, Bismuth, Sodium bicarbonate, Carbolic acid, Thymol, Sulphurous acid, the Sulphites, Charcoal, Opium, the Bromids, Nux vomica, Cerium oxalate, Ipecac (minute doses), Fowler's solution, Counterirritation) . . 182

Carminatives—(Asafetida, Eucalyptus, Ether, Capsicum, Pepper, Cinnamon, Nutmeg, Mace, Cloves, Allspice, Ginger, Cardamom, Aromatic powder, Aromatic fluid extract, Oil of cajuput, Calamus, Oil of gaultheria, Oil of lavender-flowers, Peppermint, Spearmint, Oil of rosemary, Pennyroyal, Horehound, Sage, Oil of thyme, Fennel, Caraway, Anise, Coriander, Orange-peel, Orange-flowers, Vanilla, Oil of turpentine) 183–189

Cathartics—(Tamarind, Manna, Cassia fistula, Frangula, Cascara sagrada, Castor oil, Sulphur, Rhubarb, Juglans, Aloes, Senna, Leptandra, Euonymus, Mercurials, Magnesia, Magnesium carbonate, Epsom salt, Effervescent magnesium sulphate, Magnesium citrate solution, Glauber's salt, Sodium phosphate and pyrophosphate, Potassium sulphate, Potassium bitartrate, Rochelle salt, Seidlitz powder, Manganese sulphate, Jalap, Bryony, Podophyllum, Iris, Scammony, Colocynth, Gamboge, Compound cathartic pills, Vegetable cathartic pills, Elaterin, Croton oil, Enemata) 189–201

Anthelmintics—(Spigelia, Chenopodium, Santonica and Santonin, Aspidium, Pomegranate and Pelletierin, Cusso, Pumpkin-seed, Kamala, Oil of turpentine, Calomel, Thymol, Sulphur, Infusion of quassia, Sodium chlorid, Naphtol, Tannin, Alum-water, Lime-water, Injections of sweet oil) 201–204

PAGES

MEDICINES ACTING ON THE BODY BY THEIR EFFECT ON THE VARIOUS SECRETIONS AND EXCRETIONS . . 204–247

Diuretics—(Solution of potassa, Potassium carbonate, Potassium bicarbonate, Potassium citrate, Potassium acetate, Cream of tartar, Potassium nitrate, Potassium chlorate, Lithium carbonate, Lithium citrate, Lithium benzoate, Sodium acetate, Strontium lactate, Squill, Digitalis, Caffein, Theobromin, Theophyllin, Sodiotheobromin salicylate, Apocynum, Broom, Dandelion, Sweet spirit of niter, Mercurials, Buchu, Pareira, Uva ursi, Chimaphila, Triticum, Oil of juniper, Oil of erigeron, Oil of santal, Corn-silk, Turpentine, Copaiba, Cubeb, Matico, Cantharides, Hexamethylene, Methylene blue) 204–220

Diaphoretics—(Ipecac, Dover's powder, Antimonials, Aconite, Veratrum, Salicylic acid, Potassium citrate, Spirit of Mindererus, Sweet spirit of niter, Pilocarpus) 220–223

Expectorants—(Ipecac, Apomorphin, Tartar emetic, Pilocarpin, Lobelia, Grindelia, Ammonium chlorid, Senega, Quillaja, Quebracho, Eriodictyon, Garlic, Sanguinaria, Ammoniac, Benzoin, Peruvian balsam, Balsam of tolu, Tar, Terpin hydrate, Terebene, Squill, Turpentine, Eucalyptus, Serpentaria, Prunus Virginiana) 223–231

Astringents—(Tannic acid, Gallic acid, Nutgall, Gambir, Catechu, Kino, Krameria, Logwood, White oak bark, Geranium, Witch-hazel, Red rose, Sumach, the Lead salts, Alum, Aluminum hydroxid, Aluminum sulphate, the Salts of copper, of zinc, of silver, and of bismuth, Cerium oxalate) 231–245

Antacids—(Solution of potassa, Spirit and aromatic spirit of ammonia, Solution of sodium hydroxid, Monohydrated sodium carbonate, Sodium bicarbonate, Sodium citrate, Lime-water, Carron oil, Syrup of lime, Precipitated calcium carbonate, Prepared chalk and its preparations) 245–247

TOPICAL MEDICINES 247–274

ANTISEPTICS—(Solution of hydrogen dioxid, Potassium permanganate, Chlorin water, Chlorinated lime, Labarraque's solution, Mercuric chlorid, Bromin, Iodin, Mercuric oxid, Iodoform, Aristol, Europhen, Iodol, Losophan, Nosophen, Sulphurous acid, the Sulphites and sulphids, Boric acid and the borates, Carbolic acid and the Sulphocarbolates, Cresol, Creosote, Benzoic acid and the benzoates, Naphtalin, Betanaphtol, Formaldehyd, the Antipyretics, Antiseptic oils, Thymol) 247–260

IRRITANTS 260–266

Rubefacients—(Mustard, Capsicum, Oil of turpentine, Ammonia) 260–262

PAGES

Vesicants—(Cantharides, Potato fly, Ammonia) 262, 263

Suppurants—(Croton oil, Antimonial ointment) 264

Escharotics—Potassium hydroxid, sodium hydroxid, Arsenous acid, Bromin, Zinc chlorid, Acid nitrate of mercury, Corrosive sublimate, Potassium dichromate, Chromic acid, the Mineral acids, Organic acid, Silver nitrate, Copper sulphate, Alum) 264-266

DEMULCENTS—(Water, Acacia, Tragacanth, Slippery-elm bark, Marshmallow, Flax-seed, Sassafras pith, Licorice-root, Irish moss, Starch, Kaolin, Talc, Lycopodium) . . 267-270

EMOLLIENTS—(Lard, Lanolin, Wool-fat, Suet, Spermaceti, Wax, Oleic acid, Glycerin, Glycerinated gelatin, Cacao butter, Cotton-seed oil, Petrolatum, the Demulcents) . 270-272

PROTECTIVES—(Plasters, Ointments, Plaster of Paris, Collodion, India-rubber) 272, 273

COLORING AGENTS—(Cochineal, Red saunders) 273

SWEETENING AGENT—(Saccharin) 273

SERUM THERAPY—(Diphtheria antitoxin) 274

ORGANOTHERAPY—(Suprarenal gland, Thyroid gland) . . . 274

Index 275

ESSENTIALS OF

MATERIA MEDICA AND THERAPEUTICS.

What is meant by the term "materia medica"?

Materia medica is that division of medical science which treats of all that relates to the medicines employed in the treatment of disease. It embraces the study of the source of remedies, their physical and chemic properties, their action in medicinal doses on the human body both in health and in disease, their poisonous effects and the means by which they may be antagonized, and the methods of preparing and administering them. It is closely allied to botany, mineralogy, zoölogy, chemistry, physiology, and pathology.

How may this knowledge be subdivided?

Into *materia medica proper, pharmacy, pharmacology,* including *toxicology* and *therapeutics.*

What is materia medica proper?

By materia medica proper is understood a description of the source and the physical and chemic characteristics of remedies.

What is pharmacy?

Pharmacy (*φάρμακον*, a medicine) relates to the preparation and combination of remedies.

What is pharmacology?

Pharmacology (*φάρμακον*, a medicine, and *λόγος*, a discourse), though originally meaning a "treatise on drugs" or "on pharmacy," is now usually applied only to the study of the action of drugs on the body. It embraces toxicology (*τοξικόν*, poison with which arrows are smeared, and *λόγος*, a discourse), which deals with poisons and their antidotes.

What is therapeutics?

Therapeutics (θεράπευω, I take care of, or cure) deals with the application of remedies to the cure of or relief from disease, and may be either *empirical* or *rational.*

How does empirical differ from rational therapeutics?

When a remedy is given in any disease because it has succeeded in similar cases before, although the manner in which it acts is often not understood, it is given empirically. When a remedy is prescribed because, from a knowledge of its action on the body, it is likely that it will antagonize or overcome a particular pathologic condition, it is administered on the rational plan. Rational therapeutics is the more scientific, and is the outgrowth of pharmacology.

What are remedies?

Remedies are the agents employed in the treatment of disease.

How may remedies be classified?

Remedies are subdivided into *mechanical, physical, dietetic, hygienic,* and *pharmaceutic* agents. The first four classes are usually treated of in works especially devoted to such subjects.

What are mechanical remedies?

Venesection; local blood-letting by means of leeches, cups, scarifications, incisions, or punctures; bandages; splints; sutures; ligatures; acupressure needle and forceps; acupuncture; aspiration; frictions; massage; stomach and colon washing, etc., are mechanical remedies.

What are physical remedies?

When Röntgen rays, light, heat, cold, electricity, galvanism, or other of the physical forces are used in the treatment of disease, they are spoken of as *physical remedies.* They are treated of at length in works on physics and in books devoted to them exclusively.

What is meant by dietetic remedies?

All relating to the food of the sick [1] or to special plans of diet are included under this head.

[1] In many diseases the diet is of equal importance to, or of more importance than, medication—*e. g.*, in diabetes mellitus and in various forms of dyspepsia.

What are hygienic remedies?

The clothing, bathing, and cleanliness of the sick, the ventilation of the sick-room, etc., belong to this subdivision, and will be found in works on practice of medicine, but more particularly in those relating to hygiene.

What are pharmaceutic remedies?

Pharmaceutic remedies or "medicines are substances not essentially alimentary, which, when applied to the body, so alter or modify its vital functions as to be rendered applicable to the treatment of diseases."[1] It is preëminently with this subdivision that materia medica deals.

What is meant by "official" preparations?

This term is applied to such remedies as are authorized (*officialis*) by the pharmacopeia.

How does a pharmacopeia differ from a dispensatory?

A *pharmacopeia* (φάρμακον, a medicine, and ποιέω, to make) is a book containing directions for the preparation of medicines with the object of securing uniformity of nomenclature, preparation, and strength. The United States Pharmacopœia has been decennially revised since 1820, when it was first authorized by a representative convention of druggists and physicians held at Washington. It is an authoritative list of remedies, with formulas for such preparations as may be in general use. "A *dispensatory* differs from a pharmacopeia in containing the physical and medical history of the various substances." It "contains the whole of the pharmacopeia" "with additions by the author, under whose authority alone it usually appears" (Dunglison). It is a commentary on the pharmacopeia, and treats also of the therapeutics, modes of administration, and doses of the various drugs, while the pharmacopeia is restricted to determining the identity and quality of drugs, and the method of preparing them for use.

How may the official preparations be classified?

They may be classified, according to their physical state, into *solids*, *semisolids*, and *liquids*.

Name the official solid and semisolid preparations.

Extracts, powders, triturations, masses, pills, troches or

[1] Biddle's *Materia Medica*, eleventh ed., 1889, p. 46.

lozenges, confections, plasters, papers, granular effervescent salts, ointments, cerates, oleates, and suppositories.

Mention the official liquid preparations.

Solutions, mixtures, waters, infusions, decoctions, tinctures, spirits, wines, glycerites, fluid extracts, honeys, syrups, vinegars, and oleoresins.

What are extracts?

Extracts (*extracta*) are made by evaporating solutions of vegetable substances (or in some cases the juices expressed from plants) to a pilular or dry consistence. They are called aqueous or watery, alcoholic, and acetous extracts, according to the menstruum used as a solvent.

What are powders?

Powders (*pulveres*) are dry mixtures of drugs in powder form.

What are triturations?

Triturations (*triturationes*) consist of 1 part of a medicinal substance and 9 parts of sugar of milk thoroughly mingled and reduced to a fine powder in a mortar.

What is a mass?

A mass (*massa*) is a plastic mixture designed for the manufacture of pills, etc., and made by incorporating drugs with an adhesive substance.

What are pills?

Pills (*pilulæ*) are preparations of such size that they can be conveniently swallowed whole. They usually contain some excipient to give the proper degree of tenacity to their particles, and are rolled into a spheric or oval form.

What are lozenges?

Lozenges or troches (*trochisci*) are dry, flat, lozenge-shaped bodies, made of powders incorporated usually with mucilage and sugar, and intended to be slowly dissolved in the mouth.

What is a confection?

Confections or conserves (*confectiones*) are remedies made into a soft mass with sugar, honey, etc., which render them more pleasant to the taste.

What is a cataplasm?

A cataplasm (*cataplasma*) is a poultice, and is intended for external application.

What is a plaster?

A plaster (*emplastrum*) is a solid mixture which becomes plastic and adhesive on warming. It is usually spread on linen, muslin, silk, or sheep-skin for application to the body-surface.

What are papers?

Papers (*chartæ*) are made by soaking bibulous paper in medicinal solutions (*e. g.*, charta potassii nitratis), or by spreading medicinal mixtures on paper (*e. g.*, charta sinapis).

What is a granular effervescent salt?

A granular effervescent salt (*sal granulatus effervescens*) is made by mixing the medicinal substance with tartaric acid and sodium bicarbonate, moistening with alcohol, and passing through a sieve to form coarse granules. These effervesce when added to water.

What are ointments?

Ointments or unguents (*unguenta*) are medicaments incorporated with some fatty substance, and intended for external use. They are of the consistence of lard, and soften or melt at body-temperature.

What are cerates?

Cerates (*cerata*) are unctuous preparations intended for external application, made with wax, spermaceti, or resin, which gives them a firmer consistence than an ointment and prevents them from melting at the temperature of the body.

What are oleates?

Oleates (*oleata*) are semisolid solutions in oleic acid of metallic salts or alkaloids, and are applied externally.

What is a suppository?

A suppository (*suppositorium*) is a globular, cone-shaped, or elongated solid, which retains its shape at normal temperature, but fuses when inserted into an orifice of the body. The base is usually cocoa-butter (oil of theobroma). Vaginal suppositories are globular or oviform, and weigh 10 grams; rectal are conical and weigh 2 grams; and urethral are pencil-shaped and weigh 2 to 4 grams.

What are solutions?

Solutions (*liquores*) are preparations in which a non-volatile substance is entirely dissolved in the menstruum (usually water).

What are waters?

Waters (*aquæ*) are aqueous solutions of gaseous or volatile substances.

What are mixtures?

Mixtures (*misturæ*) are aqueous preparations containing insoluble matter.

What are infusions?

Infusions (*infusa*) are aqueous preparations obtained by *pouring* hot or cold water on vegetable substances, and allowing to remain sufficiently long to extract the virtues of the drug, and then straining.

What are decoctions?

Decoctions (*decocta*) are aqueous preparations obtained by *boiling* vegetable substances in water, allowing them to cool in closely covered vessels, and then straining.

What are tinctures?

Tinctures (*tincturæ*) are alcoholic solutions, usually of non-volatile substances. Alcohol or diluted alcohol is generally used as a solvent, but occasionally the aromatic spirits of ammonia is employed, the product being called an *ammoniated tincture.*

What are fluid extracts?

Fluid extracts (*fluidextracta*) are alcoholic, hydro-alcoholic, or acetic acid liquid preparations of uniform strength, 1 c.c. of which represents 1 gm. (about 1 minim to the grain) of the crude drug.

What are spirits?

Spirits (*spiriti*) are alcoholic solutions of gaseous or volatile substances.

What are wines?

Wines (*vina*) are tinctures made with wine as the vehicle.

What are glycerites?

Glycerites (*glycerita*) are medicinal substances mixed with or dissolved in glycerin.

What are honeys?

Honeys (*mellita*) are medicines mixed with or dissolved in honey.

What are syrups?

Syrups (*syrupi*) are composed of *medicinal* substances or of *flavoring* ingredients, with sugar and water. *Simple syrup* is a concentrated solution of sugar in water.

What are vinegars?

Vinegars (*aceta*) are medicinal solutions in diluted acetic acid.

What are liniments?

Liniments (*linimenta*) are oleaginous or alcoholic preparations intended for external application with friction.

What are emulsions?

Emulsions (emulsi) are mixtures in which oil or resin is held in suspension in, and rendered miscible with, water by means of some adhesive or viscid material.

What are oleoresins?

Oleoresins (*oleoresinæ*) are concentrated extracts consisting chiefly of the resin dissolved in the oil of the drug from which they are obtained.

May medicines be prescribed in forms other than those referred to above?

Medicines are often administered in *capsules* (small, elongated gelatin boxes with rounded ends, which dissolve readily in the stomach), *granules* or *parvules* (very minute pills), *enemata* (liquids injected into the rectum for their local or systemic effect), or *injections* (liquids forced by a syringe into the mucous passages or cavities, under the skin, or into a blood-vessel). *Inhalations* of vapors may be employed for their local effect on the bronchopulmonary tract or for their influence on the system at large, and *gargles* may be used as sedative, astringent, or disinfecting and deodorizing applications to the buccal and pharyngeal mucous membranes. Externally, *poultices* (simple or medicated), *lotions* (washes), and *fomenta-*

tions (hot lotions applied on flannel or cloth and allowed to remain in contact with the surface) are also often used.

What weights and measures are used in prescribing and dispensing medicines?

Troy or *apothecaries' weight* is used in dispensing solids, while *wine* or *apothecaries' measure* is employed for liquids; or the *metric system* is used in prescribing solids and liquids.

What is apothecaries' weight?

In apothecaries' weight the pound is divided into ounces, drams, scruples, and grains, as follows:

20 grains (gr.) = 1 scruple (℈).
60 grains or 3 scruples = 1 dram (ʒ).
480 grains or 24 scruples or 8 drams = 1 ounce (℥).
5760 grains or 288 scruples or 96 drams or 12 ounces = 1 pound (℔).

What is wine measure?

In wine measure the gallon is divided into pints, fluidounces, fluidrams and minims, thus:

60 minims (♏) = 1 fluidram (fʒ).
480 minims or 8 fluidrams = 1 fluidounce (f℥).
7680 minims or 128 fluidrams or 16 fluidounces = 1 pint (O).
61440 minims or 1024 fluidrams or 128 fluidounces or 8 pints = 1 gallon (C).

The minim (♏), fluidram (fʒ), fluidounce (f℥), and the pint (O) are used in prescriptions.

Describe the metric system of weights.

In the *metric* or *decimal system* the gram is multiplied or divided by ten, Greek prefixes denoting the multiplication, and Latin the subdivisions of the unit; thus:

10 milligrams (mg.) = 1 centigram (cg.).
100 milligrams, or 10 centigrams = 1 decigram (dg.).
1000 milligrams, or 100 centigrams, or 10 decigrams = 1 gram (gm.).
10,000 milligrams, or 1000 centigrams, or 100 decigrams, or 10 grams = 1 decagram.
100,000 milligrams, or 10,000 centigrams, or 1000 decigrams, or 100 grams, or 10 decagrams = 1 hectogram.
1,000 000 milligrams, or 100,000 centigrams, or 10,000 decigrams, or 1000 grams, or 100 decagrams, or 10 hectograms = 1 kilogram (kilo.).

In writing prescriptions in the metric system the abbreviation is *preceded* by *Arabic figures* or decimals denoting the amount of the drug (*e. g.*, 10.0 gm., 0.02 gm., etc.).

What is a gram?

The gram is the weight of a cubic centimeter (c.c.) of distilled water at 4° C. (39.5° F.).

What is a centimeter?

A centimeter ($\frac{4}{10}$ of an inch) is the $\frac{1}{100}$ of a meter (39. 37 inches), which is the ten-millionth part of a quarter of a meridian of the earth (or of the distance from the pole to the equator).

What relation does the metric system of weights bear to apothecaries' weight and measure?

1 gram = 15.5 grains; 1 decigram (0.1 gm.) = 1.5 grains; 1 centigram (0.01 gm.) = 0.15 (or $\frac{1}{6}$) grain; 1 milligram (0.001 gm.) = 0.015 (or $\frac{1}{64}$) grain; 1 grain (gr. j) = 0.06 gram; 1 dram (ʒj) = 4 grams (approximately); 1 ounce (℥j) = 32 grams (approximately).

The following table gives the value of grains in the metric system. (The fractions have not been carried out beyond the fourth decimal point.)

Grains.	Grams.	Grains.	Grams.
$\frac{1}{100}$ =	0.0006	3 =	0.194
$\frac{1}{50}$ =	0.0013	4 =	0.259
$\frac{1}{25}$ =	0.0027	5 =	0.324
$\frac{1}{8}$ =	0.008	10 =	0.648
$\frac{1}{4}$ =	0.016	30 or ʒss =	1.944
$\frac{1}{2}$ =	0.032	60 or ʒj =	3.888
$\frac{3}{4}$ =	0.049	120 or ʒij =	7.775
1 =	0.065	240 or ℥ss =	15.551
2 =	0.13	480 or ℥j =	31.103

As the weight of a cubic centimeter of fluid depends upon its density, 1 gm. of a light liquid (*e. g.*, alcohol) will measure more than the same weight of a heavy liquid (*e. g.*, glycerin). Approximately, however, ♏j = 0.06 gm.; fʒj = 4 gm. (a little less), and f℥j = 32 gm. (a little less).

The following table gives the value of minims (of water at 4° C. *in vacuo*) in the metric system. For ordinary purposes these values may be used without correction.

Minims.	Grams.	Minims.	Grams.
1 =	0.06161	20 =	1.232
2 =	0.123	30 or fʒss =	1.848
3 =	0.185	60 or fʒj =	3.696
4 =	0.246	120 or fʒij =	7.393
5 =	0.308	240 or f℥ss =	14.786
10 =	0.616	480 or f℥j =	29.573
15 =	0.924	960 or f℥ij =	59.147

What approximate measurements are used in medicine?

Medicines are sometimes ordered in *drops* instead of in minims. As the size of the drop depends on a variety of circumstances, this is a bad practice. A *teaspoonful* is often used for fʒj, or 4 c.c.; a *tablespoonful* for f℥ss, or 15 c.c.; a *wineglassful* for f℥ij; but these are uncertain measures, and should be employed only when an excess of the quantity intended would be harmless. Graduated medicine glasses are easily obtained and are much more reliable.

May a physician prescribe formulas other than those contained in the Pharmacopeia?

The physician often extemporizes formulas to meet the requirements of the individual case.

For what purposes are different remedies often combined in a single prescription?

Remedies are combined to increase or to moderate the effects of some single medicine, or to overcome some action which it is undesirable to produce; to procure the simultaneous action of drugs having different effects upon the body, or to form a new chemic compound, often differing in its action from those of the substances forming it; for convenience in administering, or for rendering nauseous drugs more palatable.

What precautions should be used in prescription writing?

The physician should be careful while writing the prescription—

1. To bear constantly in mind the object for which the medicine is wanted, in order that he may better combine his remedies to accomplish his purpose.

2. The writing should be clear and distinct, and the words not so abbreviated as to be unintelligible or susceptible of more than one meaning. Attention to these points will prevent the occurrence of mistakes in compounding the medicine.

3. The doses should be neither large enough nor close enough together (in the case of powerful medicines) to cause injurious effects. It is better to give too little than too much.

4. Medicines which form poisonous compounds (as calomel and sodium chlorid) should not be combined in the same prescription.

5. Remedies should not be combined (except for particular purposes) which are physiologic antagonists—*i. e.*, which by their actions on the body render each other inert.

6. Remedies which are chemically incompatible—*i. e.*, which will decompose or precipitate each other—should not be combined for internal administration. Sometimes, however, the chemic change is desired.

7. The prescription should be as simple as possible, and contain as few ingredients as the nature of the case will allow.

8. It is better not to order a larger quantity of medicine than the patient will probably require.

9. Never send out a prescription without having carefully reread it, to be certain no mistake has been made.

10. Never give a patient a prescription which has been corrected. If a mistake has been made, rewrite the prescription entirely.

11. Place name of patient and date on the prescription.

Of what parts does a prescription consist?

A prescription consists of four parts:

1. The *superscription* (*super*, "over," and *scribo*, "I write"), which consists of the sign ℞ (which is possibly an abbreviation for recipe, "take"), and in some cases the name and address of the patient, with the date.

2. The *inscription*, the body of the prescription, containing the names of the drugs which are to be used, with the amount of each.

3. The *subscription* (*sub*, "under," and *scribo*, "I write"), the directions to the apothecary regarding the preparation of the medicine.

4. The *signature*, commencing with *S.* or *Sig.* (*Signa*, "write"), and including directions for taking the medicine, the physician's name, and frequently the date, which may be placed here instead of at the beginning of a prescription.

It is customary to write the superscription and signature in English and the inscription and subscription in much abbreviated *medical Latin*.

The *inscription* formerly consisted almost universally of a *basis* (the principal medicine), an *adjuvant* (to aid its action), a *corrective* (to prevent unpleasant effect), and a *vehicle*.

Although inscriptions thus formed are still sometimes seen, particularly in purgative prescriptions, yet the tendency to simplicity in prescribing is increasing daily, and prescriptions are often found containing only the basis and the vehicle.

Is a knowledge of Latin necessary in writing a prescription?

A very limited knowledge of Latin is sufficient for ordinary prescription writing, because, owing to the common practice of abbreviating, the last syllable of the Latin words, which varies with the case, is generally omitted.

Describe the method of writing a prescription.

Having written the superscription,[1] the physician places the names of the drugs which he wishes to administer in a vertical column under the sign ℞, writing them in Latin and in the genitive case. He next determines how many doses he wishes to prescribe, and multiplying the single dose of each drug by the total number of doses in the prescription, he sets the amount opposite the corresponding medicine, expressing the quantity by the proper signs and numerals if it is written in apothecaries' weight and measure, or by Arabic figures and abbreviations if written in grams. Thus, having determined to prescribe an iron mixture containing 24 doses, he might write—

℞	Tincturæ ferri chloridi, . . .	fʒij	or	8	gm.
	Acidi acetici diluti, ...	fʒj		4	"
	Liquoris ammonii acetatis, . .	f℥j		32	"
	Elixir aromatici, ...	fʒxiij		52	"

Next come the directions to the druggist, which in this case are simply to mix the medicines together, and which are expressed by the Latin word *misce*, usually abbreviated to M.

Then follows Sig. or S. (signa), which means the druggist must write what follows on the label, as a direction for the patient—"Take one teaspoonful in water three times a day after eating"—ending the prescription with the physician's name.

May the above prescription be written in any other way?

Instead of writing "Elixir aromatici f ʒxiij," he may write "Elixir aromatici *quantum sufficiat* ad f℥iij," which means

[1] The patient's name and address and the date are often omitted.

"as much of the aromatic elixir as will suffice (to make the whole mixture measure) f℥iij," or q. s. ad ℥iij. As in America liquids are measured and solids are weighed, it is superfluous, when prescribing liquids, to precede the quantity by the letter *f* (indicating fluid measurement).

Why are the titles of the drugs written in the genitive case?

The verb "*recipe*" (℞, "take thou") governs not the drug, but the quantity to be taken, which is placed consequently in the accusative case ("take thou two drams"); the name of the drug *limits* the meaning of the quantity expressed, and, according to rule, is placed in the genitive case and governed by the amount ("take thou two drams"—of what?—"of the tincture of the chlorid of iron").

Given a prescription containing a number of doses of different ingredients, how may a single dose of any one drug be ascertained?

Calculate the number of doses in the mixture and divide the quantity of any ingredient by the number; the result is a single dose.

Thus, the above prescription is a f℥iij mixture, of which the dose is a teaspoonful, or fʒj. As fʒviij = f℥j, there are 3 times fʒviij or fʒxxiv in the mixture, consequently 24 doses To ascertain the amount of tincture of chlorid of iron in each dose, convert the quantity of the tincture to minims and divide by 24: ♏60 = fʒj, therefore ♏120 = fʒij; ♏120 ÷ 24 = ♏v, the quantity of the tincture in a single dose of the mixture.

How many doses should a mixture contain?

A physician should avoid prescribing more of a medicine than his patient will probably want. As a general rule, 24 doses is a sufficient amount, and forms a prescription in which the single doses of the ingredients are easily calculated.

Thus, if the dose be a teaspoonful (fʒj), 24 doses would make a f℥iij mixture (see above); if, however, the dose is a dessertspoonful (fʒij), 24 doses would be twice as much—f℥vj. As ♏iiss × 24 = ♏60 or fʒj, the latter amount represents 24 doses of ♏iiss each, and consequently, if an entire mixture contains 24 doses, fʒj of any of its components will contain 24 doses of ♏iiss.

As solids, when in a thorough state of solution, are equally diffused throughout the menstruum, if ʒj or 60 grains of any solid is dissolved in

24 doses of a solution, each dose will contain gr. iiss of the solid. Hence in prescribing, first write—

For a f℥iij mixture if the dose is to be a teaspoonful (fʒj), or
" f℥vj " " " " dessertspoonful (fʒij);

in either case the mixture will contain 24 doses.

Second, recollect that if each dose of such a mixture is to contain gr. iiss or ♏iiss of any substance, there should be ʒj or fʒj of the substance in the mixture.

If each dose should contain gr. v or ♏v, there should be ʒij or fʒij.
" " " gr. x or ♏x, " " ℥ss or f℥ss.
" " " gr. xx or ♏xx, " " ℥j or f℥j.

These rules simplify prescription-writing for beginners.

Can any general rule be formulated for dosage of official preparations?

As a general rule, the *fluid extracts* may be prescribed in ♏x doses. (*Exceptions* (the poisons), the fluid extracts of aconite, ♏ss–ij; belladonna, ♏j–ij; colchicum root, ♏ij–v; colchicum seed, ♏ij–x; digitalis, ♏j–ij; nux vomica, ♏j–v; sanguinaria, ♏j–v; squill, ♏j–ij; stramonium, ♏j; veratrum viride, ♏j–iv.) *Infusions* and *decoctions* in f℥ss–ij doses. (*Exception*, infusion of digitalis, fʒj–iv.) *Syrups*, fʒj–ij doses. (*Exceptions*, syrup of the iodid of iron, ♏v–xxx; compound syrup of squill, ♏x–xxx.) *Tinctures*, ♏v–fʒj doses. (*Exceptions* (the poisons), tinctures of aconite, ♏ij–iij; belladonna, ♏viij–xxx; colchicum, ♏v–xxx; digitalis, ♏v–x; iodin, ♏j–x; ipecac and opium, ♏v–xv; nux vomica, ♏j–x; opium, ♏ij–x; deodorized opium, ♏ij–x; physostigma, ♏v–xv; squill, ♏v–xxx; stramonium, ♏v–xv; veratrum viride, ♏ij–x.) *Powders*, gr. ij–x. *Volatile oils*, gtt. j–ij.

Many preparations can be administered in larger doses than indicated by this general rule.

Mention some circumstances which, by modifying the effects, will influence the dose of medicines.

As the activity of a drug is increased or lessened by the age, sex, idiosyncrasy, constitution, and habits of the patient, as well as by the condition of the digestive and absorbent systems, disease, and manner of administration, these circumstances must be considered in relation to dosage.

How does age influence the activity of a drug?

Children and old persons are more readily influenced by most drugs, particularly narcotics, than adults in the prime of life; but, as a rule, they bear larger *proportionate* doses of purgatives. No scheme for calculating the doses from the age of the patient alone can be relied on in practice.

What is Dr. Young's rule for calculating the dose for children?

Convert the child's age into a fraction by using the age itself as a numerator, and the age + 12 as a denominator, the result being the proportion of the adult dose which should be administered to the child. Thus, at three years $\frac{3}{3+12} = \frac{3}{15} = \frac{1}{5}$ of that of the adult. At twenty-one years of age the full dose is given.

What is Dr. Cowling's rule?

Dr. Cowling proposed to divide the patient's *next birthday* by 24; thus, at three years the dose would be $\frac{4}{24} = \frac{1}{6}$ of that of the adult.

How may the dose for a child be more easily calculated in the metric system?

Dr. Lauder Brunton proposes to multiply the next birthday by 4 and divide the result by 100; or, what is the same thing, to multiply the full dose by the child's next birthday, then by 4, and remove the decimal point two places to the left. Thus, if the dose for an adult be 1 gm., that for a child of three years will be $\frac{1 \times 4 \times 4}{100} = 0.16$ gm.

How do sex, idiosyncrasy, constitution, and habits influence medicinal effects?

Men generally bear larger doses of medicines than women. Many persons manifest idiosyncrasies with respect to certain drugs; thus, some are very susceptible to the poisonous effects of even minute doses of arsenic; others cannot take quinine, opium, belladonna, or the iodids, and in others very dilute solutions of cocaine applied to the mucous membranes may cause alarming symptoms. As a rule, the larger and more robust the individual, the less easily is he influenced by drugs. When a medicine is habitually taken, the system becomes tolerant to it, and larger doses are required to produce any effect. This is especially the case with opium and purgatives.

In what way does the condition of the digestive and absorbent systems modify the effects of medicine?

During digestion larger amounts of medicine are borne than can be taken fasting. In certain conditions of the alimentary canal, as in the third stage of yellow fever and of cholera, during a congestive chill of the gastro-enteric variety, or during profound opium narcosis, absorption from the stomach if it take place at all is slow.

What effect does disease have upon the influence of medicines on the system?

In certain diseases great tolerance is manifested to medicine; thus, in peritonitis and cerebrospinal fever enormous doses of opium are taken with advantage; in typhoid fever the tolerance to alcohol is marked.

Does the method of administration modify the effect of medicines?

It does: diuretics act more powerfully when much diluted; saline purgatives, when concentrated. Usually medicines act more rapidly and powerfully when given by the mouth than when administered by the rectum; still more so when injected under the skin, and most powerfully when injected into the blood.

How may medicines be administered?

Medicines may be administered by the *skin*, being applied either without friction (*enepidermic method*) or with friction (*epidermic method*), or else directly to the derma, which has been denuded by means of a blister (*endermic method*). They may also be given *hypodermically*, by means of a small syringe armed with a long, hollow needle. When thus administered, the dose should be from one-half to two-thirds of that which is required by the mouth, and the medicine should be in a thorough state of solution. Medicines are also applied to all the *mucous tracts* in the form of solutions, vapors (by atomization), powders (by insufflation), etc. The gastro-intestinal tract is most generally used when a systemic effect is desired, and the remedy is given either by the mouth or by the rectum. Suppositories and ointments are occasionally used per vaginam for their influence on the system. The broncho-pulmonary mucous membrane is utilized for the inhalation of vapors, as ether. *Intravenous injection* is rarely practised except as a last resort.

How are medicines classified?

Medicines are usually classified according either to their physiologic action or to their therapeutic uses. The latter is the better arrangement.

The difficulty of grouping medicines is increased by the fact that even as yet the study of pharmacology is in its infancy, so that the exact physiologic group to which many of them belong is not definitely determined. The action of most medicines, also, is complex, affecting different organs at the same time, and in many instances varying much according to the dose and the manner of administration.

They may be divided accordingly into—

GROUP 1.—SYSTEMIC MEDICINES.

Class 1.—Medicines acting on the body at large by their influence on digestion, nutrition (tissue waste and repair), and calorification.

Order I. Digestants. *Order. II.* Tonics. *Order III.* Alteratives. *Order IV.* Antipyretics.

Class 2.—Medicines acting on the body by their effect on its various organs.

A. On the Nervous System:

Order I. Hypnotics. *Order II.* Mydriatic Anodynes. *Order III.* Anesthetics. *Order IV.* Antispasmodics. *Order V.* Excitomotors. *Order VI.* Depressomotors.

B. On the Organs of Circulation:

Order I. Stimulants. *Order II.* Sedatives.

C. On the Sexual Organs:

Order I. Aphrodisiacs. *Order II.* Anaphrodisiacs. *Order III.* Oxytocics. *Order IV.* Uterine Sedatives. *Order V.* Emmenagogues.

D. On the Alimentary Canal:

Order I. Emetics. *Order II.* Gastric Sedatives. *Order III.* Carminatives. *Order IV.* Cathartics. *Order V.* Anthelmintics.

Class 3.—Medicines Acting on the Various Secretions:

Order I. Diuretics. *Order II.* Diaphoretics. *Order III.* Expectorants. *Order IV.* Astringents. *Order V.* Antacids.

GROUP 2.—TOPICAL MEDICINES.

Class 1.—Antiseptics.

Class 2.—Irritants.

Order I. Rubefacients. *Order II.* Vesicants. *Order III.* Suppurants. *Order IV.* Escharotics.

Class 3.—Demulcents.

Class 4.—Emollients.

Class 5.—Protectives.

Class 6.—Coloring Agents.

SYSTEMIC MEDICINES.

Medicines Acting on the Body at Large by their Influence on Digestion, Nutrition (Tissue Waste and Repair) or Calorification.

DIGESTANTS.

What are digestants?

Digestants are animal or vegetable substances given to aid digestion when the normal alimentary secretions are insufficient for this function.

Name the digestants.

1. *Pepsinum (pepsin)*, a proteolytic ferment obtained from the glandular layer of fresh stomachs from healthy pigs, and capable of digesting 3000 times its own weight of coagulated and disintegrated egg-albumen.

2. *Ingluvin* (not official), a preparation from the gizzard of the domestic chicken.

3. *Pancreatinum (pancreatin)*, a mixture of the enzymes naturally existing in the pancreas of warm-blooded animals, usually obtained from the fresh pancreas of the hog (*sus scrofa*).

4. *Papain* (not official), a ferment obtained from the fruit of *Carica papaya* (*Fam.* Papayaceæ), a tree of South America.

5. *Extractum malti* (*extract of malt*), prepared from *maltum* (malt), consists of maltose, dextrin, proteids, and the ferment *diastase*, which is capable of changing starch to maltose.

What are the physiologic actions of these substances?

1. *Pepsin* (when combined with an acid) digests albumin, which it converts into albumose and peptone.

2. *Ingluvin* also aids the digestion of albumin, this action being probably due to a bitter principle which it contains and which stimulates the gastric glands.

3. *Pancreatin* (in neutral or alkaline solutions) converts albumin into albumose and starches into glucose, and aids in saponifying and emulsifying fats.

4. *Papain* digests albumin in acid, neutral, or alkaline media.

5. *Diastase* and *extract of malt* digest starch.

What are the therapeutic uses of the digestants?

1. *Pepsin* is useful when the secretion of the peptic glands is not sufficient for the purposes of digestion, as in *atonic dyspepsia, apepsia of infants, anemia, chlorosis, gastric ulcer, cancer,* and *infantile diarrhea.* It has been used for the relief of *reflex vomiting,* as that of *pregnancy.* It is an invaluable addition to nutritive enemata, and has been *injected into tumors* to arrest their growth and aid in their absorption.

2. *Ingluvin* is used chiefly for the relief of *vomiting of pregnancy,* also in *indigestion accompanied with flatulency,* and in *acute dyspepsia.*

3. *Pancreatin* is used in *intestinal indigestion,* and to aid in emulsifying fats. It is also added to nutritive enemata.

4. *Papain* is sometimes used in *dyspepsia,* to aid the digestion of albuminous foods, but more frequently for its solvent action on *false membranes* and *tenia.*

Pepsin, pancreatin (under the name of *trypsin*), and *papain* have been successfully used to *dissolve the membranes of croup and diphtheria.* They are used in solution, either in the form of spray or applied by a brush to the part.

5. *Extract of malt* is given to aid starch digestion.

What are the preparations and doses of the digestant ?

Pepsinum (pepsin), the average dose of which is 0.25 gm. (4 grains).

Ingluvin (not official) may be given in doses of gr. v–xv (0.3–1.0 gm.).

Pancreatinum (pancreatin), in doses of gr. v–xv (0.3–1.0 gm.).

Papain (not official), in doses of gr. j–v (0.06–0.3 gm.).

Extractum malti (extract of malt), in doses of ℥iv (15 c.c.).

Name some of the substances which are incompatible with the digestants.

Alcohol and many of the *mineral salts* destroy their properties.

Alkalis, when sufficiently powerful, interfere with the action of pepsin and ingluvin, while materially aiding that of pancreatin.

Acids retard and finally destroy the action of pancreatin, while aiding that of pepsin and of ingluvin.

How and at what time should the digestants be given ?

Pepsin and ingluvin should be given with meals, in solution with an acid or in capsules, powder, or compressed pill.

Often they are combined with sodium bicarbonate, to which bismuth is sometimes added, and administered before eating.

Pancreatin is usually given from two to four hours after meals, combined with an alkali.

Papain is taken after meals, in powder, capsule, or compressed pill.

TONICS.

What are tonics ?

Tonics are remedies which, in conditions of debility, impart a gradual and permanent increase of vigor to the body or its various parts, restoring the energy and strength which were wanting.

How may tonics be divided ?

They may be divided into *vegetable* and *mineral tonics.*

Vegetable Tonics.

What subdivisions of vegetable tonics are made?

VEGETABLE TONICS are divisible into *simple or pure bitters, aromatic bitters, and peculiar bitters.*

Simple Bitters.

Mention the simple bitters.

1. QUASSIA, the *wood* of *Picrasma excelsa* and of *Quassia amara* (*Fam.* Simarubaceæ), a lofty tree of the West Indies.

2. GENTIANA (*gentian*), the rhizome and roots of *Gentiana lutea* (*Fam.* Gentianaceæ), a plant of the mountainous portions of central and southern Europe.

3. CALUMBA, the *root* of *Jateorrhiza palmata* (*Fam.* Menispermaceæ), a plant of the southeastern coast of Africa.

4. CHIRATA, *Swertia chirayita* (*Fam.* Gentianaceæ), a plant of India.

5. BERBERIS, the rhizome and roots of *Berberis aquifolium* and other species of *Berberis* (*Fam.* Berberidaceæ).

What are their chief chemic constituents?

1. *Quassia-wood* contains *quassin*, a neutral bitter principle.

2. *Gentian*, an acid, *gentisic acid* (gentisin), a fixed oil, and a bitter principle, *gentianin* or *gentiopicrin*.

3. *Calumba*, an alkaloid, *berberine* (which is found in many other plants, and has been used as a tonic and febrifuge), a bitter principle, *calumbin*, and an acid, *calumbic acid*.

4. *Chirata*, a neutral bitter principle, *chiratin*, and an amorphous bitter acid, *ophelic acid*.

5. *Berberis*, the alkaloid, *berberine*.

What are the physiologic actions of the simple bitters?

The simple bitters increase the secretions and impart tone to the mucous membranes; increase the appetite and digestion, and thus promote nutrition and improve the condition of the blood, but when taken continuously for too long a time, they disorder digestion and cause gastric catarrh. Gentian in full doses, by increasing the intestinal secretion, acts as a mild laxative.

Calumba is least likely to disorder the stomach.

What are the therapeutic uses of the simple bitters?

They are given: (1) To *increase secretion* and *promote appetite* in *atonic dyspepsia*, in *chronic gastric catarrh*, and during *convalescence* from acute diseases. Calumba is the mildest, and, being best adapted to weak stomachs, may be used in *vomiting of pregnancy* and in *sea-sickness*; quassia, gentian, and chirata are well adapted to cases of dyspepsia with relaxation or torpor of the mucous membrane and resulting constipation. (2) *To give tone to the mucous membranes*, in *diarrhea* and in *accumulations of flatus* in the bowel from a relaxed condition, calumba may be used. (3) *As vehicles* for the administration of other medicines, as acids or alkalis. (4) *To destroy pin-worms* an infusion of quassia may be used as an enema.

What are the preparations and doses of these substances?

1. EXTRACTUM QUASSIÆ (*extract of quassia*), dose, gr. j–v (0.06–0.3 gm.), principally used as an excipient.

FLUIDEXTRACTUM QUASSIÆ (*fluid extract of quassia*), dose, ♏v–xxx (0.3–2.0 c.c.).

TINCTURA QUASSIÆ (*tincture of quassia*), dose, ʒj–ij (4–8 c.c.).

Quassin (not official), dose, gr. ¼–½ (0.016–0.032 gm.).

2. EXTRACTUM GENTIANÆ (*extract of gentian*), dose, gr. j–xxx (0.06–2.0 gm.).

FLUIDEXTRACTUM GENTIANÆ (*fluid extract of gentian*), dose, ʒss–j (2–4 c.c.).

TINCTURA GENTIANÆ COMPOSITA (*compound tincture of gentian*), dose, ʒss–ij (2–8 c.c.).

3. FLUIDEXTRACTUM CALUMBÆ (*fluid extract of calumba*), dose, ʒss–j (2–4 c.c.).

TINCTURA CALUMBÆ (*tincture of calumba*), dose, ʒss–ij (2–8 c.c.).

Berberine (not official), dose, gr. j–x (0.06–0.6 gm.), as a sulphate or hydrochloride.

4. FLUIDEXTRACTUM CHIRATÆ (*fluid extract of chirata*), dose, ♏x–xx (0.6–1.3 c.c.).

5. FLUIDEXTRACTUM BERBERIDIS (*fluid extract of berberis*), dose, ʒss–ij (2–8 c.c.).

What medicines should not be prescribed with gentian?

The salts of silver and of lead are incompatible with gentian. Iron salts produce a dark color but do not impair the efficiency of the drug.

How and at what time should the simple bitters be given?

The simple bitters are given before eating, either alone or combined with other medicines in pills or in mixtures or solutions. They are more efficient in liquid form.

Aromatic Bitters.

How do the aromatic differ from the simple bitters?

The aromatic bitters are more *stimulating* to the mucous tract than the simple bitters, because of the aromatic volatile oils which they contain; they also contain tannic or gallic acid, which renders them more or less *astringent.*

Mention the aromatic bitters.

1. SERPENTARIA (*Virginia snakeroot*), the *rhizome* and *roots* of *Aristolochia Serpentaria* and of *A. reticulata* (*Fam.* Aristolochiaceæ), indigenous plants.

2. EUCALYPTUS, the *leaves* of *E. globulus*, or blue gum-tree (*Fam.* Myrtaceæ), a tree of Australia.

3. PRUNUS VIRGINIANA, the *bark* of *P. serotina*, or wild cherry (*Fam.* Rosaceæ), an indigenous tree.

4. ANTHEMIS, the *flower-heads* of *A. nobilis*, or chamomile (*Fam.* Compositæ), a native of Europe.

5. MATRICARIA, the *flower-heads* of *M. Chamomilla*, or German chamomile (*Fam.* Compositæ).

6. EUPATORIUM, the *leaves* and *flowering tops* of *E. perfoliatum*, boneset or thoroughwort (*Fam.* Compositæ), a common indigenous plant.

CASCARILLA and ABSINTHIUM are no longer official.

What are the chief chemic constituents of the aromatic bitters?

They all contain a *volatile oil*, a *bitter principle*, *resin*, and *tannic acid*.

The *volatile oil of eucalyptus* is composed of two terpenes, cymol and eucalyptol; that of *Prunus Virginiana* contains hydrocyanic acid, and is formed by the reaction in water of a peculiar ferment (emulsin) existing in the bark, with the bitter principle; that of *absinthium* contains absinthol.

The *bitter principle of serpentaria* is called *aristolochin;* that of *anthemis, anthemic acid;* that of *eupatorium, eupatorin;* that of *cascarilla, cascarillin;* and that of *absinthium, absinthin.*

What are the physiologic actions of the aromatic bitters?

Owing to the bitter principles which they contain, their action on digestion, nutrition, and secretion is similar to that produced by the simple bitters. They have, in addition, a stimulating influence on the mucous membranes, due to the volatile oils (which are eliminated by the bronchial mucous membrane, skin, and kidneys, and by increasing their secretions are somewhat expectorants, diaphoretics, and diuretics), and an astringent effect, owing to their tannic acid. In large doses they are emetic and laxative. *The oil of eucalyptus* destroys germs and is an irritant when applied locally. It quickens the pulse and respiration and lowers the blood-pressure. In large doses it causes diarrhea. From the hydrocyanic acid which is developed in it *Prunus Virginiana* has a sedative influence over the pneumogastric nerve, and thus quiets cough. *Absinthium* in large doses, or when habitually used in the form of the *liqueur* (*absinthe*), produces epileptiform convulsions.

What are the therapeutic uses of the aromatic bitters?

They are used for the same purposes as the simple bitters.

Serpentaria is used as a *cardiac stimulant* and *tonic* in low fevers, and occasionally as a *stimulating expectorant* in capillary bronchitis and low pneumonias. *Eucalyptus* is used in *chronic catarrhal conditions* of the gastric, bronchopulmonary, and genito-urinary mucous membranes, and from its *destructive influence on germs* it is of benefit in vomiting due to Sarcina ventriculi. As an *antimalarial* agent, it is far inferior to cinchona, but sometimes proves useful where the latter has failed. As a *local* application it is employed in stomatitis, and with liquid albolene as a spray in nasal or pharyngeal catarrh. *Prunus Virginiana* is also used as a *stomachic tonic*, but is especially employed as a *cough-relieving agent* in bronchial catarrh and in phthisis.

What are the preparations and doses of these substances?

1. FLUIDEXTRACTUM SERPENTARIÆ (*fluid extract of serpentaria*), dose, ʒss–j (2–4 c.c.).

TINCTURA SERPENTARIÆ (*tincture of serpentaria*), dose, ʒj–ij (4–8 c.c.).

TINCTURA CINCHONÆ COMPOSITA (*compound tincture of cinchona*) contains 2 per cent. of serpentaria; dose, ʒss–ij (2–8 c.c.).

2. FLUIDEXTRACTUM EUCALYPTI (*fluid extract of eucalyptus*), dose, ʒss–j (2–4 c.c.).

OLEUM EUCALYPTI (*oil of eucalyptus*), dose, ♏v–xv (0.3–1.0 c.c.), in capsules or in emulsion.

EUCALYPTOL, a neutral body obtained from the volatile oil of *Eucalyptus globulus* and of some other species of Eucalyptus; dose, ♏v–xv (0.3–1.0 c.c.). It enters into the *liquor antisepticus*.

3. FLUIDEXTRACTUM PRUNI VIRGINIANÆ (*fluid extract of Prunus virginiana*), dose, ʒj–ij (4–8 c.c.).

INFUSUM PRUNI VIRGINIANÆ (*infusion of Prunus virginiana*), dose, ℥ss–ij (15–60 c.c.).

SYRUPUS PRUNI VIRGINIANÆ (*syrup of Prunus virginiana*), dose, ʒj–℥ss (4–15 c.c.).

4, 5. There are no official preparations of *anthemis and matricaria*, the latter of which is not much used in this country. They are usually given in infusion (chamomile tea) in doses of ℥ij (60 c.c.) t. i. d., as a stomachic tonic.

6. FLUIDEXTRACTUM EUPATORII (*fluid extract of eupatorium*), dose, ʒss–j (2–4 c.c.).

7, 8. *Cascarilla* and *absinthium* may be given in infusion.

At what time should the aromatic bitters be administered?

They should be given shortly before meals when intended

to promote appetite and digestion, but when given for their effects on the bronchial or vesical mucous membranes or for their action on the heart, they should be given between meals.

Peculiar Bitters.

What are the peculiar bitters?

They are such bitters as, owing to peculiarity of action, cannot be classed with either of the preceding groups.

Name the peculiar bitters.

Cinchona and hydrastis.

CINCHONA.

What is cinchona?

Cinchona is the bark of *Cinchona Calisaya*, *Cinchona Ledgeriana*, *Cinchona officinalis*, and of hybrids of these with other species of *Cinchona* (*Fam.* Rubiaceæ). It must contain not less than 5 per cent. of total alkaloids and at least 4 per cent. of ether-soluble alkaloids. *Cinchona rubra* is the bark of *Cinchona succirubra*, and contains not less than 5 per cent. of total alkaloids.

What is the habitat?

The cinchona trees are natives of the mountainous regions of the western parts of South America, from 22° south latitude to 10° north latitude, but have been successfully cultivated in India, Ceylon, Java, the West Indies, and other parts of the world. Cinchona is known as "yellow or Calisaya bark," Cinchona rubra, as "red bark."

How is the bark obtained?

The bark was formerly obtained by stripping the trees, but as this killed them and threatened to extinguish the genus, the present method has been adopted: One-fifth the circumference of the tree is denuded of bark in longitudinal strips each year, in the dry season, for five years, at the end of which time the bark has again grown over the portion first denuded. The process is then repeated.

What are the chemic constituents of cinchona?

The most important constituents are the alkaloids *quinine*

and *cinchonine*, of which the former is found to preponderate in the yellow bark, the latter in pale barks, and both exist in about equal proportions in red bark. Other important alkaloids are *quinidine* and *cinchonidine*. Combined with these alkaloids are *kinic*, *kinovic*, and *cinchotannic acids*. *Quinicine* and *cinchonicine* are amorphous modifications of quinine and cinchonine. Red bark contains more tannic acid and less quinine than does calisaya.

Describe a chemic test for the cinchona alkaloids.

If *quinine and quinidine, or their salts*, are treated with fresh chlorin-water, an emerald-green precipitate will form when ammonia-water is added. When the same test is applied to *cinchonine*, *cinchonidine*, *or their salts*, a white precipitate results; solutions of quinine and quinidine are fluorescent.

What are the physiologic effects of cinchona and its alkaloids?

Locally, cinchona and its alkaloids are irritant and antiseptic, destroying minute organisms or inhibiting their movements.

Internally, it acts on the *alimentary canal* as a simple bitter; in small doses it is a tonic, increasing the appetite and digestion. If long continued in large dose, it produces indigestion and gastric catarrh. In ordinary doses cinchona constipates. In excessive doses cinchona or its alkaloids irritate the mucous membrane and cause vomiting and diarrhea.

Nutrition is stimulated and the excretion of waste-products increased by small doses; large doses, however, diminish the amount of urea and uric and phosphoric acids in the urine. In malarial fever the products of waste tissue are much increased.

In the *blood* it interferes with the oxygen-carrying function of the red corpuscles, and diminishes the number, inhibits the movements, and prevents the migration of the white corpuscles, both in health and in disease.

Circulation.—In small doses the cardiac action is increased; large doses, by acting on the cardiac motor ganglia, depress the heart, sometimes causing it to intermit, and finally arrest it in diastole; the blood-pressure is lowered.

The *temperature* in health is very slightly, if at all, influenced; in fevers a rapid decline takes place, due to the action on the blood and circulation.

Nervous System.—Small doses stimulate the cerebral functions; large doses cause *cinchonism—i. e.*, a constricted feeling in the forehead; giddiness and tinnitus aurium, with impairment of hearing and sometimes of vision; after toxic doses these symptoms are aggravated, and delirium, weak pulse, coma (sometimes convulsions), and in rare cases death, supervene. It probably reduces the reflex excitability of the spinal cord, and although it never causes, may energize, uterine contractions when present. *Elimination* takes place chiefly by the urine, the greater portion escaping from the system within eight hours.

Cutaneous eruptions, as erythema, urticaria, or herpes, are produced in some subjects by even small doses of cinchona or its alkaloids.

What are the therapeutic uses of cinchona and its alkaloids?

1. *As a Tonic.*—The cinchona preparations, as well as the salts of its alkaloids, are largely used to improve the appetite and digestion in *debility*, the *latter stages of inflammations*, and in *convalescence* from acute diseases generally, also in *atonic dyspepsia* (combined with a mineral acid), in *relaxed conditions* of the alimentary mucous membrane, and in *summer complaint* of children. The alkaloids are also used as tonics to sustain the vital forces in *diphtheria, erysipelas, pyemia, septicemia*, in all *typhoid conditions*, in the *eruptive fevers*, and in *surgical shock*. In the various *neuralgias* combined with other remedies (as morphine or belladonna, iron or arsenic) it is a valuable agent. From its influence on the migration of leukocytes and on cell-proliferation it is used (in larger doses) in the *early stages of inflammation*.

2. *As an antipyretic* in all conditions of hyperpyrexia quinine may be prescribed in large doses, repeated in about six or eight hours to maintain its effects, but the newer and more powerful antipyretics have largely superseded this practice.

3. *As an antiperiodic*, cinchona has no rival in the materia medica. The salts of the alkaloids are preferred for this purpose. Quinine may be used as a *prophylactic* against

malaria in small doses, given early in the morning (gr. iij–x —0.2–0.6 gm.). In the treatment of *intermittent* (gr. x—0.6 gm.) during the sweating stage, repeated five hours before the next paroxysm is expected; *remittent* (gr. xxx—2 gm.—a day in two doses, given at any time); *hemorrhagic* and *pernicious malarial fevers* (gr. xx–ʒj—1.3–4.0 gm.), administered promptly by the mouth or rectum or even subcutaneously, it acts as a specific. It is useful also in malarial cachexia, but must often be combined or alternated with arsenic and other treatment.

4. *Locally,* quinine may be applied in solution as an astringent and antiseptic to the nares in *summer catarrh,* etc., or to the mouth in *muguet.*

What are the preparations and doses of cinchona and its alkaloids?

FLUIDEXTRACTUM CINCHONÆ (*fluid extract of* (yellow bark of) *cinchona*), dose, as a *tonic,* ʒss (2 c.c.).

TINCTURA CINCHONÆ (*tincture of* (yellow bark of) *cinchona*), dose, ʒj–iv (4–15 c.c.).

TINCTURA CINCHONÆ COMPOSITA (*compound tincture* (Huxham's) *of cinchona*), containing 10 per cent. of red bark, serpentaria, bitter orange peel, glycerin, alcohol, and water; dose, ʒj–iv (4–15 c.c.).

QUININA (*quinine*), soluble in 1750 parts of water and 0.6 part of alcohol.

QUININÆ SULPHAS (*quinine sulphate*), the basic sulphate, not very soluble in water (740 parts), but rendered more soluble by the addition of a diluted mineral acid; dose, as a *tonic,* gr. j–vj (0.06–0.4 gm.); as an *antipyretic* or antiperiodic, gr. x–xx (0.6–1.3 gm.); repeated as indicated.

QUININÆ BISULPHAS (*quinine bisulphate*), the normal sulphate, soluble in 8.5 parts of water, and containing less quinine than the basic sulphate;

QUININÆ HYDROBROMIDUM (*quinine hydrobromide*), soluble in 40 parts of water;

QUININÆ HYDROCHLORIDUM (*quinine hydrochloride*), soluble in 18 parts of water;

QUININÆ SALICYLAS (*quinine salicylate*), soluble in 77 parts of water;—are given in the same doses as quinine sulphate.

CINCHONINÆ SULPHAS (*cinchonine sulphate*), doses ⅓ larger than those of quinine.

CINCHONIDINÆ SULPHAS (*cinchonidine sulphate*), dose, gr. j–xv (0.06–1.0 gm.), according to the effects desired.

OLEATUM QUININÆ (*oleate of quinine*) contains 25 per cent. of quinine.

What medicines are incompatible with cinchona?

The *alkalies* and *alkaline earths* precipitate the alkaloids of cinchona; the *benzoates* and *salicylates*, *tannic*, *gallic*, and *tartaric acid*, the *tincture* and the *compound solution of iodin*, form insoluble compounds with them; and the *ferric salts* precipitate cinchotannic acid from the preparations of cinchona.

How are cinchona and its alkaloids administered?

The preparations of *cinchona* are frequently combined with the mineral acids or administered alone as tonics; the alkaloids are given in solution, freshly made pills or capsules, or may be made into suppositories or used subcutaneously. They are often combined with iron, arsenic, and other medicines. Saccharin and yerba santa help to disguise their unpleasant taste.

HYDRASTIS.

What is hydrastis?

HYDRASTIS is the *rhizome* and *roots* of *Hydrastis canadensis*, yellow root or golden seal (*Fam.* Ranunculaceæ), an indigenous plant, and yields not less than 2.5 per cent. of hydrastine.

What alkaloids does it contain?

It contains *hydrastine* and *berberine.*

What are its physiologic actions?

It acts on the appetite, digestion, nutrition, and secretions like the simple bitters; it increases the secretions, especially of the glandular appendages of the intestine and probably that of the liver; without increasing the heart's action it stimulates the peripheral vessels to contraction, so may be useful in uterine and other hemorrhages. When given to animals in sufficient doses, it is said to act on the nervous system like strychnine, but less powerfully, stimulating the reflex centers of the spinal cord, heightening the irritability of the motor nerves, and causing incoördination, tremor, convulsions, and, finally, death from tetanic spasm of the respiratory muscles. It is also claimed that it always provokes uterine contractions.

What are the therapeutic applications of hydrastis?

It is used as a tonic, to promote appetite, digestion, and nutrition in *atonic dyspepsia* and *chronic gastric catarrh.* From its effects on secretions it is used in *catarrhal jaundice* and in *constipation* from deficient secretion, and as a *blennorrhetic* in *chronic cystitis.* It has also been recommended internally to check *uterine hemorrhage* and as a uterine tonic. As an antiperiodic in *intermittent fever* and *chronic malaria* it is inferior to quinine.

Locally, it has been used as an application to sore mouth, fissured nipples, sores and ulcers generally, and as an injection in gleet and vaginal leukorrhea.

What are the preparations and doses of hydrastis?

FLUIDEXTRACTUM HYDRASTIS (*fluid extract of hydrastis*), dose, ♏v–ʒj (0.3–4.0 c.c.); as a *stomachic tonic,* ♏v–xv (0.3–1.0 c.c.) before meals.

TINCTURA HYDRASTIS (*tincture of hydrastis*), dose, ♏x–ʒj (0.6–4.0 c.c.).

GLYCERITUM HYDRASTIS (*glycerite of hydrastis*) is chiefly used as a local application.

HYDRASTINE (*hydrastine*), dose, gr. $\frac{1}{6}$ (0.01 gm.).

HYDRASTININÆ HYDROCHLORIDUM (*hydrastinine hydrochlorid*), a derivative of hydrastine, has been used to check *uterine hemorrhage,* and also as a *circulatory tonic* (*see* Oxytocics); dose, gr. $\frac{1}{4}$–1 (0.016–0.06 gm.).

Mineral Tonics.

Name the mineral tonics.

The mineral tonics are the *preparations of iron* and of *manganese* (which are sometimes classed separately as *hematinics* or blood medicines), *phosphorus, zinc phosphid,* the *mineral acids; lactic acid,* although of animal origin, is usually considered in connection with the latter.

FERRUM (IRON).

What is the source of iron?

Iron is the most common of all the metals, and is found widely distributed both in the metallic state and as oxid, sulphid, carbonate, phosphate, etc.

What are the physiologic effects of iron?

Metallic iron is inert, but when swallowed, it is dissolved by the acid of the stomach and forms salts. It probably enters the blood as an albuminate. A large part of the iron is probably taken from the portal circulation by the liver and excreted in the bile, without its entering the general circulation. Any iron which is not absorbed passes into the intestine, is converted into a sulphid, and colors the stools black. Iron exists normally in the red corpuscles of the blood in the proportion of 1 part of iron to 230 parts of corpuscles. When deficient in the blood, under a course of iron the number of corpuscles increases, the blood is improved in quality, and consequently the tissues are better nourished and all the functions of the body are better performed. In appropriate cases it promotes the appetite and digestion by stimulating the gastric glands, but if given for too long a time, it disorders digestion.

The *more soluble preparations* of iron, if given in large doses, cause nausea and vomiting; its *salts with the mineral acids* and *with iodin* possess more or less toxic properties.

The *sulphates*, *nitrates*, and *chlorids* of iron are astringent, diminishing the secretions of the mucous membranes, thus causing constipation, and coagulating albumin, thus proving hemostatic. Iron is eliminated by the feces, bile, and urine.

What are the therapeutic uses of iron?

1. *As a general tonic*, to improve the appetite and digestion, when it should be combined with a purgative, as aloes.

2. *To improve the condition of the blood* and aid nutrition in *anemia* and *chlorosis;* in *malarial anemia* (with quinine); in *various cachexiæ*, as the scrofulous, strumous, or syphilitic (iodids); in *amenorrhea*, *dysmenorrhea*, or *menorrhagia* associated with anemia; in *fatty degeneration* and in *dilatation of the heart;* in many forms of *neuralgia* and in many

nervous affections associated with anemia, as *epilepsy* or *chorea;* in *convalescence* from acute diseases, and after *exhausting hemorrhages.* In *erysipelas* iron is almost a specific (tincture of the chlorid, ♏xx–xxx (1.2–2.0 c. c.) every two or three hours), and in diphtheria it is also useful.

3. *As an astringent* it is sometimes used internally in *chronic diarrhea* and in dysentery. In *chronic albuminuria* it is useful both as a tonic and as an astringent.

4. *As a hemostatic* in all *passive hemorrhages* in the anemic (tincture of the chlorid), and in hemorrhages from the stomach or bowels (subsulphate, tersulphate or nitrate in drop-doses largely diluted and frequently repeated).

5. *Locally,* it is employed as a *styptic* (subsulphate) to check the *bleeding from hemorrhoids* and *leech-bites,* or to arrest *capillary oozing* from a large surface; in the form of spray in *epistaxis* and *hemoptysis,* and it is sometimes injected into the cavity of the uterus (more or less dangerous) to check bleeding from that organ. As an *astringent* it is applied to syphilitic vegetations (Monsel's solution), and as an injection (largely diluted) in gonorrhea and leukorrhea.

6. Ferrous sulphate is useful as a disinfectant for water-closets and sewers; the *hydrated oxid of iron* is the best antidote for arsenic.

What are the preparations of iron and their doses?

FERRUM REDUCTUM (*reduced iron; Quevenne's iron*), an impalpable powder of metallic iron, well borne by the stomach, and not astringent; dose, gr. j–v (0.06–0.3 gm.).

FERRI HYDROXIDUM (*ferric hydroxid*) and FERRI HYDROXIDUM CUM MAGNESII OXIDO (*ferric hydroxid with magnesium oxid*), used almost exclusively as antidotes in arsenical poisoning; dose, ℥ss (15 c.c.), every five or ten minutes.

FERRI CARBONAS SACCHARATUS (*saccharated ferrous carbonate*), dose, gr. ij–x (0.12–0.6 gm.).

MASSA FERRI CARBONATIS (*mass of ferrous carbonate; Vallet's mass*), dose, gr. iij–v (0.2–0.3 gm.).

PILULÆ FERRI CARBONATIS (*pills of iron carbonate; Blaud's pills*); each pill is intended to contain about gr. j (0.06 gm.) of ferrous carbonate, an excellent preparation in anemia and chlorosis; dose, 2 to 5 pills.

MISTURA FERRI COMPOSITÆ (*compound iron mixture: Griffith's antihectic mixture*), dose, in anemia or chlorosis, ℥ss–ij (15–60 c.c.).

FERRI SULPHAS (*ferrous sulphate; green vitriol* or *copperas*); one of the most active and astringent preparations of iron. It is irritant to the stomach, and in overdoses is a poison. It is used locally as a styptic and astringent, and in solution to disinfect privies and drains; dose (in pill), gr. ss–ij (0.03–0.13 gm.).

FERRI SULPHAS EXSICCATUS (*dried ferrous sulphate*)—ferrous sulphate deprived of its water of crystallization; dose, gr. ¼–2 (0.016–0.13 gm.).

FERRI SULPHAS GRANULATUS (*granulated ferrous sulphate*), dose, gr. j–v (0.06–0.3 gm.).

LIQUOR FERRI TERSULPHATIS (*solution of ferric sulphate*), a solution of normal ferric sulphate; rarely used except in making hydrated ferric oxid (the arsenic antidote).

LIQUOR FERRI SUBSULPHATIS (*solution of ferric subsulphate; Monsel's solution*), a solution of basic ferric sulphate. It may be given internally, largely diluted, as a hemostatic; dose, ♏j–x (0.06–0.6 c.c.). It is chiefly used locally as a styptic.

FERRI CHLORIDUM (*ferric chlorid*), rarely used internally; dose, gr. j–ij (0.06–0.13 gm.).

LIQUOR FERRI CHLORIDI (*solution of ferric chlorid*), dose, ♏ij–v (0.12–0.3 c.c.), largely diluted; externally it is used as a styptic.

TINCTURA FERRI CHLORIDI (*tincture of ferric chlorid*) is one of the best preparations of iron for internal use. It possesses diuretic properties and has an acid reaction; dose, ♏v–xxx (0.3–2 c.c.).

LIQUOR FERRI ET AMMONII ACETATIS (*solution of iron and ammonium acetate; Basham's mixture*); an excellent preparation, combining tonic and diuretic properties, very valuable in chronic desquamative nephritis and chronic dropsies generally; dose, ℥ss–j (15–30 c.c.).

SYRUPUS FERRI IODIDI (*syrup of ferrous iodid*), dose, ♏v–xxx (0.3–2 c.c.).

PILULÆ FERRI IODIDI (*pills of ferrous iodid*), dose, 1 to 3 pills.

FERRI PHOSPHAS SOLUBILIS (*soluble ferric phosphate*), dose, gr. ij–v (0.13–0.3 gm.).

FERRI PYROPHOSPHAS SOLUBILIS (*soluble ferric pyrophosphate*), dose, gr. ij–v (0.13–0.3 gm.).

FERRI HYPOPHOSPHIS (*ferric hypophosphite*), dose, gr. v–x (0.3–0.6 gm.).

FERRI CITRAS (*ferric citrate*), dose, gr. ij–x (0.13–0.6 gm.).

FERRI ET POTASSII TARTRAS (*iron and potassium tartrate; potassiotartrate of iron*) may be prescribed with alkalis; dose, gr. ij–x (0.13–0.6 gm.).

FERRI ET AMMONII TARTRAS (*iron and ammonium tartrate*), a mild preparation; dose, gr. ij–x (0.13–0.6 gm.).

FERRI ET AMMONII SULPHAS (*ferric ammonium sulphate; ammonioferric alum*) is given internally as an astringent in chronic diarrhea and dysentery; dose, gr. j–v (0.06–0.3 gm.).

FERRI ET AMMONII CITRAS (*iron and ammonium citrate*), dose, gr. ij–v (0.13–0.3 gm.).

VINUM FERRI (*wine of iron*), dose, ʒj (4 c.c.).

FERRI ET QUININÆ CITRAS (*iron and quinine citrate*).

FERRI ET QUININÆ CITRAS SOLUBILIS (*soluble iron and quinine citrate*); each contains 85 per cent. of ferric citrate and 12 per cent. of the alkaloid, and may be given in doses of gr. j–v or x (0.06–0.3 or 0.6 gm.).

VINUM FERRI AMARUM (*bitter wine of iron*), dose, ʒj–ij (4–8 c.c.).

FERRI ET STRYCHNINÆ CITRAS (*iron and strychnine citrate*) contains 1 per cent. of strychnine; dose, gr. ij–v (0.13–03 gm.).

ELIXIR FERRI, QUININÆ ET STRYCHNINÆ PHOSPHATUM (*elixir of iron, quinine, and strychnine phosphates*), dose, ʒj (4 c.c.), which contains $\frac{1}{64}$ grain (0.001 gm.) of strychnine and $\frac{1}{2}$ grain (0.03 gm.) of quinine.

GLYCERITUM FERRI, QUININÆ ET STRYCHNINÆ PHOSPHATUM (*glycerite of iron, quinine, and strychnine phosphates*), dose, ♏xv (1 c.c.)—exactly four times as strong as the syrup.

SYRUPUS FERRI, QUININÆ ET STRYCHNINÆ PHOSPHATUM (*syrup of iron, quinine, and strychnine phosphates*), dose, ʒj (4 c.c.), which contains $\frac{1}{80}$ grain (0.0008 gm.) of strychnine and $1\frac{3}{5}$ grains (0.1 gm.) of quinine. It is one-quarter the strength of the glycerite.

What medicines are incompatible with the iron preparations?

1. *The alkaline preparations of iron* are incompatible with the acids and acidulous salts.

2. *The salts formed by mineral acids with iron*, with the alkalis and alkaline earths and their carbonates.

3. *The iodids, bromids, and salts containing vegetable acids*, with the alkalis and alkaline earths and their carbonates, and with acids and (other) acidulous salts.

4. *All the iron preparations*, with substances containing tannic or gallic acids; hence they cannot be prescribed with any of the vegetable tonics except the simple bitters.

When and how should iron be administered?

The fluid preparations should all be given freely diluted. The solid preparations may be given combined with other remedies in pilular form or in solution. Iron causes less gastric irritation and enters the blood more readily if given with or immediately after meals. If gastric irritability is present in anemia, a course of bitters with the acids had better precede the administration of iron, which, as these symptoms subside, may be given in the form of the lactate, followed by the bitter wine, and finally, by the dried sulphate with arsenic in pill, or by the tincture of the chlorid. In anemia iron should be given in rapidly increasing doses until headache, flushing of the face, and some nausea supervene, when the dose should be diminished or the medicine withheld for a few days. It is important to overcome the resulting constipation by occasional laxatives.

MANGANUM (MANGANESE).

What are the sources of manganese?

Manganese is obtained from the native (impure) dioxid and also from the carbonate.

What are its physiologic actions?

Manganese exists normally in the blood, hair, bile, etc., associated with iron, the proportion to iron in the red corpuscles being as 1 to 20. Given internally in small doses, *manganese dioxid* improves the appetite, digestion, and nutrition; in larger doses it depresses the heart's action and lowers the blood-pressure; if large doses are given for some time, the effects resemble those of zinc (wasting and feebleness, staggering gait, and finally paraplegia); it increases menstruation. In toxic doses it is a gastro-intestinal irritant. The *sulphate* is an emetocathartic and cholagogue. *Potassium permanganate* is a powerful oxidizing agent, and hence an antiseptic. It increases the menstrual flow.

For what medicinal purposes is manganese used?

It has been used—(1) *to improve the condition of the blood* in *anemia* and *chlorosis* and in *various cachexiæ*, either combined with iron or as a substitute for it; (2) *to improve the appetite and digestion* in *gastrodynia* and *pyrosis;* (3) *as a cholagogue* in *jaundice* when of malarial origin (sulphate); (4) *as an antidote to snake-bites* and other animal poisons, and in poisoning by morphine (potassium permanganate internally and locally); (5) in *amenorrhea* (potassium permanganate and manganese dioxid); and (6) *locally* as a *disinfectant* and to *correct fetor* in *scarlatina* and *diphtheria* (permanganate as a gargle), or applied to *cancerous or other ulcers, abscesses, otorrhea*, etc.

What are the preparations and doses of manganese?

MANGANI DIOXIDUM PRÆCIPITATUM (*precipitated manganese dioxid*), dose, gr. j–x (0.06–0.6 gm.), in pill, powder, or capsule.

MANGANI HYPOPHOSPHIS (*manganese hypophosphite*), dose, gr. j–v (0.06–0.3 gm.).

MANGANI SULPHAS (*manganese sulphate*), dose, gr. j–v (0.06–0.3 gm.).

POTASSII PERMANGANAS (*potassium permanganate*), dose, gr. ss–ij (0.03–0.13 gm.), in distilled water, in capsule, or made into pill with kaolin.

What medicines are incompatible with manganese?

The salts of lead, silver, and mercury, and the caustic alkalis are chemically incompatible with the manganese preparations. Organic matter decomposes the permanganate.

PHOSPHORUS.

What is the source from which phosphorus is obtained?

Phosphorus is obtained from the calcium phosphate of bones

What are the physiologic effects of phosphorus?

Phosphorus exists normally in nervous tissue and in the bones. *Locally* applied, phosphorus causes inflammation, ulceration, and even gangrene of the skin. The *vapor*, when inhaled, irritates the mucous membrane, and if caries of the teeth exists, may cause caries or necrosis of the maxillæ.

In medicinal doses phosphorus increases the *appetite and digestion* (if too long continued, it disorders digestion), and causes eructations of hydrogen phosphid; increases *nutrition*, the *cardiac action*, and cutaneous circulation, *mental activity*, *sexual activity*, the formation of the *compact tissue of bone*, and the excretion of phosphates by the *urine*. It is *eliminated* by the liver, kidneys, mucous membrane, and skin.

What are the toxic effects of phosphorus?

From one to three hours after a poisonous dose has been swallowed violent *epigastric pains* occur, followed by nausea and *vomiting* (the vomited mater *smelling of phosphorus* and being *luminous in the dark*); *vomiting of blood* occurs at a later period; violent purging takes place if the phosphorus passes into the bowel. *Jaundice* may supervene after several days if the patient lives. The pulse is at first strong, soon becoming feeble and rapid. There are great thirst, restlessness, anxiety, noisy delirium or coma, and death, preceded by convulsions. The *urine* is diminished, contains albumin, blood, and (after jaundice occurs) biliary pigment. After death, acute fatty degeneration of various viscera, as the liver, kidneys, heart, and the walls of the arterioles and capillaries, is found; the red corpuscles are altered in form and the blood contains much fat.

What is the treatment of acute poisoning by phosphorus?

1. Give *cupric sulphate*, gr. v (0.3 gm.), at once as an emetic and as an antidote (forming a less soluble phosphid).

2. Give *hydrated magnesia* as a purgative.

3. Continue the use of *cupric sulphate* in small doses (gr. $\frac{1}{12}$—0.005 gm.—every fifteen or twenty minutes) as an antidote or emetic, or, better, give *turpentine* (French acid turpentine or old common, crude turpentine, which forms with phosphorus an almost insoluble spermaceti-like mass) as soon

as possible, to neutralize the poison. *Peroxid of hydrogen* forms the less active oxid of phosphorus.

4. Give *opium* to counteract the general depression.

5. If the blood is much damaged, transfusion should be resorted to.

6. Never, under any circumstances, give any oils (except turpentine) or fats, as they increase the solubility of phosphorus.

What are the medicinal uses of phosphorus?

Phosphorus is used as a *tonic to promote nutrition:* (1) In various nervous affections associated with anemia, as *cerebral exhaustion, locomotor ataxia, paralysis agitans*, and the various *neuralgias;* (2) in general disease, as, *osteomalacia, rickets*, and *pernicious anemia;* (3) in *functional impotence;* and (4) as a substitute for arsenic in certain skin diseases, as *lupus* and *psoriasis.*

What are the preparations of phosphorus and their doses?

PILULÆ PHOSPHORI (*pills of phosphorus*); each pill contains gr. $\frac{1}{100}$ (0.006 gm.) of phosphorus; dose, 1 to 5 pills, three times a day.

The unofficial *Elixir of Phosphorus*, of which each cubic centimeter contains gr. $\frac{1}{250}$ (0.00025 gm.) of phosphorus, and the *Phosphorated Oil*, containing 1 per cent. of phosphorus, are sometimes used. *Zinci Phosphidum (zinc phosphid)*—unofficial—is identical in its actions and uses with phosphorus, but not so active; dose, gr. $\frac{1}{20}$–$\frac{1}{12}$, or even $\frac{1}{2}$ (0.003–0.03 gm.), given in pill or granule.

What medicines are incompatible with phosphorus?

Hydrated magnesia, lime-water, cupric sulphate, powdered charcoal, and oil of turpentine are chemically incompatible with it.

What substances aid its absorption?

The oils and fats.

What caution should be observed in prescribing it?

Great care should be taken, especially when large doses are prescribed, that the remedy be not administered for a long period continuously for fear of causing fatty degenerations of the viscera.

Mineral Acids.

Name the mineral acids.

The mineral acids are *sulphuric, nitric, hydrochloric, nitrohydrochloric,* and *phosphoric.*

What are their physiologic effects?

Locally the strong acids are *escharotics,* abstracting water from the tissues and combining with the bases. *Sulphuric* and *phosphoric* acids penetrate the tissues more deeply than the others. *Sulphuric* produces a *black,* while *nitric* acid causes a *yellow,* eschar.

Acids *in the mouth* increase the flow of saliva and relieve thirst.

Acids *in the stomach* aid pepsin digestion, diminish the secretion of gastric juice, and reflexly increase the secretion of pancreatic juice.

Excess of acid *in the duodenum* induces closure of the pylorus, and so prevents the stomach from discharging more acid chyme until that already discharged is neutralized.

Sulphuric acid possesses an astringent influence over the secretions of the skin and bowels; nitric acid, on the contrary, appears to increase the alimentary secretions and that of the liver.

They are *eliminated* by the secretions of the kidneys, bowels, and skin. *In large doses* they act as irritant corrosive poisons.

How should poisoning by the mineral acids be treated?

1. Give *alkalis* or *alkaline earths* (tooth-powder or soap may be used) to neutralize the acid. If possible, avoid the carbonated alkalis, as they liberate too much carbon dioxid gas.
2. Give *eggs, milk,* or other *demulcents* to protect the surface.
3. Give *opium* and *nutritive* and *stimulating enemata* or *intravenous injection* of ammonia, to counteract the resulting depression.
4. As stricture of the esophagus often follows in these cases if they survive, the passage of an esophageal bougie should be practised within three or four months after the poisoning.

What are the therapeutic uses of the mineral acids?

1. *For their Effects on Digestion and Nutrition.*—To prevent

excessive formation of acid diluted hydrochloric or phosphoric acid is given before meals; or in *atonic dyspepsia* and *indigestion* due to deficient acid, they may be taken after meals (often combined with pepsin). *In fevers* they are used to aid digestion and allay thirst (by stimulating the secretions of the mouth and fauces, thus keeping these parts moist).

2. *For their Effects on Secretion.*—Diluted nitric or nitro-hydrochloric acid is used internally to increase the secretions, and as a bath (℥iij to water Cj), in *chronic hepatic congestions* and *inflammations*, in *malarial* and *catarrhal jaundice*, and in *duodenal catarrh*. As an *astringent in diarrheas, dysentery*, and *cholera*, diluted sulphuric acid is given combined with opium; and to arrest profuse sweating, diluted or aromatic sulphuric acid may be temporarily employed.

3. *As a hemostatic* the same agent is often used in uterine or intestinal hemorrhage and occasionally in purpura.

4. *In the treatment of, or as a preventive to, lead-poisoning* diluted sulphuric acid is administered (forming an insoluble lead sulphate).

5. *Locally, as an escharotic*, fuming nitric acid may be applied to *chancroids, phagedenic ulcers, hospital gangrene*, or *gangrene in wounds*. It is also used to remove *warts*, and as an intra-uterine application in various forms of *endometritis*. As a *stimulating lotion* to *unhealthy granulations*, and to check bleeding from hemorrhoids, weak solutions of nitric acid are used.

What are the preparations of the mineral acids, and what are their doses?

1. ACIDUM SULPHURICUM (*sulphuric acid; oil of vitriol*) contains not less than 92.5 per cent. of *absolute* sulphuric acid, and is too strong for internal use.

ACIDUM SULPHURICUM DILUTUM (*diluted sulphuric acid*) contains 10 per cent. by weight of the *official sulphuric acid*, and is used internally as a *tonic, refrigerant, astringent*, and *hemostatic;* dose, ♏ij–xx (0.12–1.2 c.c.), freely diluted.

ACIDUM SULPHURICUM AROMATICUM (*aromatic sulphuric acid; elixir of vitriol*) contains 20 per cent. by weight (11.1 per cent. by volume) of the *official acid* with alcohol, tincture of ginger, and oil of cinnamon. It is used as a pleasant substitute for the preceding preparation and is given in the same doses.

2. Acidum Nitricum (*nitric acid*) contains 68 per cent. of the *absolute* acid, and is not employed internally.

Acidum Nitricum Dilutum (*diluted nitric acid*) contains 10 per cent. by weight of *absolute* nitric acid; dose, ♏ij–xx (0.12–1.2 c.c.), freely diluted.

3. Acidum Hydrochloricum (*hydrochloric acid; muriatic acid*) contains nearly 32 per cent. by weight of *absolute* acid; dose, ♏ij–v (0.12–0.3 c.c.), freely diluted.

Acidum Hydrochloricum Dilutum (*diluted hydrochloric acid; diluted muriatic acid*) contains 10 per cent. of the absolute acid. It is probably a normal constituent of the gastric juice, and is used as an aid to digestion; dose, ♏v–xx (0.3–1.2 c.c.), freely diluted.

4. Acidum Nitrohydrochloricum (*nitrohydrochloric acid; nitromuriatic acid; aqua regia*) is used as a stomachic tonic and to increase the secretions of the liver and intestine; dose, ♏ij–x (0.12–1.2 c.c.), freely diluted. It contains *nitrosyl chlorid.*

Acidum Nitrohydrochloricum Dilutum (*diluted nitrohydrochloric acid; diluted nitromuriatic acid*), dose, ♏ij–xx (0.12–1.2 c.c.), freely diluted. It should be freshly prepared as it does not keep long.

5. Acidum Phosphoricum (*phosphoric acid*) contains 85 per cent. by weight of absolute orthophosphoric acid, and is not used internally.

Acidum Phosphoricum Dilutum (*diluted phosphoric acid*) contains 10 per cent. by weight of absolute orthophosphoric acid, and is chiefly used as an aid to digestion; dose, ♏v–xxx (0.3–2.0 c.c.), freely diluted.

Acidum Hypophosphorosum (*hypophosphorous acid*) contains 30 per cent. by weight of absolute hypophosphorous acid, and is used, well diluted, as an antiseptic in gastric fermentation. Dose, ♏v–x (0.3–0.7 c.c.).

What medicines are incompatible with the mineral acids?

1. Alkalis and their carbonates and the salts of lime and lead are incompatible with the mineral acids, which also decompose salts of the vegetable acids, uniting with their bases.

2. The mercurial salts should not be given during the administration of hydrochloric or nitrohydrochloric acids or their

preparations, as they may react with the mercury and form corrosive sublimate.

How and when are these acids administered?

They are administered before or after meals, according to the indications present, and may be given freely diluted with water either alone or with glycerin and syrup, or with some of the bitters.

They should be taken through a glass tube to prevent injury to the teeth, or the mouth may be washed out immediately after their use with some weak alkaline solution.

ACIDUM LACTICUM (LACTIC ACID).

What is lactic acid?

Lactic acid is a syrupy liquid, formed by the souring of milk.

What are its effects and uses?

In *medicinal doses* it increases the appetite, aids digestion, and stimulates nutrition. In *large doses* (ʒj) or *long continued* it disorders digestion, causing flatulency and epigastric pain. *Injected into the peritoneal cavity* (dog's) it produces endocarditis, and when given for a very long time (in diabetes) it has caused acute rheumatism. *Lactic acid is used* to *diminish the acidity* of the gastric juice or to *replace the deficiency of the acid;* to aid digestion and nutrition in *oxalic, phosphatic,* or *uric* acid *diathesis;* in *diabetes,* and *locally* as a solvent for the false membranes of croup and diphtheria. It has been claimed that it is a hypnotic in *insomnia* due to nervous excitement, but this is still *sub judice.* It has been much used as a local application to tuberculous ulcers of pharynx and larynx.

What are its preparations and doses?

ACIDUM LACTICUM (*lactic acid*) contains 75 per cent. of absolute lactic acid. Dose, ♏v–xxx (0.3–2.0 c.c.), freely diluted and often prescribed in a mixture with pepsin.

ALTERATIVES.

What are alteratives?

Alteratives are medicines which, without exerting any very perceptible action on any particular organ, so modify the nutritive processes as to enable nature to restore healthy action in many diseased conditions.

Mention the principal alteratives.

The preparations of mercury and of gold; iodin and the iodids; the arsenical preparations; cod-liver oil; the phosphates and hypophosphites; the chlorids of ammonium and calcium; colchicum; sarsaparilla; guaiac; and perhaps mezereon; calendula; sassafras; stillingia; and lappa.

HYDRARGYRUM (MERCURY).

What is mercury?

Mercury is a liquid metal principally obtained from the native sulphid or cinnabar.

What are the physiologic effects of mercury?

Metallic mercury (quicksilver) in large quantities passes mechanically through the alimentary tract, but in small quantities is readily absorbed by mucous membrane or skin. Most of the salts are irritating, corrosive sublimate being so to the greatest degree and calomel to the least degree. Mercury is administered by mouth, by hypodermic injection, by inunction through the skin, or by inhalation of the vapor. Unlike most metals, mercury quickly enters the circulation and unites with the tissues.

Mercury and its salts possess the properties of an alterative, stimulating the secretions, promoting absorption of morbid products, and improving the nutrition. They increase the flow of bile, probably by acting on the duodenal mucous membrane, for direct action on the liver-cells has not been demonstrated, and they stimulate peristalsis and intestinal and pancreatic secretion, and so produce catharsis. They are partly retained in the body, being fixed in the tissues, and partly eliminated by the kidneys and large intestine.

Externally they are antiseptic and antiparasiticide, especially corrosive sublimate, white precipitate, and blue ointment.

The first symptoms of overdosage are usually profuse salivation, tender gums, offensive breath, and a metallic taste. These effects are less frequent if a gargle of potassium chlorate is used or if potassium iodid is given with the mercury. Continued usage induces loss of nutrition, ulceration of the gums, loosened teeth, diarrhea, albuminuria, and grave nervous symptoms. In syphilis mercury is well borne in large doses.

What are the symptoms and treatment of poisoning by corrosive sublimate?

The symptoms are violent gastro-enteritis with vomiting and purging, bloody stools, abdominal pain and tenderness, albuminous urine, and death from collapse. The treatment consists in—(1) Giving an antidote (*albumin* is the best, *white of eggs,* milk or wheat flour); (2) giving an emetic; and (3) the free use of opiates and demulcents.

What are the therapeutic uses of mercury?

Mercury is used—(1) As an *antisyphilitic,* by the mouth (yellow iodid, calomel, blue-mass, corrosive sublimate), fumigation (calomel), inunction (mercurial ointment or oleate), or hypodermic injection (albuminate, peptonate, or even calomel or corrosive sublimate). It is of most use in secondary syphilis, the iodids (alone or combined with the red iodid or corrosive chlorid) giving better results in tertiary syphilis.

(2) As an *antiplastic and sorbefacient* in *acute glandular affections, iritis,* and the *latter stages of inflammations* after plastic effusion has occurred. In *diphtheria* and *membranous croup* calomel is advantageously given in repeated doses, guarded by minute doses of opium, or its vapor inhaled. In the latter disease the subsulphate is often used as an emetic. Mercurials are useful in ileocolitis of infants (gray powder) and in acute dysentery. (3) As an *indirect tonic* and to *stimulate secretions,* calomel, gray powder, or blue-mass is used in dyspepsia attended with constipation and torpid liver and in the early stages of acute diseases. (4) As a *purgative* calomel and blue-mass are often used, followed by some saline cathartic. (5) *Locally* as *antiseptics* mercuric chlorid is almost indispensable in surgical practice, used in solutions of 1: 10,000 to 1: 1000. It is very corrosive, precipitates albumin, and may produce a slough over a wounded area. It attacks steel instruments. Various preparations are used locally in various *skin diseases,* especially of parasitic origin, and to *promote*

absorption in *goiter, enlarged spleen, chronic epididymitis, orchitis,* and other glandular swellings. The ointments are also used in conjunctivitis.

What are the preparations of mercury and their doses?

MASSA HYDRARGYRI (*mass of mercury; blue-mass*), dose, as a *laxative,* gr. v–xv (0.3–1.0 gm.); as an *alterative, anti-syphilitic,* or *sorbefacient,* gr. ss–iij (0.03–0.2 gm.), t. i. d., guarded by opium, and often combined in the treatment of syphilis with iron, quinine, or iodids.

UNGUENTUM HYDRARGYRI (*mercurial ointment*)—not used internally—contains 50 per cent. of mercury and 2 per cent. of oleate of mercury. Used externally for *inunction* in syphilis, as a *sorbefacient,* to *destroy pediculi,* and as a dressing to *syphilitic ulcers.*

UNGUENTUM HYDRARGYRI DILUTUM (*blue ointment*) contains 67 per cent. of *mercurial ointment.*

EMPLASTRUM HYDRARGYRI (*mercurial plaster*), used locally as a *sorbefacient.*

HYDRARGYRUM CUM CRETA (*mercury with chalk; gray powder*) contains mercury, 38 parts, with prepared chalk and clarified honey, and is used as an *alterative* and *antisyphilitic;* dose for an adult, gr. j–v (0.06–0.3 gm.); for a child, gr. ¼ (0.02 gm.), t. i. d.; as a mild laxative, gr. v–xv (0.3–1.0 gm.); for a child, gr. iij–v (0.2–0.3 gm.).

HYDRARGYRI OXIDUM RUBRUM (*red mercuric oxid*) and
HYDRARGYRI OXIDUM FLAVUM (*yellow mercuric oxid*) are rarely used except in the form of—

UNGUENTUM HYDRARGYRI OXIDI RUBRI (*ointment of red mercuric oxid; red precipitate ointment*) and

UNGUENTUM HYDRARGYRI OXIDI FLAVI (*ointment of yellow mercuric oxid*), each containing 10 per cent. of mercuric oxid. They are applied in *granular* and other forms of *conjunctivitis* and in *corneal ulcers.*

OLEATUM HYDRARGYRI (*mercurial oleate*) contains 25 per cent. of the yellow oxid dissolved in oleic acid. Used chiefly for inunction in syphilis.

HYDRARGYRI CHLORIDUM MITE (*mercurous chlorid; calomel*), dose, as a *purgative* or *anthelmintic,* gr. ss–j–x (0.03–0.06–0.6 gm.) at bedtime; as an *antisyphilitic,* gr. $\frac{1}{10}$–j

(0.006–0.06 gm.), t. i. d., with opium; as an *alterative* and *absorbent*, gr. ss–j (0.03–0.06 gm.), every two or three hours; for its effect on *secretions*, gr. ss–j (0.03–0.06 gm.), t. i. d.; to *arrest vomiting*, gr. $\frac{1}{10}$–j (0.006–0.06 gm.), combined with sodium bicarbonate and frequently repeated; to *abort pneumonia*, gr. xx (1.2 gm.) are sometimes given at one dose. It is used externally as a dusting-powder to the conjunctiva and as an ointment in various skin affections. It is also used by *fumigation* in syphilis and acute laryngeal troubles.

Hydrargyri Chloridum Corrosivum (*mercuric chlorid; corrosive sublimate*), used as an *alterative* and *antisyphilitic;* dose, gr. $\frac{1}{16}$–$\frac{1}{8}$ (0.004–0.008 gm.) by the mouth, gr. $\frac{1}{48}$–$\frac{1}{16}$ (0.001–0.004 gm.) by hypodermic injection. Locally, in weak solutions as an injection in vaginitis, in *gonorrhea* after the more acute stage has passed (gr. $\frac{1}{12}$–$\frac{1}{8}$–℥viij—0.005–0.008–240 c.c.), in diphtheria as a throat irrigation or as a *parasiticide* in ringworm, etc., or for the destruction of pediculi. As an *antiseptic*, gr. viiss to hot water Oij – 1 : 2000.

Hydrargyri Iodidum Flavum (*mercurous iodid* or *protoiodid*), dose, as an *antisyphilitic*, gr. $\frac{1}{8}$–j (0.008–0.065 gm.), combined with opium in pill. Used also locally, in the form of ointment, to syphilitic ulcers.

Hydrargyri Iodidum Rubrum (*mercuric iodid*), dose, as an *alterative* or *antisyphilitic*, gr. $\frac{1}{16}$–$\frac{1}{4}$ (0.004–0.015 gm.). It is often combined with potassium iodid in the treatment of tertiary syphilis, and is used locally in the form of ointment to promote the absorption of glandular swellings, goiter, enlarged spleen, etc. As an *antiseptic* it is used in solution of gr. iv–viiss (0.25–0.5 gm.) to hot water Oij (1000 c.c.). Potassium iodid increases its solubility.

Hydrargyrum Ammoniatum (*ammoniated mercury; white precipitate*) is used only externally as—

Unguentum Hydrargyri Ammoniati (*ointment of ammoniated mercury*), which contains 10 per cent. of ammoniated mercury, and is used especially in parasitic skin diseases and to destroy pediculi.

Unguentum Hydrargyri Nitratis (*ointment of mercurial nitrate; citrine ointment*), used externally (usually diluted with other ointment) in various skin affections, especially those of parasitic origin, to destroy pediculi and as a dressing for venereal ulcers.

LIQUOR HYDRARGYRI NITRATIS (*solution of mercuric nitrate; acid nitrate of mercury*), used as an *escharotic.* Diluted with water, it forms a useful stimulating application to indolent ulcers.

HYDRARGYRI SUBSULPHAS FLAVUS (*turpeth mineral*) is not official, but is employed as an *emetic* in croup, in dose of gr. j–v (0.06–0.3 gm.), repeated two or three times at ten-minute intervals, or till vomiting ensues.

What substances are incompatible with the mercurial preparations?

The *metallic preparations* and *calomel* are incompatible with the chlorids, hydrochloric and nitrohydrochloric acids, which are apt to form with them corrosive sublimate. *Calomel* is also incompatible with the alkalis, their carbonates, alkaline earths, soap, and the hydrosulphates. *Corrosive sublimate* is decomposed by nearly everything, and *yellow mercurous iodid* is converted into the more active red mercuric iodid by combination with iodin and other iodids.

AURUM (GOLD).

What are the physiologic effects of the salts of gold?

Locally they are caustic. *Internally* in *small doses* they increase the appetite, digestion, glandular secretions, and excretions of urine and perspiration; they stimulate the nervous system, and particularly the spinal cord; they stimulate the sexual organs, and in women (probably) increase the menstrual flow. In *larger doses* or after prolonged use they disorder digestion, cause salivation without ulceration of the gums, diminish the oxygen-carrying function of the red globules, and stimulate the lymphatic system, thus causing rapid wasting. In *overdoses* they are gastro-intestinal irritants, the *symptoms* and *antidote* being the same as those of poisoning by corrosive sublimate.

What are the medicinal uses of the gold salts?

They are used as substitutes for corrosive sublimate in the

treatment of *tertiary syphilis*; as *alteratives* in scrofula, chronic Bright's disease, myelitis, chronic ovarian inflammations, and neuralgia; and as *aphrodisiacs* in functional impotence.

The so-called "*bichlorid of gold*" or "*Keeley cure*" does not consist in the administration of gold bichlorid, as no such salt is known.

What are the preparations and doses of the gold salts?

AURI ET SODII CHLORIDUM (*gold and sodium chlorid*) is the only official preparation; dose, gr. $\frac{1}{30}$–$\frac{1}{10}$ (0.002–0.006 gm.), in pill or capsule.

IODUM (IODIN).

What is iodin?

Iodin is a non-metallic element, obtained from the ashes of sea-weed.

What are the physiologic effects of iodin and the iodids?

Iodin is a *disinfectant* and *antiseptic*. *Locally* applied, it is an *irritant caustic* to the skin and mucous membranes, staining the former yellow and causing superficial inflammation and desquamation, and sometimes even vesication. The *vapor*, when inhaled, is irritant to the air-passages. In sufficient amounts it is a gastro-intestinal irritant. It enters the blood readily, and, combining with sodium or potassium, corresponds, in its constitutional effects, to the *iodids*. They *stimulate* the *lymphatic system* and cause the *absorption* especially of newly formed tissues and diseased cells, thus removing indolent swellings, inflammatory and syphilitic deposits, and various metallic poisons, as lead, mercury, etc., which may have been deposited in the tissues. When *too long administered*, they cause great emaciation and depression of the vital powers. They are rapidly *eliminated* by the mucous membranes (irritating them in their passage), salivary glands, and kidneys.

Given in *large quantities*, they cause *iodism*—*i. e.*, malaise, some fever, frontal headache, coryza, lacrimation, sore throat, difficult swallowing, various eruptions on the face and shoulders, and anaphrodisiac effects, sometimes permanent. The susceptibility varies greatly in different persons, but these symptoms may in great measure be prevented by copious drafts of water frequently taken during the course of treatment and by the administration of arsenic.

What is the treatment of acute poisoning by free iodin?

A decoction of starch is the *antidote*, followed by emetics and opium and demulcents.

What are the therapeutic use of iodin and the iodids?

They are employed as *alteratives* and *absorbents* in the active manifestations of *tertiary syphilis* (iodids chiefly), in the treatment of *scrofulous and glandular enlargements*, in the early stages of *cirrhosis* of the liver or kidneys, in the various forms of *sclerosis* of the nervous centers, and in *chronic poisoning* by mercury, lead, and other metals; to aid the absorption of *lingering pneumonic consolidation* and of *plastic* and *serous* inflammatory *exudations*, in *aneurysms*, in *chronic rheumatism*, and in *malaria*.

For their effects on the *mucous secretions* the iodids are given in *chronic bronchitis*, *spasmodic asthma*, *catarrhal pneumonia*, *acute catarrh*, *hay-fever*, and *duodenal catarrh*. Iodin has been used to check the *vomiting of pregnancy*. *Locally*, *iodin* is used by inhalation in *catarrh*, *coryza*, and *hay-fever*, and is applied to *aid absorption* and as a *counterirritant* to *chronic inflammations* and *chronic glandular* and other *swellings*. *The tincture* is *injected* undiluted into the serous cavity after the removal of the fluid in empyema, hydrocele, etc., and is applied to the uterine cavity in various forms of *endometritis*.

What are the preparations and doses of iodin and the iodids?

LIQUOR IODI COMPOSITUS (*compound solution of iodin; Lugol's solution*), containing iodin (5 parts), potassium iodid (10 parts), and water (85 parts); dose, ♏ v–xv (0.3–1.0 c.c.), t. i. d.

TINCTURA IODI (*tincture of iodin*), containing 7 per cent. of iodin and 5 per cent. of potassium iodid; dose, ♏ ij–xv (0.12–1.0 c.c.), t. i. d. It is chiefly used externally.

UNGUENTUM IODI (*iodin ointment*) contains iodin (4 parts), potassium iodin (4 parts), glycerin (12 parts), and benzoinated lard (80 parts).

Potassii Iodidum (*potassium iodid*), dose, gr. ij–xv–ʒj (0.13–1.0–4.0 c.c.), t. i. d.

Unguentum Potassii Iodidi (*ointment of potassium iodid*) is much less powerful than iodin ointment.

Ammonii Iodidum (*ammonium iodid*), dose, gr. ij–xv (0.13–1.0 gm.).

Sodii Iodidum (*sodium iodid*), dose, gr. v–xxx (0.3–2.0 gm.).

Sulphuris Iodidum (*sulphur iodid*) is but little used; dose, gr. ss–j (0.03–0.6 gm.).

Strontii Iodidum (*strontium iodid*) is supposed to be as efficacious as the other iodids and to be less likely to cause iodism; dose, gr. v–x (0.3–0.6 gm.).

Acidum Hydriodicum Dilutum (*diluted hydriodic acid*) is of 10 per cent. strength; dose, ♏v–x (0.3–0.7 c.c.).

Syrupus Acidi Hydriodici (*syrup of hydriodic acid*) is of 1 per cent. strength; dose, ʒss–ij (2–8 c.c.).

The *mercurial iodids* and *iron iodid* have already been mentioned. *Arsenic, zinc, and lead iodids* will be described in their appropriate places.

What are the incompatibilities of these preparations?

The *iodids* are incompatible with the acids and acidulous salts; with the soluble metallic salts generally; with most of the alkaloids, and with sweet spirits of niter. Iodin is precipitated from the *tincture* on the addition of water.

How are iodin and the iodids administered?

Lugol's solution may be given in syrup and water. The iodids may be administered in compressed pill or capsule, or they may be given dissolved in water flavored with orange syrup, or in one of the bitter tinctures, or in compound syrup of sarsaparilla. Nothing effectually disguises their unpleasant taste.

ARSENUM (ARSENIC).

What is arsenic?

Arsenic is a metallic element found in various ores combined with other metals as an arsenid.

Mention some of the tests for arsenic.

When *in powder*, if heated with charcoal in a small test-tube, it sublimes and condenses in the form of a brilliant steel-gray ring of minute octahedral crystals, soluble in sodium or calcium hypochlorite. When in *solution*, the addition of sulphureted hydrogen or ammonium sulphid produces a lemon-yellow arsenic trisulphid, insoluble in diluted hydrochlorid acid, but soluble in a solution of ammonium carbonate; also the addition of ammonia-water, followed by a solution of silver nitrate, gives a canary-yellow silver arsenite. Marsh's and Reinsch's test should also be used.

What are the physiologic effects of arsenical preparations?

Metallic arsenic is inert, but when swallowed may be converted into arsenous acid and cause poisoning. No matter how administered, it has a selective action on the gastro-intestinal and bronchopulmonary mucous membranes. *Locally*, arsenous acid is a painful *caustic*, and when in sufficient amount, produces so much inflammation that absorption cannot take place. The *inhalation* of arsenical fumes (as from wall-papers) has caused chronic poisoning. Given *internally in small doses*, it improves the appetite, digestion, nutrition, and condition of the blood, stimulates the secretions of the alimentary canal, and increases peristalsis; slightly stimulates the respiratory and circulatory centers and the cerebral functions; lessens the excretion of carbonic acid and urea. *In larger doses* (not toxic), or when *taken for some time continuously*, it irritates the mucous membranes, disorders digestion, gives rise to *epigastric pain*, *nausea*, vomiting, *diarrhea*, tenesmus, and sometimes dysentery, palpitation, oppressed breathing, *edema of the eyelids*, albuminuria, cutaneous eruptions, tremor, and disordered sensation. It is *eliminated* by the mucous membranes, liver, kidneys, and skin. *Tolerance* is sometimes established, and very large doses may be taken without poisonous effect.

What are the symptoms, pathologic anatomy, and treatment of acute arsenical poisoning?

The symptoms of the gastro-intestinal variety of poisoning are *intense* burning pain in the epigastrium, radiating over the abdomen, violent vomiting, great thirst, bloody and offensive stools, strangury, bloody urine, rapid feeble heart, oppressed breathing, and collapse, sometimes simulating cholera.

Those of the cerebral variety are sudden—profound insensibility and coma with collapse.

Pathologic Anatomy.—*Alimentary mucous membrane* congested, eroded, softened, and ecchymotic; *bronchopulmonary mucous membrane* and lungs congested; fatty degeneration of the *liver, kidneys, heart,* and other organs.

Treatment.—(1) Give a *prompt emetic* or use the stomach-pump; (2) give as antidotes *hydrated ferric oxid* or the *hydrated ferric oxid with magnesia,* and continue the emetics; (3) mucilaginous drinks to protect the surfaces; (4) large amounts of diluents to favor elimination.

Prognosis.—Death often results long afterward, from the pathologic conditions produced by the poison.

What are the medicinal use of the arsenical preparations?

Arsenic is used as a *tonic* and *alterative* in *anemia* and *chlorosis,* persistent *malaria, rheumatoid arthritis,* and *chronic rheumatism,* and to delay the formation of connective tissue in the various *scleroses* and the growth of *carcinomata.* In minute doses it is used as a gastric tonic in *irritative dyspepsia, gastric ulcer,* and *cancer,* and in *gastralgia* and *enteralgia* (Fowler's solution). In *emphysema, chronic bronchitis,* and *phthisis* it is of value. For its nervous action it is used in *chorea, neuralgias, paralysis agitans,* and *melancholia.* In *chronic skin diseases,* as psoriasis, eczema, and acne, it is of the greatest service, and in *diabetes* and *sexual debility* it is highly recommended. *Locally,* arsenous acid has been used as a caustic in *lupus, onychia maligna, cancer,* and to destroy the nerves of carious teeth; it causes intense pain. Cigarettes made of bibulous paper saturated with a solution of sodium arsenate are smoked for the relief of *asthma.*

What are the preparations and doses of arsenic?

ARSENI TRIOXIDUM (*arsenous acid; white arsenic*), dose, gr. $\frac{1}{16}$–$\frac{1}{12}$ (0.004–0.005 gm.) in pills, t. i. d.

LIQUOR POTASSII ARSENITIS (*solution of potassium arsenite; Fowler's solution*) contains arsenous acid gr. $\frac{6}{10}$ in each ʒj of solution; dose, ♏j–x (0.06–0.6 c.c.), freely diluted.

LIQUOR ACIDI ARSENOSI (*solution of arsenous acid*), dose, ♏j–x (0.06–0.6 c.c.), freely diluted.

SODII ARSENAS (*sodium arsenate*) is milder in its action than the foregoing preparations; dose, gr. $\frac{1}{12}$–$\frac{1}{4}$ (0.005–0.016 gm.).

SODII ARSENAS EXSICCATUS (*dried sodium arsenate*) is sodium arsenate deprived of its water of crystallization. It is about double the strength of sodium arsenate; dose, gr. $\frac{1}{20}$–$\frac{1}{8}$ (0.003–0.008 gm.).

LIQUOR SODII ARSENATIS (*solution of sodium arsenate*), dose, ♏ij–x (0.12–0.6 c.c.), freely diluted.

ARSENI IODIDUM (*arsenic iodid*), dose, gr. $\frac{1}{8}$ (0.008 gm.), t. i. d.

LIQUOR ARSENI ET HYDRARGYRI IODIDI (*solution of arsenic and mercuric iodid; Donovan's solution*) contains 1 per cent. each of arsenic iodid and of mercuric iodid, and is used in obstinate syphilis and in papular and squamous skin-diseases; dose, ♏ij–x (0.12–0.6 c.c.), freely diluted.

What medicinal substances are incompatible with these preparations?

The *salts of iron, magnesium,* and *calcium*, and the *astringents* are chemically incompatible with the preparations of arsenic. *Fowler's solution* should not be prescribed with infusions or decoctions of cinchona nor *Donovan's solution* with the alkalies or the salts of the alkaloids.

How and when is arsenic administered?

As individual susceptibility to arsenic varies greatly,[1] it is better to give a small dose at first. When it is determined that the patient can take arsenic, large doses should be given until some constitutional symptoms occur, when the medicine is discontinued for a few days; or full doses of the liquid preparations gradually decreased to the minimum and as gradually increased may be given when it is desirable to continue the medicine for some time. Arsenic is less likely to disorder the stomach when freely diluted and taken after eating.

[1] The author has seen gastro-enteric symptoms follow the administration of one dose of Fowler's solution of ♏j.

OLEUM MORRHUÆ (COD-LIVER OIL).

What is cod-liver oil?

Cod-liver oil is a *fixed oil* obtained from the fresh *livers* of *Gadus morrhua*, or codfish, and of other species of *Gadus*.

What are its principal chemic constituents?

It contains various fatty acids, several biliary principles, *gaduin*, *iodin*, *chlorin*, and traces of *bromin*.

What are its physiologic effects?

Cod-liver oil is more of a *food* than a *medicine*. It is readily absorbed, whether rubbed into the skin or taken internally. Oil is digested in the intestines (not in the stomach), and is readily assimilated, increasing the deposit of fat in the tissues and the number of corpuscles in the blood. In suitable doses it *improves* the *appetite* and *digestion* and *increases nutrition*. In large doses or in very hot weather it causes nausea and diarrhea.

What are its therapeutic applications?

Cod-liver oil is used as a *nutrient* in chronic wasting diseases, particularly in *phthisis* (the earlier it is given, the more pronounced are its effects), also in *rickets*, *scrofula*, *chlorosis*, *rheumatoid arthritis*, *chronic rheumatism*, *chronic bronchitis*, *emphysema*, and *chronic intestinal diseases* leading to malnutrition.

It is applied *locally for its constitutional effects* when it cannot be taken internally, and also in squamous skin affections.

What is the dose of cod-liver oil, and how should it be administered?

OLEUM MORRHUÆ (*cod-liver oil*) is given in doses of ʒj–℥ss (4–15 c.c.), t. i. d., and preferably one-half to two hours after meals. The *pure oil* is the best form for administration. If it nauseates, it may be given in emulsion with the hypophosphites or with mucilage of acacia and oil of lemon. The addition of a few drops of ether renders it more easy of digestion.

EMULSUM OLEI MORRHUÆ (*emulsion of cod-liver oil*)

contains 50 per cent. of cod-liver oil with acacia, syrup, oil of gaultheria, and water; dose, ℨij–iv (8–15 c.c.).

EMULSUM OLEI MORRHUÆ CUM HYPOPHOSPHITIBUS (*emulsion of cod-liver oil with hypophosphites*) contains in addition the *hypophosphites of calcium, potassium, and sodium.*

THE PHOSPHATES AND HYPOPHOSPHITES.

What is the chemic difference between a phosphid, a phosphate, and a phosphite?

A *phosphid* is formed by the direct union of *phosphorus;* a *phosphate,* by the union of *phosphoric acid;* and a *phosphite,* by the union of *phosphorous acid* with a base.[1]

What are the physiologic actions of the phosphates and hypophosphites?

They increase the nutrition of the body.

Calcium phosphate exists normally in all the tissues of the body, and hence is an important nutrient. It is to this salt that bone owes its hardness.

What are the medicinal uses of these substances?

They are used as *alteratives* and *nutrients* in diseases of malnutrition, especially when these salts are wanting in the system, as in *rickets, mollities ossium, caries* and *necrosis, delayed union* of fractures, *superlactation, prolonged suppuration, anemia, chronic diarrhea,* and *chronic phthisis.* The *hypophosphites* have been lauded in the treatment of phthisis, but probably act only as nutrients.

What are the preparations of these salts and their doses?

CALCII PHOSPHAS PRÆCIPITATUS (*precipitated calcium phosphate*) is a very insoluble preparation, and may form intestinal concretions; dose, gr. v–x (0.3–0.6 gm.). It may be given in milk.

[1] In other words, whenever a salt ends in *id*, it is formed by the union of an element with a base (thus, iron ox*id*, iron and oxygen; iron phosph*id*, iron and phosphorus; iron iod*id*, iron and iodin; iron sulph*id*, iron and sulphur); when a salt ends in *ate*, it shows the union of an *acid ending in ic* with a base (thus iron phosph*ate*, iron and *phosphoric acid;* iron sulph*ate*, iron and *sulphuric acid;* iron nitr*ate*, iron and *nitric acid*); when a salt ends in *ite*, it is composed of an *acid ending* in *ous* and a base (thus, sodium sulph*ite*, sodium and *sulphurous acid;* amyl nitr*ite*, amyl and *nitrous acid*, etc).

Syrupus Calcii Lactophosphatis (*syrup of calcium lactophosphate*); the addition of lactic acid renders the calcium phosphate much more soluble; dose, ʒj–iv (4–15 c.c.), t. i. d.

Calcii Hypophosphis (*calcium hypophosphite*); Potassii Hypophosphis (*potassium hypophosphite*); Sodii Hypophosphis (*sodium hypophosphite*), may each be given in doses of gr. x–xxx (0.6–2.0 gm.), t. i. d. Usually administered as—

Syrupus Hypophosphitum (*syrup of hypophosphites*); dose, ʒj–ij (4–8 c.c.), t. i. d.

Syrupus Hypophosphitum Compositus (*compound syrup of hypophosphites*) contains about $\frac{1}{150}$ gr. (0.00046 gm.) of strychnine and $\frac{1}{15}$ gr. (0.0044 gm.) of quinine in each teaspoonful. Dose, ʒj–ij (4–8 c.c.), t. i. d.

Elixir Ferri, Quininæ et Strychninæ Phosphatum (*elixir of the phosphates of iron, quinine, and strychnine*) and

Glyceritum Ferri, Quininæ, et Strychninæ Phosphatum (*glycerite of the phosphates of iron, quinine, and strychnine*); and

Syrupus Ferri, Quininæ et Strychninæ Phosphatum (*syrup of the phosphates of iron, quinine, and strychnine*) have been considered under Iron (see page 51).

The *ferric phosphates* and *hypophosphite* have also been considered under Iron; *sodium phosphate* will be mentioned with the Cathartics.

CALCII CHLORIDUM (CALCIUM CHLORID).

What are the effects, uses, and doses of this salt?

Calcium chlorid is a gastro-intestinal irritant, and is supposed to possess *alterative* powers in *strumous affections, glandular enlargements, uterine fibroid,* and *ovarian tumors.* It increases the coagulating power of blood, and enhances the action of the gastric juice in coagulating milk. Dose, gr. x–xx (0.6–1.2 gm.) in milk or water.

AMMONII CHLORIDUM (AMMONIUM CHLORID).

In addition to the general effects of the ammonium salts (*q. v.*), it is an alterative and expectorant (see under Expectorants).

COLCHICUM.

What is colchicum?

Colchicum is the *corm* and *seed* of *C. autumnale* or meadow saffron (*Fam.* Liliaceæ), a native of Europe.

What alkaloid does it contain?

It contains *colchicine*, which is converted by mineral acids into *colchicein*.

What are its physiologic effects?

Locally applied it is *irritant. Internally, colchicum or its alkaloid in small doses* increases the secretions generally, particularly the urine, in gout increasing greatly the amount of urea and uric acid eliminated; in *larger doses* it causes nausea and vomiting, frequent purging, and depresses the heart's action; in *excessive doses* it acts as an irritant poison, producing violent vomiting and purging, great depression, collapse, and death by failure of respiration.

How should poisoning by colchicum be treated?

(1) Give emetics and cathartics; (2) tannic acid, as a partial antidote; (3) demulcents, to protect the surfaces; (4) opium and stimulants, to counteract the resulting depression.

What are the therapeutic uses of colchicum?

Colchicum is used as an *alterative* and *diuretic* in *acute gout* (often combined with magnesia and magnesium sulphate (Scudamore's draft) or with potassium iodid or other alkali) and in *rheumatism*. As a *diuretic* it is employed in ascites and other varieties of dropsy. As a *cholagogue* it is given in congestions of the portal circulation.

What are the preparations and doses of colchicum?

EXTRACTUM COLCHICI CORMI (*extract of colchicum corm*), dose, gr. j–ij (0.06–0.13 gm.) in pill.

FLUIDEXTRACTUM COLCHICI SEMINIS (*fluid extract of colchicum seed*), dose, ♏ij–vj (0.12–0.4 c.c.).

TINCTURA COLCHICI SEMINIS (*tincture of colchicum seed*), dose, ʒss–j (2–4 c.c.).

VINUM COLCHICI SEMINIS (*wine of colchicum seed*), containing 10 per cent. of the fluid extract; dose, ℳv–xxx (0.3–2 c.c.)—the best preparation.

COLCHICINA (*colchicine*), dose, gr. $\frac{1}{128}$ (0.005 gm.).

SARSAPARILLA.

What is sarsaparilla?

Sarsaparilla is the *root* of *Smilax medica, Smilax ornata, Smilax papyracea,* and of Honduras sarsaparilla, probably *Smilax officinalis* (*Fam.* Liliaceæ), prickly vines of Mexico, Central and South America.

What special chemic principle does it contain?

A glucosid, called *smilacin* or *parillin,* which resembles saponin.

What are its effects and uses?

It has a very slight diaphoretic action, and in large doses is emetic and purgative. It is popularly supposed to depurate the blood. It has been used as an alterative in tertiary syphilis, and in chronic rheumatism and various cachectic conditions.

What are its preparations and doses?

FLUIDEXTRACTUM SARSAPARILLÆ (*fluid extract of sarsaparilla*), dose, ʒss (2 c.c.), t. i. d.

FLUIDEXTRACTUM SARSAPARILLÆ COMPOSITUM (*compound fluid extract of sarsaparilla*), containing also sassafras, mezereum, and glycyrrhiza; dose, ʒj (4 c.c.).

SYRUPUS SARSAPARILLÆ COMPOSITUS (*compound syrup of sarsaparilla*), containing the fluid extracts of sarsaparilla, licorice, and senna, and the oils of sassafras, anise, and gaultheria; dose, ℥ss–j (15–30 c.c.), t. i. d.

GUAIACUM (GUAIAC).

What is this substance?

Guaiacum is the resin of the *wood* of *G. officinale* and *G. sanctum* (*Fam.* Zygophyllaceæ), evergreen trees of South America, and is composed of *guaiaconic, guaiacic* and *guaiaresinic acids, guaiac beta-resin, guaiac yellow,* and *guaiacin.*

What are the effects, uses, preparations, and doses of these substances?

Guaiac wood and *resin* slightly increase the secretions of the skin and mucous membranes, and in large doses prove emetic and cathartic. They have been used as *alteratives* in syphilis and chronic rheumatism, and also as *emmenagogues* in amenorrhea and congestive dysmenorrhea. In *tonsillitis* the tincture (ʒss (2 c.c.) every three or four hours) or the lozenges (unofficial) are of value.

The preparations are TINCTURA GUAIACI (*tincture of guaiac*) and TINCTURA GUAIACI AMMONIATA (*ammoniated tincture of guaiac*); dose of either, ʒss–ij (2–8 c.c.), three or four times daily, in milk. *Guaiac wood* enters into the *compound decoction* and the *compound syrup of sarsaparilla.*

MEZEREUM (MEZEREUM).

What is mezereum?

It is the *bark* of *Daphne mezereum* and other European species of Daphne (*Fam.* Thymelæaceæ), and contains daphnin (a bitter glucosid) and an acrid resin. *Locally* it is highly irritant; *internally in medicinal doses* it increases the secretions, especially of the salivary glands, skin, and kidneys; *in overdoses* it is an irritant poison and may cause death. It is *used* (generally with sarsaparilla) as an alterative in chronic rheumatism, tertiary syphilis, and strumous affections, and as a *masticatory* it has been chewed in paralysis of the muscles of the tongue and deglutition. For external application as a counterirritant it is an ingredient of the compound liniment of mustard.

FLUIDEXTACTUM MEZEREI (*fluid extract of mezereum*), dose, ♏x (0.6 c.c.).

What is calendula?

Calendula is the *dried ligulate florets* of *C. officinalis* or marigold (*Fam.* Compositæ). It contains *calendulin*, and is supposed to be *diuretic, diaphoretic,* and *alterative.* It is not much used.

TINCTURA CALENDULÆ (*tincture of calendula*); dose, ʒss–j (2–4 c.c.). It may be used externally (diluted) as an application to wounds and contusions.

What is sassafras?

Sassafras is the *bark* of the *root* of *S. variifolium* (*Fam.* Lauraceæ), and contains a *volatile oil.* It is supposed to be a mild *alterative* and *diaphoretic*, and is used in combination with sarsaparilla. The *oil* is used as a flavoring ingredient and as a perfume.

OLEUM SASSAFRAS (*oil of sassafras*), dose, ♏j–v (0.06–0.3 c.c.).

What is stillingia?

It is the *root* of *S. sylvatica*, or Queen's Delight (*Fam.* Euphorbiaceæ), and contains a *volatile oil* and a *resin.* It increases all the secretions and excretions, slightly stimulates the cardiac action, and is believed to be alterative. It has been used in *secondary* and in *tertiary syphilis, scrofula,* and *chronic rheumatism.*

FLUIDEXTRACTUM STILLINGIÆ (*fluid extract of stillingia*), dose, ʒss (2 c.c.).

What is lappa?

Lappa, or burdock, is the *root* of *Arctium Lappa* and other species of Arctium (*Fam.* Compositæ). It contains a bitter extractive, perhaps a glucosid, tannin, resin, etc., and possesses tonic, laxative, and slight diuretic, diaphoretic, and alterant properties. It is used in chronic rheumatism, syphilis, and "scrofulous affections," and occasionally in chronic cutaneous diseases, as psoriasis and prurigo. Locally it is used as an application to contusions.

FLUIDEXTRACTUM LAPPÆ (*fluid extract of lappa*), dose, ♏xv–ʒj (1–4 c.c.).

ANTIPYRETICS.

What are antipyretics, and how do they act?

Antipyretics are remedies which reduce temperature in fever, but in medicinal doses have little or no effect upon it in the normal condition. The temperature may be lowered: (1) By *lessening the production of heat*, or (2) by *increasing the loss of heat.* Heat-production may be diminished either —(1) By *depressing nutrition* (*i. e.*, by retarding oxidation and cell-proliferation); (2) by *depressing the circulation of the part* (as by local abstraction of blood, etc.), or of the system (cardiac sedatives); while the loss of heat may be increased—(1) By *increasing evaporation* from the surface (diaphoretics; (2) by *increasing heat radiation*, through dilatation of the cutaneous vessels (amyl nitrite, alcohol, etc.); (through *direct withdrawal of heat* from the surface (cold applications, etc.). The antipyretics both lessen the production and increase the loss of heat.

Mention the principal antipyretics.

Antipyrin; acetanilid (antifebrin); phenacetin; phenocol; quinine; salicin; salicylic acid and the salicylates; salol; salophen; guaiacol; resorcin.

ANTIPYRIN.

What is antipyrin?

ANTIPYRIN (*antipyrin; phenyldimethyl pyrazolon*), obtained by the condensation of phenyl-hydrazine with aceto-acetic ether, and methylation of the product, has the chemic properties of an alkaloid.

What are the physiologic effects of antipyrin?

Locally antipyrin is *analgesic* and *hemostatic.* Internally its most noteworthy effect is a marked *depression of febrile temperature.* The temperature may drop several degrees to normal, or even a degree or two below normal, and there are depression and sweating. It seems to act on the heat-regulating apparatus of the nervous system. It is sedative to the cerebrum, sometimes inducing sleep, but it increases reflex irritability. The heart and respiration are at first accelerated, later are slow and irregular; tremors, convulsions, collapse, and paralysis may ensue; untoward effects, not uncommon, are giddiness, vomiting, cardiac weakness, restlessness, and a general erythema. It may produce cyanosis by the formation of methemoglobin. It is eliminated by the kidneys, and when the perspiration is slight, increases the urine.

What are the symptoms of poisoning by this drug?

When an overdose is taken, there are often nausea and vomiting, a sense of fulness in the head, tinnitus aurium, relaxation of the muscular system, muscular weakness, cyanosis, cutaneous eruptions, sweating, rapid breathing, feeble pulse, convulsions, and collapse. Occasionally the reflexes are absent. Consciousness is retained.

How should these symptoms be treated?

The treatment consists in keeping the patient in a recumbent position; maintaining the body-heat; administering alcoholic and diffusible stimulants; giving atropine hypodermically, and, if the cyanosis is marked, inhalations of alcohol.

The profuse sweating which is sometimes seen is best combated by giving atropine or agaricin.

The cutaneous eruptions rapidly disappear when the drug is discontinued.

What are its therapeutic uses?

It is used as an *antipyretic* in all cases of *hyperpyrexia*, as in *typhoid fever*, in *sunstroke* with high temperature, in the *exanthemata*, *surgical fever*, *pneumonia*, *erysipelas*, and *influenza*. In *acute rheumatism* it not only lowers temperature, but relieves the pain. It is not an antiperiodic, but may be used to reduce the temperature in *malarial fevers*.

As an *analgesic* it is much employed in *neuralgias*, the "lightning pains" of *locomotor ataxia*, *muscular rheumatism*, *myalgia*, *dysmenorrhea*, to allay the pains of the first stage of *labor*, and in *influenza*. It has been used with success in *chorea* and *whooping-cough*. In *acute coryza* and in *tuberculous laryngitis* it is useful as a spray (4 per cent. solution), as it lessens the hyperemia.

In 10 to 25 per cent. solution it is a valuable *hemostatic* in nose-bleed and other superficial hemorrhages. It does not produce a slough like the iron styptics.

What is the dose of antipyrin, and how may it be administered?

The dose is gr. v–xv (0.3–1.0 gm.), repeated in from one to four hours, if necessary.

It is given in capsules or in solution. As it is non-irritating, it may be used hypodermically.

It is incompatible with calomel and with sweet spirits of niter, tannates, iodids, and solutions of chloral, mercury, arsenic, and carbolic acid.

ACETANILIDUM (ACETANILID).

What is acetanilid?

Acetanilid or *antifebrin* is a neutral chemic product, obtained by the action of glacial acetic acid and heat on anilin. It is an acetyl derivative of anilin, and is known chemically as phenylacetamid (C_6H_5NH,C_2H_3O).

What are its physiologic actions?

Like antipyrin, *acetanilid* is markedly *antipyretic* and *analgesic.* As an antipyretic *in fevers* it acts more slowly than antipyrin, influencing the temperature in the same manner and being attended with the same symptoms and with more marked cyanosis. As the temperature declines the pulse becomes slower and stronger and the arterial tension is elevated. Gastric and intestinal disturbance and other unpleasant concomitants rarely result. Given to *healthy men* in ordinary doses, it produces no apparent effect. In *decided doses* acetanilid lessens the conductivity of nerves, depresses the reflex centers, and acts as a hypnotic. In *poisonous amounts* it causes motor and sensory paralysis. Its effects are chiefly expended upon the sensory cord and nerves. Given to animals *in toxic doses,* beside cyanosis it causes general prostration, stupor, rapidly lowered temperature, with primary stimulation and afterward depression of the heart and respiration, coma, convulsions, and death. It is eliminated by the kidneys as para-amidophenol sulphate.

What are its uses?

It is used as an *antipyretic* in all cases of high temperature, as *typhoid fever, acute rheumatism, scarlatina, phthisis, influenza, pneumonia,* and *acute sepsis.* As an *anodyne* it is employed, also, in the same diseases in which antipyrin is indicated, and has been found useful in *epilepsy,* particularly in the lesser attacks (*petit mal*). It is also used *locally* as an *antiseptic.*

How may it be administered, and in what doses?

The dose of acetanilid is from gr. ij–v (0.12–0.3 gm.). It is nearly insoluble in water, and is better given in capsules or in powder.

Pulvis Acetanilidi Compositus (*compound acetanilid powder*) contains acetanilid 70, caffeine 10, and sodium bicarbonate 20 parts; dose, gr. v–x (0.3–0.7 gm.).

ACETPHENETIDIN (PHENACETIN).

What is phenacetin?

Acetphenetidin or *phenacetin* is an acetyl derivative of para-amidophenetol.

What are its physiologic effects?

It is a nervous sedative, acting principally upon the sensory portions of the spinal cord. It is less energetic than acetanilid or antipyrin but is considered safer.

In small doses it has no effect upon the circulatory system. Large doses produce a general cyanosis due to the formation in the blood of methemoglobin.

It slightly depresses normal temperature, and reduces markedly that of fever, usually causing but slight diaphoresis. When administered in the evening, its effects upon febrile temperature appear to be more marked than when given in the morning. After large doses, cyanosis, vomiting, incoördination, hurried breathing, and somnolence may occur.

What are its therapeutic uses and doses?

As an *antipyretic* and sedative to the nervous system in febrile conditions generally, as in *typhoid fever, pneumonia, pleurisy, tuberculosis, influenza, acute rheumatism*, etc.

As an *analgesic* in *migraine, headache* from any cause, *myalgia*, etc. It is better to administer this, as well as the other coal-tar products, cautiously in all cases of weak heart. Dose, gr. ij–v (0.12–0.3 gm.), repeated if necessary.

PHENOCOLL.

What is phenocoll?

Phenocoll (not official) or *amidophenacetine* is a coal-tar product prepared by the action of glycocoll, which is amido-acetic acid, upon phenacetine.

It is a white crystalline powder and is soluble in 16 parts of water. It is incompatible with the alkalis.

It is said to reduce febrile temperature very rapidly by diminishing the heat-production without affecting the heat-radiation, and to have no unpleasant sequelæ, except occasionally profuse perspiration.

It should be used with care, however, in all cases of prostration, as it may then produce cyanosis and cardiac depression. It has been used as a hydrochlorid for its *antipyretic* effect in various febrile conditions, as an *analgesic* in *acute rheumatism* and in *neuralgia*, and as a *sedative* in *whooping-cough.* Dose of the hydrochlorid, gr. v–xv (0.3–1.0 gm.).

QUININE.

Is quinine used as an antipyretic?

Quinine (see p. 42) was formerly much used for this purpose, but at the present time it has been largely superseded by other agents.

As an antipyretic it is given in doses of gr. x–xx (0.6–1.3 gm.), repeated as required.

SALICIN, SALICYLIC ACID, AND THE SALICYLATES.

What are these substances, and whence are they obtained?

Salicin is a glucoside obtained from several species of *Salix* and *Populus* (*Fam.* Salicaceæ). *Salicylic acid* is a derivative of salicin, is found also as a salt (of methyl) in oil of gaultheria, and has been prepared synthetically by combining pure carbolic acid with dry carbon dioxid by means of heat. The *salicylates* are the salts formed by the union of this acid with bases.

What are the physiologic effects of these substances?

The effects of *salicin* resemble those of salicylic acid, but its action is slower and less powerful. It is *antipyretic, tonic, antifermentative, antiseptic,* and, to a slight extent, *antiperiodic.* It does not depress the heart nor upset the stomach to the same extent as does salicylic acid, and is much less toxic. It is eliminated by the urine (chiefly as salicylic and salicyluric acids) and by the perspiration.

Salicylic acid, when *locally* applied, is *antiseptic* and *anti-*

fermentative, like carbolic acid, to which it is closely related. Administered *internally in full doses*, it lowers the temperature in fevers, causes profuse, sometimes exhausting, sweats, and produces symptoms similar to those of *cinchonism*, such as tinnitus aurium, partial deafness, headache, etc., due largely to congestion of the internal ear. After very *large doses* these symptoms are all increased, and dyspnea, depression of the heart and nervous system, and dilated pupils are observed. If a *toxic dose* be given, delirium, irregular respiration, involuntary evacuations, stupor, and death from respiratory failure occur. In healthy subjects salicylic acid in full doses at first stimulates the heart and respiration, but soon depresses them, producing weak heart action and dyspnea, often causes nausea and vomiting, inhibits the movements of the leukocytes, is a diaphoretic, and does not affect the normal temperature. It is eliminated chiefly by the urine as salicyluric acid. The urine frequently contains albumin.

The salicylates administered internally are less irritant to the stomach than is salicylic acid; in other respects their effects are identical.

What are the medicinal uses of these substances?

Salicin is not much employed. It has been used as an *antipyretic*, especially in rheumatism, for which purpose gr. iij–xv (0.2–1.0 gm.) may be given every few hours.

Salicylic acid has been given as an *antipyretic* in various fevers, but is now little used for this purpose except in *acute rheumatism* in robust subjects, where it not only lowers the temperature and moderates the pain, but materially aids in the elimination of uric acid. It is also used in *pleurisy with effusion* and as an *anthelmintic*. *Externally* it is applied for the removal of corns and warts; to check sweating of the feet and hands; in eczema; and as an *antiseptic* to wounds and ulcers.

The *salicylates* are used internally as *antipyretics* and *sedatives* in *acute rheumatism*, and as *antizymotics* to prevent *fermentation* of food in the stomach.

What are the preparations and doses of these remedies?

SALICINUM (*salicin*), dose, gr. x–ʒj (0.6–4.0 gm.). In acute *rheumatism*, gr. iij–xv (0.2–1.0 gm.) may be given every two or three hours.

ACIDUM SALICYLICUM (*salicylic acid*), dose, gr. x–ʒj (0.6–4.0 gm.). In *acute rheumatism*, gr. x (0.6 gm.) may be administered every hour until six doses are taken. If more is necessary, decrease the frequency of the dose.

SODII SALICYLAS (*sodium salicylate*) is more soluble and less apt to cause vomiting than the acid, and hence is preferred for internal use.

LITHII SALICYLAS (*lithium salicylate*) is used for the same purposes and in the same doses.

STRONTII SALICYLAS (*strontium salicylate*) has the same use and dose.

Phenyl salicylate will be described under a separate heading.

Ammonium, physostigmine, and *quinine salicylates,* and *bismuth subsalicylates* will be spoken of in connection with their respective bases.

What other official preparations are used for the salicylate which they contain?

OLEUM GAULTHERIÆ (*oil of gaultheria*), a volatile oil distilled from *Gaultheria procumbens*, or wintergreen. It contains *methyl salicylate,* and acts similarly to salicylic acid upon the system. In large doses it is toxic. It is administered for the same purposes as are the salicylates, in doses of ♏x–xv (0.6–1.0 c.c.) in capsules, repeated as required, but tends to irritate the stomach, and to cause "repeating." It may be used to paint over painful joints.

OLEUM BETULÆ (*oil of betula; oil of sweet birch*), a volatile oil obtained by maceration and distillation from the bark of *Betula lenta* (*Fam.* Betulaceæ). It is nearly identical with methyl salicylate and with oil of gaultheria.

METHYLIS SALICYLAS (*methyl salicylate; artificial* (or synthetic) *oil of wintergreen*) is a product obtained by the distillation of salicylic acid or its salts and methyl-alcohol in the presence of sulphuric acid. It is an oily liquid, and is the principal ingredient of *oil of gaultheria* and *oil of betula.*

What should be done if, during the use of these medicines, tinnitus aurium or other symptoms of intoxication should occur?

The dose should immediately be decreased or the medicine discontinued.

PHENYL SALICYLATE (SALOL).

What is phenyl salicylate or salol?

Phenyl salicylate (*salol*) is the salicylic ester of phenol and occurs as a white, crystalline, slightly aromatic, and nearly tasteless powder, insoluble in water, but soluble in alcohol.

What are its physiologic effects?

Locally it is *antiseptic*. *Internally* it lowers febrile temperature and produces sweating. The circulation is practically uninfluenced; the respirations increase in frequency and become shallow; tinnitus aurium and other salicylic acid symptoms sometimes occur. It is somewhat analgesic. It is not absorbed from the stomach, but in the intestine the pancreatic juice converts it into salicylic and carbolic acids, which render antiseptic the remainder of the alimentary canal. It seems to make the bile more watery. It is eliminated chiefly in the urine, which, after its use, resists decomposition and becomes darker in color.

What are its uses and doses?

As an *antipyretic* it is used in *acute rheumatism*, in *typhoid* and other *fevers;* in *phthisis* and in *pneumonia;* as an *intestinal antiseptic* in *duodenal catarrh, catarrhal jaundice, typhoid fever*, and *cholera;* to *prevent decomposition of urine* in *cystitis* and *pyelitis*, and as an *analgesic* in *neuritis, neuralgia, nervous headache*, etc. It is also employed in *pharyngitis* and in *chronic sore throat* depending upon the uric-acid diathesis. It may be given in any stage of *gonorrhea* for its influence on the urine. It is also said to be useful in diabetes.

Locally it is used as an antiseptic in surgical dressings. Dose, gr. v–ʒj (0.3–4.0 gm.) in pills, capsules, or in solution in alcohol or oil. It should be administered cautiously in disease of the kidneys, because of the carbolic acid which it yields.

SALOPHEN.

What is salophen?

Salophen (not official) is acetylpara-amidophenol salicylate. Like salol it is decomposed in the intestine by the pancreatic juice, being split into salicylic acid and acetylpara-amidophenol, which is harmless, thus possessing an advantage in point of safety over salol. It is chiefly eliminated under these forms in the urine, a small quantity passing unchanged in the stools. It is an *antipyretic, intestinal antiseptic,* and *analgesic.* Its most marked antipyretic effect is seen in *acute rheumatism.* It has also been used as an *intestinal antiseptic* in *typhoid fever, cholera,* and *dysentery,* and as an *analgesic* in *sciatica, migraine,* and *neuralgia.* It appears to be non-toxic. Dose, gr. x–xv (0.6–1.0 gm.) in compressed pill or capsule every two hours until gr. xc (6 gm.) are taken in twenty-four hours.

GUAIACOL (GUAIACOL). GUAIACOLIS CARBONAS (GUAIACOL CARBONATE).

What are guaiacol and guaiacol carbonate?

Guaiacol, or methylpyrocatechin, is a colorless, volatile liquid, with a strong aromatic odor, prepared by the fractional distillation of beechwood creasote, of which it forms 60 to 90 per cent.

It is also prepared synthetically from *catechol* by methylating, or from *ortho-anisidin* by diazotizing and boiling.

It is soluble in 53 parts of water, in 1 part of glycerin, and freely in alcohol and ether.

Guaiacol carbonate is made "by decomposing guaiacol in a solution of soda with carbonyl chlorid. It is a neutral, white, crystalline powder, containing 91 per cent. of chemically pure guaiacol in combination with 9 per cent. of carbonic acid." Insoluble in water, it dissolves in 48 parts of cold alcohol, readily in ether, in chloroform, and in boiling alcohol, and sparingly in the fixed oils and in glycerin. A number of other guaiacol compounds have been introduced, among which are the *phosphate, valerianate,* and *benzoate (benzosol).*

What are their effects?

When guaiacol is given internally or administered hypodermically to healthy persons it produces no effects beyond slight depression and slight diaphoresis. When given in suitable doses to febrile patients, a gradual *reduction of the febrile temperature* takes place, the fever declining for from two to four hours. When the lowest point has been reached, the temperature rises rather rapidly to its former height, half the time being occupied in the ascent which was required for the decline of the temperature. As the temperature falls, the patient often complains of much depression, but in ordinary doses the effects upon the respiration and pulse are evanescent.

It is eliminated by the lungs and kidneys as guaiacosulphonic ether, giving a dark color to the urine when a large dose has been taken.

There is but one case of poisoning on record. *When applied locally,* it is *antipyretic* and *analgesic.*

It appears to lower the temperature by direct action on the thermogenetic centers. Guaiacol is also an *antiseptic.*

The carbonate, when given internally, is antipyretic, and, being decomposed in the small intestine into pure guaiacol and carbonic acid, acts as a local antiseptic upon the alimentary canal.

For what purposes are they employed?

They are much used as substitutes for creasote in the treatment of *pulmonary tuberculosis,* acute or chronic, especially in the first and second stages of the disease. In suitable cases it lessens the fever, improves the appetite and digestion, moderates the cough, and lessens night-sweats and diarrhea.

As an *antipyretic* it has been employed in typhoid fever, pneumonia, influenza, etc., and in typhoid fever also as an intestinal antiseptic.

Locally it has been applied to relieve the pain, and as an antiphlogistic in *sciatica, neuralgia, arthritis deformans,* and *acute rheumatism;* but especially is it painted over the abdomen in tuberculous peritonitis, over the chest in tuberculous pleurisy, and over the scrotum in epididymitis.

It has also been recommended as a *local anesthetic* in dental and minor surgical procedures.

It is used as an *inhalation* in *fetid bronchorrhea* and in *gangrene of the lung.* Dose of guaiacol, ♏iij–v (0.2–0.3 c.c.) four times a day in capsule, pill, or in solution in oil or alcohol.

Locally, ♏v–xl (0.3–2.0 c.c.) may be employed. When

used in this manner, the skin should be thoroughly cleansed and the guaiacol applied with a camel's-hair pencil and rubbed in until absorbed. The surface should then be covered with oiled silk or paraffin paper to prevent evaporation.

As an inhalation, ℳ v–x (0.3–0.6 c.c.) in a pint of hot water may be used, or an oxygen inhaler may be employed, or a few drops of a mixture of guaiacol, chloroform, and alcohol may be dropped upon the sponge of a zinc respirator.

Guaiacol carbonate is preferable for internal administration, as it is free from the odor and taste of guaiacol, which are objectionable to many persons, and does not irritate the alimentary canal. It is used in *tuberculosis* and *typhoid fever.* Dose, gr. v (0.3 gm.), t. i. d. in capsules increased gradually until gr. xlv (3 gm.) are taken in divided doses in twenty-four hours.

RESORCINOL (RESORCIN).

Resorcin and its isomers, hydroquinon and pyrocatechin, are antiseptic and antifermentative.

Internally they reduce febrile temperature and cause profuse diaphoresis, followed by a more or less well-marked chill and gradual return of the fever. Fulness of the head or headache, flushed face, and tinnitus aurium accompany these effects; the pulse and respiration are at first accelerated, but soon depressed. Large doses given to animals cause tremor, epileptiform convulsions, weak and rapid pulse, and finally failure of respiration. They are eliminated by the urine.

Hydroquinon and pyrocatechin are not employed in medicine. *Resorcin* is used in the stomach and externally as an antiseptic, its ready solubility permitting it to be used as an irrigation for nose, throat, ears, or vagina. It is also added to lotions and ointments for the scalp. Internal dose, gr. v–xxx (0.3–2.0 gm.).

Chinolin, kairin, and *thallin* are antipyretic, but have been replaced by new and less dangerous drugs.

Medicines Acting on the Body by their Effects on the Various Organs.

ON THE NERVOUS SYSTEM.

HYPNOTICS.

What are hypnotics?

Hypnotics are remedies which are administered to induce sleep. Most of them are *narcotics*, or remedies which, by a stupefying effect on the nerve-centers, diminish our relationship with external nature; and many of them are also *anodynes*, or remedies which, by lessening the excitability of the nerves and nerve-centers, tend to relieve pain.

How do hypnotics act?

As *during sleep* the functional activity of the brain is depressed, while the nutritive function is active, and as it is necessary for the nutrition of an organ that the blood should pass through the capillaries in a slow, steady, and continuous stream, removing the waste-products and giving up substances capable of replacing the tissue destroyed, while *during functional activity* the blood is in larger amount, hurried through the vessels (which are dilated) in a tumultuous manner, and does not remove the waste as fast as it accumulates in the tissues, therefore a medicine to cause sleep must *depress the cerebral functions* or *regulate the blood-supply* to the brain either by contracting its vessels or by determining more blood to other portions of the body.

Name the principal hypnotics.

Opium and its alkaloids; chloral; chloralamide; the bromids; hyoscine; sulphonal; trional; tetronal; paraldehyd; urethan; cannabis indica; humulus, and lactucarium.

OPIUM.

What is opium?

Opium is the *concrete milky exudation* obtained by incising the unripe capsules of *Papaver somniferum* (*Fam.* Papaveraceæ), a native of Persia, but cultivated throughout the civilized world.

What are its principal chemic ingredients?

Its important *alkaloids* are: Morphine, codeine, narcotine, papaverine, and paramorphine (thebaine); in addition it contains narceine, pseudomorphine, laudamine, hydrocotarnine, cryptopine, porphyroxine, meconine, and others.

These are in combination with meconic, lactic, and sulphuric acids.

What are the chemic tests for the presence of opium?

With even very diluted *solutions of opium, ferric chlorid or sulphate* produces a blood-red ferric meconate. With *morphine and its salts, ferric chlorid or sulphate* give rise to a blue color which rapidly fades, while *concentrated nitric acid* strikes with them a rich orange-red, slowly fading to yellow.

What are the physiologic actions of opium?

Opium is hypnotic, anodyne, antispasmodic, and diaphoretic. It also depresses the circulation and respiration. The first feeling is one of stimulation, due to depression of the higher centers of self-control, will, judgment, etc., then, in succession, if the dose be sufficient, follow a dreamy, drowsy condition, sleep, stupor, coma, and death. Appreciation of external conditions is diminished, and noises, lights, and even blows may fail to arouse the sleeper; the sensory centers are depressed, and if the dose be toxic, finally paralyzed, death occurring from paralysis of the respiratory center. The pupil is contracted from stimulation of the third nerve center. It depresses the *cardiac* motor ganglia, the pulse becoming slower and fuller, and the arterial tension elevated. *Respiration* is slowed. The *secretions* are all diminished, except that of the skin, which is increased. Peristalsis is retarded. *Elimination* takes place chiefly through the kidneys. Occasionally, intense itching of the skin, and sometimes cutaneous rashes occur. Headache, nausea, and constipation commonly follow a medium dose of opium.

What are the symptoms and treatment of opium-poisoning?

The *symptoms* of acute opium-poisoning may be divided into three stages:

The first stage,—not always present, and when present, usually of short duration,—in which there are mental exhilaration or excitement, with some confusion of ideas; a sensation of heat and often itching of the nose and face; a dry skin; and sometimes nausea and vomiting. This quickly passes into—

The second stage, in which there are overpowering drowsiness, passing into stupor; contraction of the pupils; dryness of the mouth and throat; sweating; full, regular respirations, diminishing in frequency as the poisoning proceeds; slow, full pulse; and congested face. The patient can be aroused, but at once relapses into a stuporous sleep. This stage gradually passes into—

The third stage, with deepening coma; minutely contracted pupils (pin-point pupils); very slow, stertorous breathing; abolition of reflexes; pale, cyanosed face; rapid, feeble circulation, and death from respiratory failure.

Before death occurs, the pupils often become widely dilated.

Death has resulted, in an adult, from morphine, gr. $\frac{1}{4}$, hypodermically (rare), and from opium, gr. ivss (rare). Children are very susceptible to its action.

Treatment.—(1) Remove any poison present in the stomach by the stomach-pump or emetics (zinc sulphate, gr. xx–xxx, or cupric sulphate, gr. v–x in a glass of tepid water, or apomorphine, gr. $\frac{1}{10}$, hypodermically); or wash out the stomach with large quantities of a 1 : 5000 solution of potassium permanganate (strongly recommended in recent years as a chemic antidote); (2) catheterize the patient to prevent resorption of the opium from the urine; (3) maintain respiration and circulation by hypodermics of atropine sulphate, gr. $\frac{1}{60}$, repeated in half the amount at the end of fifteen to thirty minutes if necessary, the guide to its administration being the respiration. Strychnine, caffeine, and cocaine are also recommended. Faradization, cold affusions, and artificial respiration are useful.

Postmortem examination shows no characteristic changes in the organs.

In *chronic opium poisoning,* which is induced either by smoking or swallowing opium or by the hypodermic injection of morphine, there are marked digestive disturbances; diarrhea or constipation, great nervousness and irritability, and mental and moral weakness.

How does the action of its alkaloids differ from that of opium?

The action of *morphine* differs from opium in that the former is less constipating, less of a diaphoretic, and more powerful in other respects. *Codeine* is uncertain as an anodyne and hypnotic but is more sedative to the respiratory mechanism. It is also less constipating, tends less to upset the stomach, and does not induce the formation of a vicious habit, like the morphine habit. It quiets cough and bronchial irritation. The results of experiments with the other alkaloids are so conflicting that no reliance can be placed on them.

In what diseases is opium used medicinally?

As an *anodyne*, opium or morphine is used in almost all diseases of which pain is a prominent and persistent symptom, and is contraindicated only when acute inflammation of the brain is present.

As a *hypnotic* in *delirium tremens* (often combined with the bromids or chloral) and in *sleeplessness* of fevers and other acute diseases; to *allay irritation*, especially when accompanied with *painful spasm*, as in the various forms of *colic* or in *asthma* (morphine hypodermically); in cough; in *severe acute vomiting* (by suppositories); to *check morbid discharges* or *restrain peristalsis*, as in *cholera, diarrhea, dysentery*, and *enteritis*. In *peritonitis* for the latter effect and as an *anodyne* large doses are required, a tolerance to opium being established.

In *puerperal septicemia*, to *support the system* and as an *anodyne* it is of great value. As a *motor depressant* in *cerebrospinal fever* very large doses are tolerated; also in *uremic convulsions* (dangerous if the renal structure is much diseased), *puerperal eclampsia, tetanus, hydrophobia*, and other affections with increased excitability of the reflex centers. In the *early stages of various inflammations*, for its influence on the circulation and tendency to retard effusion and relieve pain, and as a *diaphoretic* (Dover's powder) in muscular rheumatism, the early stages of acute catarrhs, etc., it is much employed. In *diabetes* opium and codeine are most reliable drugs to decrease the amount of sugar in the urine. *Great caution* should be exercised in prescribing opium in chronic diseases, as the *opium-habit* is almost certain to result. *Locally*, opium is applied in solution as anodyne and sedative.

What are the preparations and doses of opium and its alkaloids?

OPII PULVIS (*powdered opium*) contains not less than 12 nor more than 12.5 per cent. of morphine; dose, gr. ss–ij (0.03–0.13 gm.).

OPIUM DEODORATUM (*deodorized opium*) and OPIUM GRANULATUM (*granulated opium*) are each of the same strength as *opii pulvis;* dose, gr. ss–ij (0.03–0.13 gm.).

PILULÆ OPII (*opium pills*)—each pill contains of powdered opium gr. j (0.065 gm.).

EXTRACTUM OPII (*extract of opium*) contains 20 per cent. of morphine; dose, gr. ss (0.03 gm.).

EMPLASTRUM OPII (*opium plaster*) contains the extract with adhesive plaster.

TROCHISCI GLYCYRRHIZÆ ET OPII (*troches of glycyrrhiza and opium; Wistar's cough lozenges*)—each lozenge contains of powdered opium gr. $\frac{1}{12}$ (0.005 gm.). Very useful in laryngeal and pharyngeal coughs.

PULVIS IPECACUANHÆ ET OPII (*powder of ipecac and opium; Dover's powder*) is a diaphoretic and anodyne; dose, gr. x (0.6 gm.), containing of opium and ipecac each gr. j (0.06 gm.) with sugar of milk.

TINCTURA OPII (*tincture of opium; laudanum*), dose, ♏xij or 24 drops (0.75 c.c.).

TINCTURA OPII DEODORATI (*tincture of deodorized opium*), dose, ♏xij (0.75 c.c.).

TINCTURA OPII CAMPHORATA (*camphorated tincture of opium; paregoric*) contains opium, diluted alcohol, oil of anise, benzoic acid, glycerin, and camphor; dose, ʒj–iv (4–15 c.c.). To a young child, ♏ij–xx, or 4 to 40 drops (0.1–1.3 c.c.), according to age.

TINCTURA IPECACUANHÆ ET OPII (*tincture of ipecac and opium*)—this is Dover's powder in a fluid form; dose, ♏xij (0.75 c.c.).

ACETUM OPII (*vinegar of opium; black drop*), dose, ♏xij (0.75 c.c.).

VINUM OPII (*wine of opium; Sydenham's laudanum*), dose, ♏xij (0.75 c.c.).

MORPHINÆ SULPHAS (*morphine sulphate*); MORPHINÆ HYDROCHLORIDUM (*morphine hydrochloride*); MORPHINÆ ACETAS (*morphine acetate*).—The salts are preferred to the pure alkaloid because they are more soluble. Dose of either, gr. $\frac{1}{8}$ (0.008 gm.) is equal to opium gr. j (0.06 gm.). They are well adapted to hypodermic use.

PULVIS MORPHINÆ COMPOSITUS (*compound powder of morphine; Tully's powder*) contains of morphine sulphate 1.5 per cent., with camphor, licorice, and calcium carbonate; dose, gr. v–xv (0.3–1.0 gm.).

Magendie's solution (not official) contains of morphine 16 grains to the ounce. It is sometimes used hypodermically, but it is better to make a fresh solution of morphine for each injection, as bacteria frequently develop in solutions of the alkaloids when kept for some time, and also because otherwise there is some risk of confusion, as the French Magendie's solution contains about 12½ grains to the ounce. Also the solutions of morphine official in the British Pharmacopœia do not correspond in strength to either of the above solutions.

CODEINA (*codeine*), dose, gr. ¼–ij, or even gr. v (0.016–0.13–0.3 gm.).

CODEINÆ PHOSPHAS (*codeine phosphate*) and

CODEINÆ SULPHAS (*codeine sulphate*) have the same uses and doses as *codeine*.

What medicines are incompatible with opium?

The alkalis precipitate morphine from solutions of opium, and vegetable infusions containing tannic acid form a less soluble tannate of morphine; many mineral salts are also decomposed by solutions of opium.

How is opium administered?

Opium is often administered in the form of the official

preparations, either alone or combined with other substances. The bromids, chloral, or other hypnotics are often added to increase its soporific influence; belladonna, etc., to enhance its anodyne effects; lead or other astringent, to act more powerfully in intestinal disorders; potassium nitrate or minute doses of antimony to increase, while atropine is often combined with morphine to diminish, its action as a diaphoretic. It may be administered by the mouth or rectum (suppositories or laudanum enemata), and its alkaloids may also be given hypodermically.

CHLORALUM HYDRATUM (CHLORAL).

What is chloral?

Anhydrous chloral is an oily liquid made by saturating absolute alcohol with dry chlorin gas, and is *trichloraldehyd*. By uniting with water, a hydrate, the *official chloral hydrate*, is formed, which occurs as a crystalline solid.

What are its physiologic effects?

Locally applied, chloral is antiseptic and irritant. Given *internally*, it is a hypnotic, motor depressant, and cardiac sedative. In *medicinal doses* it causes quiet, natural sleep, contraction of the pupil, and deep, regular breathing. After *large doses* the sleep is deeper and may even pass into coma, respiration is slowed, the cardiac action is weakened and diminished, the temperature falls, and sensibility and reflex action are depressed. It is not an anodyne. Nausea and vomiting sometimes occur from its irritant action on the mucous membrane, and in some persons excitement and even delirium may take the place of the sleep which it usually produces. The *continued use* of chloral causes *chloralism* or the *chloral habit*, and produces an anemic condition, with weak, irregular heart, irritable temper, and loss of self-control: a state similar to delirium tremens has been observed.

What are the symptoms and treatment of chloral poisoning?

After toxic doses, profound narcosis, great muscular relaxation, slow and very weak pulse, diminished frequency of breathing, marked contraction of the pupil, and lividity of surface, with great reduction of body heat, occur. Death is due to paralysis of respiration or to sudden failure of the heart from paralysis of its motor ganglia.

The smallest recorded fatal dose is gr. xxx (2 gm.).

The *treatment* for chloral poisoning consists in—(1) Maintaining the temperature by artificial heat; (2) maintaining the cardiac action by *atropine* in small doses, repeated as required; and (3) maintaining the respiration (partly by the atropine or by morphine, and partly by artificial manipulations). While chloral is the best antidote for strychnine poisoning, the converse does not hold good.

What are its therapeutic uses?

As a *hypnotic*, chloral is employed in *insomnia, hysterical* or *maniacal excitement*, and in *delirium tremens* and *mania-a-potu*, but is *contraindicated* in any condition where the heart is weak or has undergone fatty degeneration. As a vasodilator in nephritis and as a *motor depressant* in *uremic, infantile*, or *puerperal convulsions*, in tetanus, and in poisoning by *strychnine*, it is of great service. It has been used in *whooping-cough* and *chorea*. It is also recommended in sea-sickness (gr. v, t. i. d.) and to relax a rigid cervix during the first stage of labor. *Locally*, in dilute solution, it has been used as an *anodyne and antiseptic* dressing, and, triturated with equal parts of camphor, it forms a valuable liniment in neuralgic and muscular pains.

How is chloral administered?

The dose of chloral is gr. ij–xx (0.13–1.2 gm.), which may be repeated in an hour or two if sleep is not produced. It is better given in syrup. It should not be given with alkalis, which decompose it, chloroform and formic acid being formed, nor with alcohol, with which it forms "knock-out drops."

What is croton-chloral hydrate?

Croton-chloral hydrate (not official), or butyl-chloral hydrate, is made by the action of chlorin gas on ethylic aldehyd, and occurs in small, glittering crystals. Its *effects* and *uses* are similar to those of chloral, and as it possesses a very decided anesthetic influence over the filaments of the trigemini, it is used in the neuralgias affecting the branches of these nerves. Dose, gr. v–xx (0.3–1.2 gm.), in glycerin or syrup.

CHLORALFORMAMIDUM (CHLORALAMID).

What is chloralamid?

Chloralamid is a compound prepared by the action of formamid upon chloral. It is soluble in water, but more so in alcohol. *Its action* is similar to that of chloral, but it is not so certain a hypnotic, and neither depresses the heart nor irritates the stomach and kidneys to the same extent as does the latter drug. It is excreted as urochloralic acid.

Occasionally, after the exhibition of large doses, it causes *slight poisoning*, the symptoms being chilliness, followed by a sensation of heat, sweating, arhythmia, nausea, and sometimes vomiting, with respiratory depression. These symptoms are rarely severe, and usually pass off rapidly.

It is used as a *hypnotic* and *nervous sedative* in the same conditions for which chloral is prescribed, and is especially useful in *insomnia* due to nervous causes, but fails usually when *insomnia* is due to pain. It is also recommended in sea-sickness.

Dose, gr. x–xxx (0.6–2.0 gm.), given in capsule or solution one hour before its effects are desired. It may be administered by the rectum.

THE BROMIDS.

What are the physiologic effects of the bromids?

The *bromids* are hypnotic and depressors of the reflex spinal centers. Applied *locally* to the pharynx, they diminish its reflex irritability. Given *internally* they cause drowsiness and permit sleep by lessening sensitiveness to external influences; they depress the reflex spinal centers and the functions of the end-organs of peripheral nerves, thus lessening nervous irritability, reflex activity, and cutaneous sensibility. They also depress the functious of the sympathetic nervous system. In very large doses *potassium bromid* lessens the cardiac frequency and force, lowers the arterial tension, and finally, in animals, paralyzes the heart in diastole. This seems to be due to the potassium only (which is a muscle and nerve poison), for the other bromids do not arrest the cardiac action. They slow the respiration and lower the temperature of the body. They are eliminated by the kidneys, skin, and mucous membrane, and in large or frequent dosage may irritate the skin so as to produce an acneiform eruption.

What is bromism?

When taken for a long time, bromids induce a condition known as *bromism*, the symptoms of which are acne, anemia, drowsiness, defective memory, malaise, impaired reflexes, malnutrition, loss of sexual power and desire, and often a tendency to melancholia. These symptoms pass away when the drug is discontinued. No case of *acute poisoning* is on record.

What are the medicinal uses of the bromids?

They are used as *hypnotics* in all forms of *insomnia due to* nervous irritability. In the early stages of *delirium tremens* they are of great service. They are also given as *depresso-motors* in local or general convulsions, as *chorea, uremic, puerperal, hysterical,* or *infantile convulsions, tetanus,* and as an *antidote* to *strychnine poisoning* (inferior to chloral). In the treatment of *epilepsy* they rank among the best remedies. In reflex vomiting, as of sea-sickness or pregnancy, they are of use. In *whooping-cough* ammonium bromid is often efficacious. In *migraine* they are sometimes beneficial. For their *influence over the sexual functions* they are used to control *nymphomania, priapism,* and *masturbation.* Conjoined with ergot they are used to decrease the uterine blood supply in *menorrhagia,* and are of utility in *subinvolution of the uterus.* Strontium bromid is said markedly to diminish the amount of sugar in the urine in *glycosuria.* Of the different bromids, the potassium bromid is most depressing to the heart and nervous system, ammonium bromid least depressing, and strontium bromid least irritating to the stomach. Zinc bromid is astringent.

What are the official bromids?

Potassii Bromidum (*potassium bromid*), dose, gr. v–ʒj (0.3–4.0 gm.).

Ammonii Bromidum (*ammonium bromid*) has less influence on the circulation, respiration, and temperature than the potassium salt; dose, gr. v–xxx (0.3–2.0 gm.).

Sodii Bromidum (*sodium bromid*), dose, gr. v–ʒj (0.3–4.0 gm.).

Calcii Bromidum (*calcium bromid*), dose, gr. v–ʒj (0.3–4.0 gm.).

Zinci Bromidum (*zinc bromid*), dose, gr. j–x (0.06–0.6 gm.) (not much used).

Strontii Bromidum (*strontium bromid*), dose, gr. iij–x (0.2–0.6 gm.).

Acidum Hydrobromicum Dilutum (*diluted hydrobromic acid*), containing 10 per cent. of the absolute acid, is said to possess similar effects to the bromids. It is chiefly used as a hypnotic, and added to quinine mixtures to prevent cinchonism. Dose, ʒss–j (2–4 c.c.).

What medicines are incompatible with the bromids?

Acids and the acidulous and metallic salts are chemically incompatible with the bromids; alkaloids are slowly precipitated. They are antagonized by cardiac and vasomotor stimulants.

How may they be administered?

They may be given in powder or in solution in syrup. Zinc bromid may be used in pilular form. They are often given together in small doses, and to enhance their hypnotic effect may be combined with opium or its alkaloids, chloral, or cannabis indica.

SCOPOLAMINÆ HYDROBROMIDUM.

What is scopolamine hydrobromid?

Scopolamine is an alkaloid obtained from plants of the *Solanaceæ*, chiefly Hyoscyamus, Scopola, and Stramonium, It is identical chemically with Hyoscine Hydrobromid, and has been used in combination with morphine as a preliminary to ether anesthesia. It is said to promote the comfort of the patient and to lessen the amount of ether required. Dose, hypodermically, gr. $\frac{1}{120}$ (0.0005 gm.).

HYOSCINÆ HYDROBROMIDUM.

What is hyoscine hydrobromid?

Hyoscine is one of the alkaloids found in *Hyoscyamus niger,* or henbane (*q. v.*). It is an efficient hypnotic when used hypodermically, and is employed in the form of *hydrobromid* in *acute mania, alcoholic delirium*, and *hysteria*. Dose, gr. $\frac{1}{80}$ (0.0008 gm.) by the mouth, or hypodermically gr. $\frac{1}{120}$ (0.0005 gm.).

PARALDEHYDUM (PARALDEHYD).

What is paraldehyd?

Paraldehyd is a colorless liquid with a disagreeable odor and taste, prepared by heating ethyl aldehyd with a mineral acid or with zinc chlorid. It is soluble in 8.5 parts of water.

What are its physiologic actions?

In medicinal doses paraldehyd produces sleep closely simulating natural sleep, without affecting the cardiac action. It depresses the reflex centers, especially those of the upper part of the cord, and in *toxic amounts* depresses and finally paralyzes the respiratory center, diminishing the amount of carbonic acid exhaled and lowering the body-temperature. It has no anodyne virtues. It often irritates the mucous membranes, and cutaneous eruptions sometimes follow its use.

What are its medicinal uses and dose?

It may be given as a *hypnotic* where sleeplessness is not induced by pain, as in *delirium tremens, hysteria*, etc. As a *reflex depressor* it has been employed in *epilepsy*, and in animals poisoned by strychnine has proved antidotal. It is given in doses of ʒj (4 c.c.), and should be freely diluted.

SULPHONMETHANUM (SULPHONAL).

What is sulphonmethane or sulphonal?

Sulphonal is a substance prepared synthetically and described chemically as diethylsulphondimethylmethane. It occurs as heavy, prismatic crystals, colorless, odorless, and nearly tasteless, and is soluble in 100 parts of cold water, but freely soluble in hot water and also in ether and alcohol.

What are its physiologic and its toxic effects?

The physiologic action of sulphonal is not thoroughly understood. It acts chiefly on the cerebral centers, depressing them and causing sleep. Sometimes, especially after large doses have been taken, it depresses the reflexes, disorders digestion, and causes cutaneous eruptions. In large doses it depresses respiration, rendering it slow, weak, and, when excessive doses have been taken, stertorous, and finally produces death by cessation of the respiratory act. It has but little effect on the circulation.

It is probably eliminated in great part by the urine, and frequently changes the color of that excretion to a reddish-brown—a change due to the presence of hematoporphyrin.

Disagreeable after-effects sometimes follow the use of sulphonal, as drowsiness, giddiness, headache, and occasionally incoördination of gait, sometimes cutaneous eruptions or disordered digestion, perhaps nausea and vomiting, occur.

Sulphonal is by no means an absolutely innocuous drug, and *death* has resulted from large doses, in many recorded cases, from respiratory failure.

The symptoms of poisoning are various, the most common being drowsiness, stupor, muscular incoördination, ptosis and edema of eyelids, mental and physical hebetude, depression of reflexes, nausea and vomiting, usually constipation, and the urine is reddish-brown.

In non-fatal cases recovery is usually rapid. Sulphonal is *cumulative* in its action. During its administration it is of the utmost importance that the bowels should be made to act daily (Schulz) and that the urinary secretion should be abundant.

If symptoms of poisoning appear, the drug should at once be discontinued; the bowels should be freely opened, saline diuretics administered, and the patient kept in the recumbent position. If there is much depression of the circulation or respiration, stimulants may be administered.

What are its therapeutic uses?

Sulphonal is much used as a *hypnotic* and *cerebral sedative* in *nervous insomnia*, and even in *melancholia, delirium tremens*, and *acute mania.* In the *insomnia* of low fevers, as that of *typhoid fever*, it sometimes gives good results.

It has been recommended as a *sedative reflex depressant* in *asthma, hiccup, trismus neonatorum*, and in *convulsions due to dentition*, and has been used even in *epilepsy* and *chorea.*

It is said that in small doses (gr. viij—0.5 gm.) it is effective in arresting the *night-sweats* of *phthisis*, and that in *diabetes* it will temporarily diminish the amount of sugar excreted in the urine.

It is said to be *contraindicated* in *angina pectoris*. Dose, gr. v–xxx (0.3–2.0 gm.), which may be given in capsules, but is better administered dissolved in hot water or milk, two hours at least before the time when its effects are desired.

As it is cumulative in its action, it is better not to give more than gr. xxx (2 gm.) in twenty-four hours.

SULPHONETHYLMETHANE (TRIONAL).

What is sulphonethylmethane or trional?

Trional is sulphonal in which one methyl (CH_3) group has been replaced by ethyl (C_2H_5). Its chemic name is diethylsulphonmethylethylmethane.

It occurs as white, odorless, almost tasteless crystals, not very soluble in cold but readily soluble in boiling water, and also in alcohol and milk.

What are its effects and uses?

Trional is a hypnotic, acting more quickly than sulphonal, being easily decomposed in the body, sometimes slightly lowering the pulse and blood-pressure, and rarely leaving any disagreeable after-effects. It is not cumulative. Occasionally after its long-continued use the urine is colored reddish-brown from the presence of hematoporphyrin.

Toxic doses given to animals cause death from respiratory paralysis.

Occasional *after-effects* are loss of appetite, epigastric pain, nausea and vomiting, vertigo, and unsteadiness of gait. These symptoms usually soon disappear.

It is supposed to act directly on the cerebral cortex.

Several cases of *acute poisoning* by trional have been reported; the symptoms are drowsiness, staggering gait, vertigo, vomiting, diarrhea, loss of muscular power, and lowered temperature, sometimes attended with rapid pulse and respiration, excitement, and collapse.

Trional is *used* as a *hypnotic* in *insomnia* due to organic cerebral affections, neurasthenia, or other functional psychosis, worry, or mental overwork. It is not anodyne.

It is a "safe and efficient hypnotic for children" when pain is not present (Claus).

It has also been recommended in *epilepsy*, either alone or combined with the bromids.

Dose, gr. xv–xxx (1–2 gm.) about half an hour before its effect is desired.

If it is administered for any length of time, it is better to intermit the dose occasionally, in order to guard against any possible cumulative effect, and it is important also to insure a daily evacuation of the bowels.

TETRONAL.

What is tetronal?

Tetronal (not official) is sulphonal in which two methyl groups are replaced by ethyl groups. It is diethylsulphon-diethylmethane. Sulphonal, trional, and tetronal differ from each other chemically only in the number of molecules of ethyl and methyl which they contain. Thus *sulphonal* contains *two* molecules each of ethyl and of methyl, and is sometimes spoken of as dional; *trional* contains *three* molecules of ethyl and one of methyl, and *tetronal* contains *four* molecules of ethyl and none of methyl.

Tetronal is formed synthetically, and occurs in colorless, shining plates, without odor or taste, soluble in about 500 parts of cold, more soluble in hot, water; soluble also in alcohol and in ether.

What are its effects and uses?

Its *effects* and *uses* are similar to those of trional, but it has a more decided sedative effect. However, it is more toxic than sulphonal or trional, and is now very little used. The dose is gr. v–xv (0.3–1.0 gm.), repeated in an hour if necessary.

ÆTHYLIS CARBAMAS (URETHAN).

What are the effects and uses of ethyl carbamate or urethan?

Urethan or ethyl carbamate is a synthetic product formed by the interaction of ethyl carbonate and ammonia, or by that of urea nitrate and ethyl alcohol, and occurs in crystalline masses readily soluble in water and alcohol. *In medicinal doses* it causes tranquil sleep, preceded by a short period of excitement. It depresses the reflex centers, at first quickens but soon slows the respiration, and somewhat reduces the temperature, and in overdoses causes, in animals, death from respiratory paralysis. The effect upon the heart is disputed. It is not analgesic. It has been *used* as a *hypnotic* in simple insomnia with varied success, and appears to be more applicable to cases where the action of chloral on the heart contraindicates the use of that agent. As a *motor depressant* it has been employed in *tetanus, infantile convulsions,* and *puerperal eclampsia.* Dose, gr. x–lx (0.6–4.0 gm.). It has been used locally as an antiseptic dressing for wounds.

CANNABIS INDICA (INDIAN CANNABIS).

What is this drug?

Cannabis Indica is the *flowering tops* of the female plant of *C. sativa* or hemp (*Fam.* Moraceæ), grown in the East Indies.

What are the active chemic constituents of hemp?

The alcoholic extract contains a *resin* (cannabin) and a volatile oil. It is claimed that several alkaloids have been discovered, but their existence is, as yet, doubtful.

What are the physiologic actions of cannabis?

In full *medicinal doses* it at first stimulates and then depresses the cerebrospinal functions without affecting respiration or circulation to any marked extent. The mental exhilaration is usually of a pleasurable kind, the pupils are dilated, ideas flow rapidly, and conception of time and space is so altered that seconds seem hours and objects a few feet off seems miles away; an active, busy delirium usually occurs, and sometimes increase of the sexual appetite; this is followed by a sense of weight in the extremities, depression of the reflexes, some loss of muscular power and cutaneous anesthesia, succeeded by sleep. It increases, but does not originate, uterine contractions. No fatal case from its use is recorded.

What are its therapeutic uses?

It is used as a *hypnotic* in *mania* and in *mania-a-potu;* as an *anodyne* in *neuralgia, migraine, dysmenorrhea, rheumatism,* and *gout,* and to relieve pain in *acute* and *chronic Bright's disease;* as an *antispasmodic* in *tetanus, chorea, hysteria,* and *spasm* of the neck of the bladder; as an *addition to cough medicines* to allay irritation of the throat, and to promote a condition of euthanasia in the later stages of phthisis. It is highly recommended in *dysentery,* and is of undoubted service in checking *uterine hemorrhages* not due to abortion or following labor. In *sexual impotence,* when functional, it is sometimes of use. In *gonorrhea* it is said to lessen the discharge and prevent chordee. As a *local application* it enters into the composition of many *corn-cures.*

What are its preparations and doses?

EXTRACTUM CANNABIS INDICÆ (*extract of cannabis Indica*), dose, gr. ¼–j (0.016–0.06 gm.).

FLUIDEXTRACTUM CANNABIS INDICÆ (*fluid extract of cannabis Indica*), dose, ♏j–x (0.06–0.6 c.c.).

TINCTURA CANNABIS INDICÆ (*tincture of cannabis Indica*), dose, ♏x (0.6 c.c.). In using a new preparation of cannabis Indica always begin with the minimum dose, as different samples vary much in strength.

HUMULUS.

What are the effects, uses, preparations, and doses of humulus?

Humulus is the *strobiles* of *H. lupulus,* or hop vine (*Fam.* Moraceæ). *Lupulin* is a yellow powder (the glandular trichomes) found near the base of the strobiles. It contains a volatile oil, *cholin* (formerly called lupulin, a strongly alkaline liquid), *lupamaric acid* (a bitter principle), resin, etc.

Hops are tonic and bitter, very feebly narcotic, anaphrodisiac, and diuretic. They are used as a *hypnotic* in mild forms of *delirium tremens,* and in *restlessness* and *sleeplessness* from overwork; as an *anaphrodisiac* in *priapism, chordee, nymphomania*, and *satyriasis*; as an *antispasmodic* and *sedative* in *hysteria* and *neurasthenia*; as a *diuretic* and *anodyne* in *irritation of the bladder*, and locally as an anodyne poultice and as a sedative injection in acute vaginitis.

Hop-pillows are a popular remedy for sleeplessness due to nervousness.

LUPULINUM (*lupulin*), dose, ʒss–ij (2–8 gm.), but not much used in this form.

FLUIDEXTRACTUM LUPULINI (*fluid extract of lupulin*), dose, ʒss–ij (2–8 c.c.).

OLEORESINA LUPULINI (*oleoresin of lupulin*), dose, gr. x–xxx (0.6–2.0 gm.).

LACTUCARIUM.

What are the effects, uses, and preparations of lactucarium?

Lactucarium is the *concrete milk-juice* of *Lactuca virosa*, the garden lettuce (*Fam.* Compositæ), and contains *lactucin*. Lactucarium is supposed to possess *anodyne* and *hypnotic* powers, and has been used as a substitute for opium when the latter is indicated, but cannot, for any reason, be given. Its action, if any, is very mild.

TINCTURA LACTUCARII (*tincture of lactucarium*), dose, ♏x–ʒj (0.6–4.0 c.c.).

SYRUPUS LACTUCARII (*syrup of lactucarium*), dose, ʒij–iv (8–15 c.c.).

MYDRIATIC ANODYNES.

What are the mydriatic anodynes?

The *mydriatic anodynes* are remedies employed as analgesics and antispasmodics, which possess no hypnotic effect, but cause dilatation of the pupil and, in large doses, a restless delirium.

What medicines are included under this head?

Belladonna, stramonium, hyoscyamus, duboisia, scopola, coca, and their alkaloids.

BELLADONNA.

What is belladonna?

Belladonna is the *leaves* and *root* of *Atropa belladonna*, or deadly nightshade (*Fam.* Solanaceæ), a European plant cultivated in this country. The leaves must yield not less than 0.35 per cent., and the root not less than 0.5 per cent. of mydriatic alkaloids.

What are the chemic constituents of belladonna?

Its properties depend upon an alkaloid called *atropine*. Both the leaves and the root also contain *belladonnine* (probably oxyatropine), *hyoscyamine* (sometimes the predominating alkaloid in the leaves and often the only alkaloid in young roots), and *atropamine*.

What are the tests for atropine?

A delicate test is the addition of hydrobromic acid, which produces a yellow, amorphous precipitate, soon becoming crystalline. The *physiologic test*—viz., the dilatation of the pupil in the lower animals after the local application of the suspected solution—should always be resorted to.

What are the physiologic effects of belladonna and its alkaloid?

Applied *locally* to the skin it is absorbed, lessens the sensibility of the sensory nerves, and produces constitutional effects. *Small doses administered internally* cause dryness of the mouth and throat, with some headache; after *larger amounts* there is difficulty in swallowing, from arrest of the mucous and salivary secretions, the pupils dilate widely, the skin becomes dry, a scarlatinoid rash appears, the cardiac action is accelerated, and an active delirium occurs. *Moderate doses* act as *cerebral excitants; larger doses* produce hallucinations and impair the excitability of the motor and sensory nerves, thus producing a peculiar delirium in which there is a great desire for constant motion, associated with lassitude. The *spinal reflex centers* are first stimulated, afterward paralyzed, if the amount taken be sufficiently large. It paralyzes the end-organs of the third nerves and stimulates the sympathetic, thus dilating the *pupil* whether used locally or internally; the power of accommodation is also paralyzed, and the intra-ocular tension is increased.

The *cardiac action* is at first slowed, if the dose be small (from stimulation of the inhibitory center), but is soon much quickened (from progressive paralysis of the peripheral filaments of the vagus and stimulation of the cardio-accelerator centers or nerves). Large doses paralyze the cardiac muscle. Atropine stimulates the vasomotor centers and raises the arterial pressure, but after toxic doses the arterioles dilate, from paralysis of their muscular walls, and the blood-pressure falls. It first stimulates and then paralyzes the respiratory center. The *temperature* rises after moderate doses, but after toxic amounts a decided fall of temperature occurs, probably from vasomotor paralysis. Small doses possibly increase *intestinal peristalsis* by depressing the inhibitory fibers of the splanchnics, while large doses paralyze the non-striated muscular fibers of the intestines and bladder. It arrests the *secretions* of the skin, mammary, salivary, and muciparous glands, and probably of the stomach, liver, and pancreas, by paralyzing the terminal filaments of the secretory nerves. The urine may be increased, but after large doses is suppressed. Atropine is eliminated principally by the kidneys.

What are the symptoms and treatment of atropine poisoning?

The pupils dilate so widely that the iris can scarcely be seen; the face and neck are flushed; the skin is hot and dry; swallowing is impossible, from dryness of the throat and mouth; the muscular system is relaxed; maniacal delirium occurs, with impaired sensation, failing pulse, quickened, followed by failing, respiration, stupor, coma, sometimes convulsions, diminished body-heat, and death, usually from asphyxia. The *treatment* consists of: (1) *Evacuation of the contents* of the *stomach* (by emetics or stomach-pump), *bowels* (by cathartics), and *bladder* (by the catheter), to prevent further absorption of the poison; (2) *giving tannic acid* freely as a chemic antidote; (3) *giving pilocarpine, physostigmine,* or *morphine* hypodermically, as partial physiologic antagonists, and (4) maintaining the circulation and respiration by electricity and artificial respiration.

What are the medicinal uses of belladonna and atropine?

As an *anodyne* in the various *neuralgias*, either locally or given by the mouth, rectum, or subcutaneously, it is of value, and is often combined with morphine. In *muscular rheumatism* and in *myalgia* it is also of service. In *conjunctivitis* and in *iritis* it is used locally, not only to dilate the pupil, but to lessen pain.

As an *antispasmodic* it is used to relax spasm and allay pain in *biliary* and *renal colic*, in *lead colic*, *spasmodic dysmenorrhea*, and *cramps* of the bowel, bladder, and urethra; also to relax the *rigid cervix uteri* in labor. In *asthma*, in *laryngismus stridulus*, and *whooping-cough* it often proves of use. In *habitual constipation* a small amount combined with purgatives modifies their griping action by relaxing spasm of the intestinal muscular layer. It is a valuable remedy in the treatment of *incontinence of urine in children* when given in doses sufficient to produce some constitutional effect.

As a *cardiac and vasomotor stimulant* in all cases of threatened collapse from *heart failure* it is advantageously employed, and has been highly recommended to contract the blood-vessels in *acute inflammatory affections* generally. *To check excessive secretion*, as in *salivation*, *excessive sweating*, especially the *night-sweats of phthisis*, and in *colliquative diarrhea*, it is of great value, and is a well-known *galactafuge*, being used internally and applied locally for this purpose. As a *respiratory stimulant* in *opium-poisoning* atropine is of great service, and may be used in cases of poisoning by other substances attended with failure of respiration.

Locally, belladonna is used as an ointment, liniment, or plaster for the relief of pain in *neuralgia*, *myalgia*, and *muscular rheumatism*; to relax the sphincter ani in painful hemorrhoids or fissure; to *relax spasmodic stricture* of the urethra (applied on a bougie or given by suppository), and as a *galactafuge*. In *ophthalmic practice* a solution of atropine, 1 : 200, may be dropped into the conjunctival sac to *dilate the pupil* and to *paralyze accommodation*, so that an examination can be readily performed or the refraction of the eye determined; the dilatation lasts for several days. In various inflammations of the ocular apparatus, as conjunctivitis, keratitis, iritis, etc., it is used to lessen pain, to diminish the blood-supply to the inflamed parts, and to keep the pupil dilated. It is contraindicated in *glaucoma.*

What are the preparations and doses of belladonna?

EXTRACTUM BELLADONNÆ FOLIORUM (*extract of belladonna leaves*), dose, gr. ⅛–ss (0.008–0.03 gm.), in pill or suppository.

FLUIDEXTRACTUM BELLADONNÆ RADICIS (*fluid extract of belladonna root*), dose, ♏j–ij (0.06–0.12 c.c.).

TINCTURA BELLADONNÆ FOLIORUM (*tincture of belladonna leaves*), dose, ♏v–xx (0.3–1.5 c.c.).

LINIMENTUM BELLADONNÆ (*liniment of belladonna*) consists of the fluid extract containing 5 per cent. of camphor.

UNGUENTUM BELLADONNÆ (*ointment of belladonna*) contains 10 per cent. of extract.

EMPLASTRUM BELLADONNÆ (*plaster of belladonna*).

ATROPINA (*atropine*), usually employed in the more soluble form of ATROPINÆ SULPHAS (*atropine sulphate*), dose, gr. $\frac{1}{120}$–$\frac{1}{60}$ (0.0005–0.001 gm.).

OLEATUM ATROPINÆ (*oleate of atropine*) contains 2 per cent. of atropine.

What substances are incompatible with belladonna?

Alkalies precipitate atropine from solutions of belladonna, and tannic acid forms with it atropine tannate, a less soluble salt.

HOMATROPINÆ HYDROBROMIDUM.

What is homatropine hydrobromid?

It is a salt of an alkaloid derived artificially from atropine. *It differs from atropine* in dilating the pupil more rapidly and much more transiently, in not causing much constitutional disturbance when used locally for this purpose, and in slowing, not accelerating, the heart's action. *It is used* in ½ to 1 per cent. solution as a substitute for atropine in ocular therapeutics.

STRAMONIUM.

What are the source, composition, action, and uses of stramonium?

Stramonium is the *leaves* of *Datura stramonium*, thorn-apple, Jamestown weed, or gypsum (*Fam.* Solanaceæ), a common indigenous plant, and must yield not less than 0.35 per cent. of mydriatic alkaloids. It contains the alkaloids *atropine* and *hyoscyamine*, and is used for the same purposes as belladonna. The leaves have been made into cigarettes and smoked to avert a threatened paroxysm of *asthma*, and it has been used externally as a poultice or an ointment in *painful wounds, external inflammations, hemorrhoids,* and *fissure of the anus.* The *official preparations* are:

EXTRACTUM STRAMONII (*extract of stramonium*), dose, gr. ss (0.03 gm.).

FLUIDEXTRACTUM STRAMONII (*fluid extract of stramonium*), dose, ♏j–v (0.06–0.3 c.c.).

TINCTURA STRAMONII (*tincture of stramonium*), dose, ♏v–xv (0.3–1.0 c.c.).

UNGUENTUM STRAMONII (*ointment of stramonium*) contains 10 per cent. of the extract.

HYOSCYAMUS.

What is hyoscyamus?

Hyoscyamus is the *leaves* and *flowering tops* of *H. niger*, or henbane (*Fam.* Solanaceæ), a native of Europe, collected from plants of the second year's growth, and yielding not less than 0.08 per cent. of mydriatic alkaloids.

What does it contain?

It contains two alkaloids, *hyoscyamine* and *hyoscine* (identical with scopolamine), both of which are isomers of atropine.

What are the physiologic effects of hyoscyamus and its alkaloids?

Hyoscyamine appears to be identical in action with its isomer atropine, but feebler and less irritant. It does not dilate the pupil so rapidly; sometimes retards, sometimes quickens, the heart's action; and at first quickens, then slows, the respiration.

Hyoscine causes dryness of the mouth and throat, flushing of the face, sleep, slow respiration, and in large doses slow, full pulse, muscular weakness, incoördination, diaphoresis, and, it is said, a rise in temperature. The treatment of poisoning by hyoscine consists in the administration of alcoholic stimulants and coffee or caffeine; in artificial respiration; in the use of faradism, and perhaps the cautious use of physostigmine.

Hyoscyamus combines the action of its alkaloids, differing from that of belladonna in proving hypnotic.

What are the uses of hyoscyamus and its alkaloids?

Hyoscyamus has been used as a substitute for belladonna in the diseases in which the latter is employed. It has also been used as a *hypnotic* in various forms of *insanity*, in *delirium tremens*, and in *hysteria*. Added to *purgatives*, it enhances their efficacy and prevents griping.

Hyoscyamine has been found useful as a *sedative* to the nervous system in *insanity;* to lessen spasm and allay pain in *vesical tenesmus* and in *irritable bladder;* and, to prevent *griping*, as an addition to purgatives. It has sometimes proved useful in *chorea*.

Hyoscine is used as a *cerebral sedative* and *hypnotic* in maniacal excitement, but should be employed only temporarily, and then only in cases where *excitement* is a prominent symptom. In melancholia it has proved useless or injurious. Cases do not do well under its continued use. It may be employed to produce sleep when morphine or chloral is contraindicated in advanced renal disease and in cases of weak heart. To produce hypnotic effects, it should be administered hypodermically. It has been found efficacious in *paralysis agitans* and in various forms of tremor. Disagreeable after-effects are rare.

What are the preparations and doses of these substances?

Extractum Hyoscyami (*extract of hyoscyamus*), dose, gr. j–ij (0.06–0.13 gm.).

Fluidextractum Hyoscyami (*fluid extract of hyoscyamus*), dose, ♏v–x (0.3–0.6 c.c.).

Tinctura Hyoscyami (*tincture of hyoscyamus*), dose, ʒss–j (2–4 c.c.).

HYOSCYAMINÆ SULPHAS (*hyoscyamine sulphate*) dose, gr. $\frac{1}{100}-\frac{1}{50}$ (0.0006–0.0013 gm.) to begin with; much larger doses may be given with impunity.

HYOSCYAMINÆ HYDROBROMIDUM (*hyoscyamine hydrobromide*), dose, gr. $\frac{1}{100}-\frac{1}{50}$ (0.0006–0.0013 gm.).

HYOSCINÆ HYDROBROMIDUM (*hyoscine hydrobromide*), dose, gr. $\frac{1}{100}-\frac{1}{80}$ (0.0006–0.0008 gm.), if given hypodermically, dose, gr. $\frac{1}{150}-\frac{1}{100}$ (0.0001–0.0006 gm.) to begin with, but much larger doses may be used.

SCOPOLA.

What is scopola?

Scopola is the rhizome of *S. Carniolica* (*Fam.* Solanaceæ), yielding not less than 0.5 per cent. of its alkaloids. It is an herb of southern Europe, and contains *atropine*, *hyoscyamine*, and *scopolamine*. Its actions are those of belladonna.

What are the preparations and doses?

FLUIDEXTRACTUM SCOPOLÆ (*fluid extract of scopola*), dose, ♏j–ij (0.06–0.12 c.c.).

EXTRACTUM SCOPOLÆ (*extract of scopola*), dose, gr. $\frac{1}{8}-\frac{1}{2}$ (0.008–0.03 gm.).

SCOPOLAMINÆ HYDROBROMIDUM (*scopolamine hydrobromide*), dose, gr. $\frac{1}{100}$ (0.0006 gm.)—see also under Hypnotics.

COCA.

What is coca?

Coca is the *leaves* of *Erythroxylon coca* and *E. Truxillense* (*Fam.* Erythroxylaceæ), yielding not less than 0.5 of the ether-soluble alkaloids of coca. It is a shrub of Peru.

What does it contain?

It contains *cocaine*, *benzoyl-ecgonine*, and *cocatannic* acid.

What are the physiologic effects of erythroxylon?

Cocaine, the active principle, is a cerebral stimulant, producing a sense of calm and well-being, followed, if the dose is large, by a pleasant, talkative delirium. It lessens the sense of fatigue and of hunger, but does not take the place of food; it will allay vomiting. It is a *cerebral* stimulant, causing delirium in large doses, followed by epileptiform convulsions and coma if the dose has been excessive. It first stimulates, then depresses, the *reflex spinal centers.* Toxic doses depress and finally paralyze the *nerves,* these effects being more marked on the nerves of sensation. The effect on the *circulation* is disputed, but in small doses it increases the strength and frequency of the cardiac contractions. It acts as a powerful stimulant upon the *respiratory* center, but in large doses paralyzes it, the heart continuing to beat after the breathing has stopped. *Injected hypodermically* into the superficial tissues, it causes local anesthesia; if a deep injection is given, a slight general lessening of sensibility, dilated pupils, a slight rise in temperature, with strong cardiac contractions, result; it is not absorbed through the unbroken skin.

Locally applied it causes marked anesthesia of the mucous membrane with which it comes in contact, with some diminution of sensibility of the deeper structures. There is at first local pallor from contraction of vessels, followed by redness. Applied to the conjunctiva, it dilates the pupil (which may, however, be contracted by eserine) transiently, lessens without entirely suspending the power of accommodation, and lowers ocular tension. It dries the cornea.

In *toxic doses* cocaine causes symptoms varying much in different persons. The most common symptoms are stimulation of the mental faculties; loquacity; incoherence; depression of temperature accompanied by profuse sweating; shallow, irregular respiration; feeble pulse; dilated pupils and disturbed vision; nausea and collapse. Sometimes there is intellectual torpor, with tonic or clonic convulsions. Sometimes the mental excitement is almost maniacal.

Respiratory disturbances are always marked, in severe cases being of the Cheyne-Stokes type, and the sufferer may die from respiratory paralysis.

Individual susceptibility to the drug varies greatly, and even persons who have used it before without inconvenience may experience a toxic effect from a dose of the same size as that which they had before taken. Even weak solutions applied to a mucous membrane occasionally produce alarming symptoms.

The *treatment of poisoning* by cocaine consists in inhalations of amyl nitrite and chloroform; ammonia should be given internally, and artificial respiration resorted to and continued for a long time.

Opium, or morphine, and chloral may be used if convulsions occur.

What are the medicinal uses of coca and its alkaloid?

Coca is not much employed in medicine. It may be given as a stomachic *tonic* in wasting diseases, as in *phthisis*.

Cocaine is principally used as a *local anesthetic* (2 to 10 per cent. solution), in operations on the various mucous membranes, particularly those of the eye, nose, mouth, pharynx, and larynx, but also to those of the vagina, rectum, and urethra. Injected into the superficial tissues, it diminishes sensation sufficiently to allow of the performance of many operations in minor surgery, particularly if its diffusion is prevented by compressing the circulation of the part. Its effects may be obtained by injection at the site of operation, or along the course of the nerves, or in the spinal canal (spinal anesthesia). By this latter method analgesia may be produced in the parts of the body supplied by the nerves which leave the spinal cord at or below the level of the injection. In ophthalmology it is useful to reduce hyperemia, to produce anesthesia, and for its rapid and transient mydriatic effect.

To *relieve pain* and *contract the blood-vessels* in the early stages of acute catarrhal inflammations, as *coryza, hay-fever, laryngitis*, and *bronchitis;* to deaden sensation and thus *lessen reflex cough* in *pertussis, influenza*, advanced *phthisis*, and *chronic laryngitis*, it may be used in spray, or directly applied to the part by a brush. It has also been used as a *hemostatic*, applied to the mucous membranes, especially to the nasal mucous membrane, previous to an operation. It is highly recommended to allay the burning and itching of rhus poisoning. *Internally* it has been employed in *gastrodynia, nervous dyspepsia*, and to check *reflex vomiting*, as that of pregnancy or of sea-sickness (by the mouth or injected into the epigastric region), as a cardiac tonic in low fevers, and as a substitute for morphine in persons accustomed to the habitual use of the latter alkaloid. When used for this purpose, the cocaine habit is apt to be formed, but can apparently be broken off suddenly without danger to the patient.

What are the preparations and doses of coca?

FLUIDEXTRACTUM COCÆ (*fluid extract of erythroxylon*), dose, ʒss–ij (2–8 gm.).

VINUM COCÆ (*coca wine*) contains 6.5 per cent. of fluid extract of coca, alcohol, sugar, and red wine; dose, ʒj–ij (4–8 c.c.).

COCAINA (*cocaine*) and COCAINÆ HYDROCHLORIDUM (*cocaine hydrochloride*), dose, gr. ¼–j (0.016–0.06 gm.).

OLEATUM COCAINÆ (*oleate of cocaine*) contains 5 per cent. of cocaine.

ANESTHETICS.

What are anesthetics?

This name is applied to a group of medicines, the vapor of which when inhaled causes a temporary loss of sensibility to painful impressions (*analgesia*), with diminution and abolition of general sensation and reflex action, and complete loss of consciousness.

Name the agents of this group.

Ether, chloroform, nitrous oxid, methylene bichlorid, ethyl bromid, bromoform, and ethyl chlorid.

ÆTHER (ETHER).

Ether is ethyl oxid, obtained by the distillation of alcohol with sulphuric acid. It is a colorless liquid, with a strong, disagreeable odor, and a hot, burning taste; it evaporates rapidly at ordinary temperatures. Its vapor is heavy—more than two and a half times as heavy as the atmosphere—and is very inflammable.

What are its physiologic effects?

When applied *locally*, ether produces a feeling of coldness by its rapid evaporation, thus obtunding the sensibility of the part, and if the application be continued, the part may be entirely frozen.

When the vapor of ether is *inhaled*, a sense of burning is experienced in the throat, followed by a feeling of suffocation and an irritative cough; then comes a *stage of stimulation*, or *intoxication*, during which the action of the higher nerve centers is more or less interfered with; there is a feeling of lightness in the head and buzzing in the ears, and the circulation is quickened; this passes into the *narcotic stage*, the patient becoming delirious and laughing, weeping, moaning, talking, singing, or fighting. The face is suffused, the eyeballs injected and often protruding, the veins turgid, sensibility is diminished, and tonic contractions of the muscles are often present. If the inhalation is continued, the *stage of anesthesia* soon supervenes, in which the functions of the spinal cord are influenced; thus, there is not only complete insensibility, but also entire abolition of the reflexes. This stage may be continued indefinitely by carefully regulating the inhalation. If, however, too much be given, the *stage of paralysis* ensues, in which the reflex centers of the medulla oblongata are paralyzed and the respiration and circulation cease. Stertorous respiration, from paralysis of the muscles of the palate, is the first indication of the approach of this stage.

During the inhalation of ether the pupils at first contract slightly, afterward slightly dilate, but always respond to light. Sudden, wide dilatation is a sign of danger.

The pulse is increased in frequency during the early stages of ether inhalation, afterward returning gradually to about the normal. The arterial pressure is increased, due principally to contraction of the peripheral capillary vessels and to the increased rapidity of the cardiac beat. During the stage of paralysis the pressure falls when respiratory failure begins.

In the first stage the respiration is increased both in frequency and in depth, becoming much more shallow in the second stage, but again becoming deep and even stertorous in the third stage, and finally ceasing if the etherization be continued into the fourth stage from paralysis of the respiratory center, the heart continuing to pulsate after the arrest of the respiratory movement.

The *after-effects* are headache, vomiting, and a taste of ether in the mouth. Some hours elapse after profound anesthesia before the patient fully regains the use of his mental faculties.

Taken *internally*, ether increases the secretions and is similar in its action to alcohol. It is rapidly eliminated by the lungs and kidneys, which it may irritate.

What are the therapeutic uses of ether?

1. As an *anesthetic*, ether is employed by inhalation for the prevention of pain during *surgical operations* and examinations, and during the passage of *renal* or *biliary calculi*. For these purposes the inhalation should be carried to the third stage—that of complete anesthesia. To alleviate suffering during labor ether is often administered, but here it should only be inhaled during the pains, and the stage of complete anesthesia is rarely required, unless some obstetric manipulations, as version, the application of the forceps, or craniotomy is necessary, or when it is desirable to prevent the patient from "bearing down," either from fear of laceration of the soft parts, or of the strain on the circulation in cardiac disease, or where thorough relaxation of a rigid cervix uteri is desired. 2. As a *reflex depressant* it is inhaled in various forms of *convulsions* during the paroxysms, and to promote the reduction of a hernia, or aid in diagnostic manipulations by relaxing tensely contracted muscles. In persistent hiccough it is sometimes successful when given internally or may be used by inhalation to check the paroxysm. 3. As a *cardiac stimulant* it may be given hypodermically or by the mouth in cases of syncope or threatened cardiac failure. 4. It is sometimes used as a *teniacide;* and, 5, it has sometimes proved useful as an *anodyne* in *neuralgia* (injected in the vicinity of the nerve), and in *nervous headache* (given internally). 6. *Locally* it is employed to relieve pain in neuralgia, myalgia, muscular rheumatism, and before the performance of minor surgical operations.

What cautions should be observed in administering ether?

As ether is highly inflammable, it should not be administered by inhalation at night near a candle or gas light, nor near an open fire or very hot stove. If a light is in the room, it should be placed as high as possible above the patient, as the vapor of ether sinks toward the floor. Ether is contraindicated in advanced pulmonary disease, and should be cautiously administered, if at all, in cases of cerebral tumors, grave renal disease, and excessive exhaustion of the nerve centers.

In cardiac diseases it is the safest anesthetic and may be cautiously employed.

How should alarming symptoms be treated?

(1) Stop the inhalation and lower the head; (2) dash cold water on the face and chest and allow the patient plenty of fresh air; (3) use artificial respiration, make rhythmic tractions of the tongue at the rate of about 20 a minute, give atropine, strychnine, or nitroglycerin hypodermically; and (4) apply the faradic current to the thoracic muscles.

What are the official preparations of ether and how are they administered?

ÆTHER (*ether, æther fortior,* U. S. P. 1880) contains about 96 per cent. by weight of absolute ether or ethyl oxid in alcohol and water; dose, ♏v–ʒj (0.3–4.0 c.c.).

SPIRITUS ÆTHERIS (*spirit of ether*) contains 32.5 per cent. of ether in alcohol; dose, ♏xv–ʒj (1–4 c.c.).

SPIRITUS ÆTHERIS COMPOSITUS (*Compound spirit of ether; Hoffmann's anodyne*) contains 32.5 per cent. of ether and 2.5 per cent. of ethereal oil in alcohol; dose, ♏xv–ʒj (1–4 c.c.).

When ether *is administered by inhalation,* the patient should be, if possible, in the recumbent position, and ℥ss (15 c.c.) may be poured on a napkin or sponge placed in a cone of stiff paper, which is then gradually approached to the patient's mouth and nose, and kept there continuously until the desired effect is produced.

The anesthetizer should pay the strictest attention to the condition of his patient, watching closely the effect on the respiration and on the circulation as shown by the pulse and by the color of the skin or conjunctival mucous membrane.

Ether inhalations are better administered on an empty stomach, or vomiting may ensue.

Spraying the nose and throat with cocaine is said to increase the safety of the patient during the anesthesia, and certainly prevents the coughing, gagging, and vomiting which otherwise usually accompany the action of the anesthetic, and lessens the vomiting, headache, and persistent taste of ether which so often follow its use.

The *spirits* are carminative, antispasmodic, and stimulant, and are employed in *flatulence, asthma, cardiac dyspnea* and *angina pectoris.*

CHLOROFORMUM (CHLOROFORM).

What is chloroform?

Chloroform is methylene chlorid or formyl terchlorid, and is obtained by distilling acetone with chlorinated lime and slaked lime.

It is a limpid, colorless, heavy liquid, having a pleasant ethereal odor and an acrid, sweetish taste; it is soluble in alcohol and the oils, and in about 200 parts of water; its vapor is not inflammable.

What are its physiologic effects?

Applied *locally*, it is to some extent anesthetic; if evaporation be prevented, it is an irritant and even a painful vesicant. It assists the absorption of organic alkaloids by the skin, which otherwise would not penetrate the epidermis. When the vapor of chloroform is *inhaled*, anesthesia and unconsciousness rapidly result.

The *stage of stimulation* is not so well marked as in the case of ether inhalation; the *narcotic stage* is usually short in duration and the struggles of the patient are, as a rule, not violent. The pulse is quickened and apparently strengthened until the *stage of anesthesia*, when, with the abolition of consciousness and sensation and muscular relaxation, it diminishes slightly in frequency and is more or less weak. The *stage of paralysis* is one of imminent danger. In addition to the symptoms of the anesthetic stage, there is stertorous breathing, entire abolition of the reflexes, with a weak and rapid pulse, and finally death, usually from cardiac paralysis.[1] When

[1] The Hyderabad Commission concluded, from their very elaborate experiments upon dogs, that death always occurs from respiratory paralysis, a conclusion which at present is not in accord with clinical observation. The author has therefore adhered to the older view as to the mode of death under chloroform.

swallowed in small doses, it stimulates the secretions and increases peristalsis. In large amounts it is an irritant, causing gastro-enteritis, and after its absorption producing anesthesia and coma. It is eliminated by the lungs and kidneys.

How do the physiologic actions of ether and chloroform compare?

Ether is the safer anesthetic; chloroform, the more rapid, more transient in its effects, which are produced by smaller amounts, pleasanter, less irritating, and with less disagreeable after-effects. It does not cause so much vomiting, and its vapor is not inflammable. Death from ether (rare) is usually the result of respiratory paralysis and is gradual, while death from chloroform (much more frequent) is usually sudden, and is due to cardiac failure.

What are the therapeutic uses of chloroform?

It has been used as an *anesthetic* by inhalation in the same range of cases in which ether is given, but its employment for this purpose is now very generally limited to diseases like puerperal eclampsia, in which it is necessary rapidly to produce anesthesia and depress reflex action. In *obstetric practice* it is largely used, but even here ether is safer. Administered *internally*, it has proved serviceable in *cholera, protracted diarrhea*, and various forms of *colic*. It has also been used as a *teniacide*. Given before the expected chill of *malarial fevers*, it frequently aborts the paroxysm. Deep *injections* in the vicinity of the affected nerve sometimes afford relief in obstinate neuralgia. *Locally* as an anodyne it is employed in the form of liniment in muscular pains and in neuralgic affections. Its *contraindications* as an anesthetic are identical with those of ether; but it is less irritating to the lungs and kidneys; *it should never be administered when any disease of the circulatory system exists or if the heart is feeble from any cause.*

How should the occurrence of dangerous symptoms be met?

Stop the inhalations; invert the patient; artificial respiration; faradization; and atropine, strychnine, or nitroglycerin hypodermically. If it has been administered internally, treat the case as one of irritant or narcotic poisoning.

What are the official preparations, and how may they be administered?

CHLOROFORMUM (*chloroform*), dose, ♏xv–ʒj (1–4 c.c.) in emulsion. As an *inhalation*, 20 drops of chloroform may be poured on a folded napkin and placed cautiously over the nose and mouth in such a manner that the vapor is freely diluted with atmospheric air. *Not more than 3½ per cent. of chloroform should be contained in the air inspired.*

AQUA CHLOROFORMI (*chloroform water*), dose, ʒj–iv (4–15 c.c.).

SPIRITUS CHLOROFORMI (*spirit of chloroform*), dose, ♏x–ʒj (0.6–4.0 c.c.).

EMULSUM CHLOROFORMI (*emulsion of chloroform*), dose, ʒj–ij (4–8 c.c.).

LINIMENTUM CHLOROFORMI (*liniment of chloroform*) contains chloroform, 30 per cent., in soap liniment.

NITROUS OXID.

What is nitrous oxid?

Nitrous oxid (not official) or nitrogen monoxid is a colorless, almost odorless gas, made by the action of heat on ammonium nitrate.

What are its physiologic actions?

When nitrous oxid is inhaled, in from one to three minutes complete anesthesia occurs, with loss of consciousness, often preceded by a stage of excitement; the face is livid and the patient presents the appearance of asphyxia. The anesthesia is probably due to diminution in the relative amount of oxygen in the blood. When the inhalation is discontinued, consciousness and sensation speedily return, and, as a rule, no after-effects are manifested. When death results, it is generally due to asphyxia.

What are the therapeutics and the mode of administration of nitrous oxid?

As an *anesthetic* in minor surgical operations of short duration, as the extraction of teeth or the opening of abscesses, it is advantageously employed, but when the operation necessitates the maintenance of anesthesia for some time, ether is a safer agent.

It is best *administered* from an india-rubber bag connected with an iron reservoir, containing at least eight gallons, furnished with a mouth-piece having two valves, so that the expired air may not pass back into the bag.

BROMOFORMUM.

What is bromoform?

Bromoform is a heavy liquid, soluble in alcohol, ether, and the oils, almost insoluble in water, and with an agreeable taste and smell. Its effects resemble those of chloroform, but are slower. It is not much used as an anesthetic. As an antispasmodic it has been used in *pertussis* in doses of ♏ij–v (0.12–0.3 c.c.), t. i. d.

ÆTHYLIS CHLORIDUM (*ethyl chlorid*), "prepared by the action of hydrochloric acid gas upon absolute ethyl alcohol," has been much employed in spray form as a local anesthetic, its volatility and rapid evaporation inducing freezing of the part sprayed. This allows small operations. It is also employed somewhat as a rapidly-acting general anesthetic.

METHYLENE BICHLORID; ETHYL BROMID.

What are these substances?

Methylene bichlorid (not official) is a neutral, colorless liquid, resembling chloroform in odor. Its vapor is inflammable. When *inhaled*, it rapidly produces anesthesia and unconsciousness, and these effects as rapidly disappear when the inhalation is discontinued. Death is due to cardiac paralysis. It is not much employed in this country.

Ethyl bromid (not official) is a colorless, neutral liquid, having an ethereal odor and a disagreeable, sweetish taste. When inhaled it is anesthetic, acting on the heart like chloroform, and apparently fully as dangerous.

LOCAL ANESTHETICS.

What are local anesthetics?

They are remedies which produce an anesthetic effect limited to the particular part to which they are applied.

What are the indications for their employment, and what are the objections to their use?

They are employed whenever it is necessary to obtund the pain in a part, either caused by disease or induced by a surgical operation, and when it is not necessary for any reason that the patient should lose consciousness.

They are generally made use of prior to minor surgical operations for the avoidance of pain, although they have also been employed for the same purpose before major operations, as amputations.

In such cases, however, it is often advantageous to have the patient unconscious, as the knowledge of what is being done, even in the absence of pain, may prove injurious by causing nervous perturbation or by allowing the patient to interfere with the operator.

They are objectionable in some cases on account of the anemia which they produce, as during the reaction the resulting hyperemia may be sufficiently intense to cause hemorrhage, or occasionally interfere with the healing process.

How is local anesthesia produced?

Either by freezing the part which it is desired to anesthetize, or by the application to, or injection into, it of an anesthetic drug.

How may a part be frozen for such a purpose, and what are the agents employed?

The part may be frozen by the direct application for a few minutes of a freezing mixture such as powdered ice and salt, or by spraying it with a very volatile liquid, such as rhigolene, ether, or ethyl chlorid.

What are these substances and how are they used?

RHIGOLENE (not official) is a very volatile and inflammable liquid, obtained in the distillation of petroleum, and is used in the ordinary hand-atomizer.

Ether has already been spoken of as a local anesthetic.

Ethyl Chlorid (not official), or *hydrochloric ether*, is a very volatile liquid, which is sold in glass bottles having a minute orifice against which a tightly fitting stopper, moved by a small lever, is kept constantly pressed by means of elastic bands. When it is desired to use it, the lever is pressed down, the orifice of the bottle passed rapidly over the part to be anesthetized at a short distance from it, and the heat of the hand volatilizing the liquid in the bottle, the part is soon frozen by the spray.

These agents are *used* as local anesthetics in all *minor surgical operations*, such as opening abscesses or felons, the extraction of ingrowing toe-nails, paracentesis thoracis or abdominis, and are sometimes used to *numb* the *pain* of headache and neuralgia.

What drugs are employed topically or by hypodermic injection for this purpose?

Cocaine (*vid. Mydriatic Anodynes*) is used locally, as has already been mentioned, applied to the conjunctival, to the nasal, and to other mucous membranes as a local anesthetic.

It is also used by injection into the skin for the same purpose. When this is desired, the part is first sprayed with ethyl chlorid, and as soon as sensibility is obtunded, the needle of the hypodermic syringe is inserted and a few drops of the cocaine solution instilled just beneath the integument. By injecting the solution in front of the point of the needle, which is then pushed further into the anesthetized area, and a few more drops inserted, it is possible gradually to anesthetize quite a large surface. By casting a ligature around the part and thus preventing the cocaine from passing out by the blood-current, this anesthetic action may be prolonged.

By this or similar means local anesthesia has been maintained for periods considerably over an hour, during which operative procedures of some magnitude have been performed. It is probably better, however, to employ general anesthesia for major surgery unless there is some contraindication to its employment, and to restrict the anesthetic use of cocaine to minor surgery.

Beta-eucaine (or Eucaine "B"), a near relative of cocaine, has a similar action, but is weaker. It also favors hyperemia, has no effect on the pupil or on accommodation, and, though toxic, is much less so than is cocaine. The hydrochlorid is soluble in 23 parts of water, and the acetate is freely soluble; both are used in 2 to 4 per cent. solution.

Alpha-eucaine, a similar compound, is not now used, as it is too irritating and too toxic.

MENTHOL (official) is a "secondary alcohol, obtained from the oil from Mentha piperita or other peppermint oils." It occurs in the form of colorless, acicular, or prismatic crystals, having a strong and pure odor of peppermint, and a warm, aromatic taste, followed by a sensation of cold when air is drawn into the mouth. It is only slightly soluble in water, but freely so in alcohol, ether, chloroform, and oils. Menthol is a superficial, local anesthetic. Given internally to animals in sufficient doses it depresses both the sensory and motor nerves, lowers the temperature, and depresses the respiration, which becomes slow and shallow. In minute doses it is a gastric sedative.

It is chiefly *used* as a *local anesthetic*, painted or sprayed on the part in ethereal or alcoholic solutions varying in strength from 10 to 50 per cent., in cases of neuralgia, toothache, and other superficial pains. The author has seen the burning pains which often follow herpes zoster quickly relieved and often permanently cured by a few applications of a 50 per cent. alcoholic solution. Urticaria and senile pruritus may be temporarily relieved by the application of a 10 per cent. solution in albolene. It is also used with lanolin as an ointment, and has been used as an antiphlogistic remedy in superficial inflammations of the skin and mucous membranes.

GUAIACOL, which has been considered among the antipyretics (*q. v.*), is also used as a *local anesthetic* in *neuralgias*, especially in *sciatica*, in rheumatic pains, and in nose and throat.

Various other remedies, among which may be mentioned *tincture of aconite* (*vid. Cardiac Sedatives*), have been used locally in neuralgia for their local anesthetic effect.

ANTISPASMODICS.

What are antispasmodics?

Antispasmodics are remedies which prevent or allay spasmodic action of voluntary or involuntary muscles, and increase the inhibiting power of the higher over the lower nerve centers. They overcome nervous and hysterical conditions.

Name the antispasmodics.

Musk, valerian, the valerianates, asafetida, camphor, ethereal oil and Hoffmann's anodyne, cypripedium, and scutellaria.

MOSCHUS (MUSK).

What is musk?

Musk is the *dried secretion* from the preputial follicles of *Moschus moschiferus*, or musk deer.

What are its effects and uses?

Musk is a mild cerebral stimulant and antispasmodic, slightly increasing the cardiac frequency. In cases of nervous exhaustion, however, it acts more powerfully, and when a pure article can be obtained, no better nervous stimulant can be employed in the later stages of *typhoid fever* with great depression of vital forces, and in *typhoid pneumonia*. It is also of use in *hysteria, hiccup*, and *chorea*.

What are the preparations of musk?

MOSCHUS (*musk*) is very expensive and is often adulterated, and imitations are not infrequently substituted for the genuine article; dose, gr. x–xv (0.6–1.0 gm.) in capsule or emulsion. It is often given per rectum.

TINCTURA MOSCHI (*tincture of musk*), dose, ʒj–ij (4–8 c.c.).

SUMBUL (SUMBUL).

What is sumbul?

Sumbul (*vegetable musk*) is the rhizome and root of an undetermined plant, probably of the family *Umbelliferæ*. It is used in hysteria and as a carminative. The official preparations are the *fluid extract* (*fluidextractum sumbul*), dose, ♏xv–ʒj (1–4 c.c.); and the *extract* (*extractum sumbul*), dose, gr. ij–v (0.12–0.3 gm.).

VALERIANA (VALERIAN).

What is valerian, and what does it contain?

Valerian is the *rhizome* and *roots* of *V. officinalis*, or wild valerian (*Fam.* Valerianaceæ). It contains a volatile oil and a colorless volatile acid (*valerianic*).

What are the effects and uses of valerian?

Large doses of valerian may cause nausea, vomiting, and sometimes colicky pains. It slightly stimulates the brain and circulation, and increases the secretions of the skin and kidneys. Its effects are more decided in nervous excitement due to depression of the cerebral functions, as in *hysteria* or "*nervousness*," and in *hypochondriasis*. It has also been used as a cerebral stimulant in the *delirium* of low fevers and in *delirium tremens*.

What are the preparations and doses of valerian?

FLUIDEXTRACTUM VALERIANÆ (*fluid extract of valerian*), dose, ♏xv (1 c.c.).

TINCTURA VALERIANÆ (*tincture of valerian*), dose, ʒj (4 c.c.).

TINCTURA VALERIANÆ AMMONIATA (*ammoniated tincture of valerian*), dose, ʒj–ij (4–8 c.c.).

AMMONII VALERAS (*ammonium valerate*) is much used in *hysteria*, *neuralgia*, and *nervous headache*; dose, gr. ij–x (0.13–0.6 c.c.), in capsules or elixir.

Zinc valerate will be noticed under the Zinc Preparations.

ASAFETIDA.

What is asafetida, and of what is it composed?

Asafetida is a *gum-resin* obtained from the *root* of *Ferula fœtida* and probably other species of *Ferula* (*Fam.* Umbelliferæ), a native of Afghanistan. It is composed of a gum-resin united to a volatile oil.

What are its effects and uses?

It is a gastric stimulant and carminative, and produces a sense of exhilaration. It increases the mucous secretions and peristalsis, and in large doses quickens the pulse and respiration. Very large doses may cause nausea and vomiting.

It is *used* as an *antispasmodic* in *hysteria* and *nervous exhaustion;* as a *carminative* in *tympanites* (by the rectum); as a *stomachic tonic* in *dyspepsia* with flatulent colic, and as an *expectorant* in *chronic bronchitis* and in *whooping-cough*, where it also acts as an antispasmodic.

What are its preparations and doses?

EMULSUM ASAFŒTIDÆ (*emulsion of asafetida; lac asafœtidæ*), dose, ℥ss–j (15–30 c.c.), or as an enema, ℥ij–iv (60–120 c.c.).

PILULÆ ASAFŒTIDÆ (*pills of asafetida*), each pill containing gr. iij (0.2 gm.) of asafetida; dose, 2 to 4 pills.

TINCTURA ASAFŒTIDÆ (*tincture of asafetida*) contains 20 per cent. of asafetida; dose, ʒss–j (2–4 c.c.).

CAMPHORA (CAMPHOR).

What is camphor?

Camphor is the dextrogyrate modification of the saturated ketone obtained from *Cinnamomum camphora*, or camphor laurel (*Fam.* Lauraceæ), an evergreen tree of China and Japan. It is obtained by boiling chips of the tree in water and skimming off the camphor as it rises to the surface. This *crude camphor* is afterward *refined* by sublimation with quicklime.

What are the physiologic effects of camphor?

Locally, camphor is a rubefacient and irritant. Internally it is carminative and antidiarrheal, anodyne, and a cerebral exhilarant, sometimes quickening the pulse and raising arterial tension, and occasionally proving aphrodisiac. It dilates the arteries of the skin. In *large doses* (gr. xx—1.3 gm.) it depresses the circulation, produces lassitude and diaphoresis, and it is also anaphrodisiac. In *toxic doses* (ʒss–j—2–4 c.c.) it causes faintness, vertigo, headache, delirium, violent epigastric pain, unconsciousness, and sometimes convulsions. No case is recorded to have proved fatal in an adult.

What are the medicinal uses of camphor?

It is employed as an *antispasmodic* in "*nervousness*," *nervous headaches, hysterical complaints, dysmenorrhea*, "*after-pains*," simple *diarrhea*, and combined with other remedies in *cholera*. It is also used in *low forms of fever*, to quiet delirium and sustain the system. As an *anaphrodisiac* to quiet abnormal sexual excitement in *chordee, nymphomania*, and *priapism*. *Externally* it is employed as a liniment in myalgia, muscular rheumatism, and sprains. Dissolved in oil of turpentine, it forms an efficient liniment in mild bronchial affections. It is an ingredient of the "Rhinitis Pill," and of the "Sun Cholera Mixture."

What are its preparations and their uses?

CAMPHORA (*camphor*), dose, gr. j–x (0.06–0.6 gm.), or even gr. xx (1.3 gm.), given in emulsion, pill, or capsule. Not much used in this form.

AQUA CAMPHORÆ (*camphor-water*) contains 1 part of camphor in 125 parts of the preparation; dose, ℥ss–ij (15–60 c.c.). It is used chiefly as a vehicle or where a mild antispasmodic is needed.

SPIRITUS CAMPHORÆ (*spirit of camphor*) contains 10 per cent. of camphor. It is used as an embrocation, and is also given internally where a stronger preparation than the water is desired; dose, ♏v–ʒj (0.3–4.0 c.c.).

LINIMENTUM CAMPHORÆ (*camphor liniment; camphorated oil*) contains 20 per cent. of camphor in cottonseed oil.

CERATUM CAMPHORÆ (*camphor cerate*) contains 10 per cent. of camphor liniment.

LINIMENTUM SAPONIS (*soap liniment*) is much used externally, either alone or combined with stronger liniments.

CAMPHORA MONOBROMATA (*monobromated camphor*), dose, gr. v–x (0.3–0.6 gm.), in gelatin-coated pill or capsule. It is useful as an antispasmodic in *hysteria*, and as an anaphrodisiac in *chordee* and *priapism*.

Hope's Camphor Mixture (not official) consists of nitrous acid ʒj (4 c.c.); laudanum ♏xij (0.8 c.c.); camphor-water ℥viij (240 c.c.). Dose, ℥ss (15 c.c.), repeated as required. Much used in diarrhea and dysentery.

ACIDUM CAMPHORICUM (*camphoric acid*), a dibasic organic acid obtained by the oxidation of camphor with nitric acid, is soluble in alcohol, but only slightly so in water. In a mild way it produces effects similar to those of camphor, but its chief uses are as a local astringent and stimulant to catarrhal mucous membranes, and internally to stop the night-sweats of tuberculosis; dose, gr. xv (1 gm.).

OLEUM ÆTHEREUM (ETHEREAL OIL).

What is ethereal oil?

Ethereal oil, or oil of wine, is made by distilling alcohol with an excess of sulphuric acid and diluting with an equal volume of ether, and is a nearly colorless, volatile liquid. It is antispasmodic, and in small doses a cardiac and vasomotor stimulant, while in large doses it paralyzes the cardiac muscle and the vasomotor nerves. It is only used medicinally as—

SPIRITUS ÆTHERIS COMPOSITUS (COMPOUND SPIRIT OF ETHER).

What is this substance?

Compound spirit of ether, or *Hoffmann's anodyne*, is a solution of ethereal oil (2.5) in ether (32.5) and alcohol (65), and is a good antispasmodic, circulatory stimulant, and carminative, especially useful in flatulency and in asthma or dyspnea, when a cardiac stimulant is required; dose, ♏xv–ʒij (1–8 c.c.) repeated as desired.

CYPRIPEDIUM; SCUTELLARIA.

What are these remedies?

Cypripedium is the *rhizome* and *roots* of *C. hirsutum* and of *C. parviflorum* (*Fam.* Orchidaceæ), indigenous plants, commonly called ladies' slipper and moccasin plant. *Scutellaria* is the *plant*, *S. lateriflora*, or skullcap (*Fam.* Labiatæ), an indigenous herb. They possess mild antispasmodic properties, and have been used as substitutes for valerian.

FLUIDEXTRACTUM CYPRIPEDII (*fluid extract of cypripedium*), dose, ♏x–xx (0.6–1.2 c.c.).

FLUIDEXTRACTUM SCUTELLARIÆ (*fluid extract of scutellaria*), dose, ʒj (4 c.c.).

EXCITOMOTORS.

What are excitomotors?

Excitomotors are medicines which, by stimulating the reflex centers of the spinal cord, excite muscular action.

Name the excitomotors.

Nux vomica and its alkaloids.

NUX VOMICA.

What is nux vomica?

Nux vomica is the *seed* of the *Strychnos Nux-vomica*, or poison nut (*Fam.* Loganiaceæ), a tree of India, and yields not less than 1.25 per cent. of strychnine.

What active principles does it contain?

In contains two alkaloids, *strychnine* and *brucine*, combined with *igasuric acid*, and also much fixed oil.

How may the presence of these alkaloids be detected?

Strychnine may be detected by the addition of a crystal of potassium bichromate to a solution of the alkaloid in concentrated sulphuric acid on a porcelain plate, when a deep, rich blue color passing through purple into red rapidly makes its appearance.

The *physiologic test* is the production of tetanic spasms in a small animal (preferably a frog) to which a minute amount of the suspected substance has been administered.

Brucine with concentrated nitric acid strikes a blood-red color, fading into yellow.

What are the physiologic effects of nux vomica?

The effects of nux vomica are identical with those of its alkaloids. The action of *brucine* is similar to, but much weaker than, that of strychnine.

In *small doses* it acts as a bitter, increasing the appetite and digestion and the peristaltic movements of the intestines. When continued for some time in small doses, it is a vasomotor stimulant, renders sight, hearing, and touch more acute, and stimulates the respiratory center. In *large doses* it causes malaise, restlessness, anxiety, muscular twitchings, and finally clonic convulsions. Strychnine acts principally on the *spinal cord*, stimulating both its motor and sensory functions. Reflex irritability is much increased, and the response to stimulus is much greater than normal. After large doses, the reflex functions are so exalted that the slightest impression conveyed by a sensory nerve produces general convulsions. It is eliminated mostly in the urine; also in sweat, saliva, and bile.

What are the symptoms and treatment of strychnine poisoning?

Sudden shuddering, quickly followed by tetanic convulsions of all the voluntary muscles, accompanied with muscular pains, opisthotonos, the *risus sardonicus* (a ghastly grin), a pale face, becoming livid from embarrassed respiration. After a time the muscles relax and an interval of quiet occurs, to be succeeded again and again by convulsions if a liberal dose has been taken and is not antagonized by antidotes, until the sufferer dies of asphyxia from fixation of the respiratory muscles during a paroxysm; or the patient may die of paralysis and collapse during one of the intervals. The mind is clear to the end.

It *differs from tetanus* in history, in clonic (not tonic) spasms, in the muscles of the jaw not being affected before other voluntary muscles.

The *treatment* consists in—(1) Evacuating the contents of the stomach by emetics or the stomach-pump before the convulsive stage, or washing out the stomach under ether or chloroform if not seen until the convulsions have commenced; (2) giving tannic acid as a chemic antidote and chloral (hypodermically) and bromids as antagonists; (3) the frequent use of the catheter to prevent resorption of the poison from the bladder; and (4) artificial respiration and the inhalation of oxygen.

What are the therapeutic uses of nux vomica and strychnine?

It is employed (1) *as an excitomotor* in all cases of *paralysis* due to depression of the spinal or other motor centers, as in *diphtheritic, alcoholic,* or *lead paralyses, paraplegia, infantile paralysis* and *hemiplegia* after the subsidence of irritation. As it stimulates the nerve centers, it is *contraindicated* whenever inflammation or excitation of these centers is present; hence, in paralyses due to the presence of blood-clots it may do great injury if too early exhibited. In *constipation* due to atony and relaxation of muscular fibers, or in *diarrhea, dysentery, impotence,* or *incontinence of urine* from the same cause, it is very useful. (2) In *amaurosis,* especially when due to the abuse of tobacco or of alcohol, and in *amblyopia* from disease, strychnine pushed to the verge of tolerance is very efficacious. It is more useful before atrophy of the optic nerve-fibers has occurred. (3) As a *circulatory* and *respiratory stimulant* in *dyspnea* depending on chronic bronchitis, emphysema, phthisis, or due to cardiac disease as fatty or dilated heart, it is of value, and is often combined or alternated with digitalis in the latter affection. (4) As a *general tonic* it is advantageously given in *atonic dyspepsia, gastric catarrh, anemia,* and *chlorosis* (combined with iron), as an adjunct to quinine in obstinate *malarial fevers,* in various *neuralgias* occurring in debilitated subjects, and in *convalescence* from acute diseases (combined with iron and other tonics). Minute doses of nux vomica (tincture) will often arrest the *vomiting of pregnancy.*

What are the official preparations and their doses?

EXTRACTUM NUCIS VOMICÆ (*extract of nux vomica*), dose, gr. ¼–j (0.016–0.06 gm.), given in pill. It is frequently combined with purgatives to enhance their effect.

FLUIDEXTRACTUM NUCIS VOMICÆ (*fluid extract of nux vomica*), dose, ♏ij–x (0.12–0.6 c. c.).

TINCTURA NUCIS VOMICÆ (*tincture of nux vomica*), dose, ♏j–xx (0.06–1.2 c.c.). Chiefly used as a bitter tonic.

STRYCHNINA (*strychnine*), preferably given as—

STRYCHNINÆ NITRAS (*strychnine nitrate*) or

STRYCHNINÆ SULPHAS (*strychnine sulphate*), dose, gr. $\frac{1}{60}$–$\frac{1}{20}$ (0.001–0.003 gm.) internally, or gr. $\frac{1}{60}$ (0.001 gm.), cautiously increased, if used hypodermically. In collapse strychnine is often given in large doses, frequently repeated. It is not safe, however, to begin with a larger dose than gr. $\frac{1}{30}$–$\frac{1}{20}$ (0.002–0.003 gm.). As a tonic, minute doses may be given in pill, alone or combined with other medicines. In nervous affections it should be given in solution, the dose being gradually increased until slight muscular twitchings are produced. *Strychnine sulphate* enters into the *compound laxative pills* or *pills of aloin, belladonna, ipecac, and strychnine*, gr. $\frac{1}{128}$ (0.0005 gm.) in each pill.

Iron and strychnine citrate and the *elixir*, *glycerite* and *syrup of iron, quinine, and strychnine phosphates* have been noticed with the Iron Preparations.

DEPRESSOMOTORS.

What are depressomotors?

They are remedies which are used to depress the functions of the spinal cord, motor nerves, or muscles, thus lessening motor activity.

Name the members of this group.

Physostigma; chloral; the bromids; the nitrites; gelsemium; prussic acid; the cyanids; oil of bitter almonds; lobelia; conium; woorara, and tobacco.

PHYSOSTIGMA.

What is physostigma, and what active principles does it contain?

Physostigma, or Calabar bean, is the *seed* of *P. venenosum* (*Fam.* Leguminosæ), a plant found on the western coast of Africa, and yields not less than 0.15 per cent. of ether-soluble alkaloids. It contains an alkaloid called *eserine* or *physostigmine*, and a second alkaloid (a tetanizing agent), called *calabarine.*

What are the physiologic effects of physostigma?

Calabar bean is a reflex depressant, causing also, in full doses, giddiness, slow and often irregular pulse, great muscular weakness, nausea, and sometimes vomiting, generally free purgation, and usually contraction of the pupils. When poisonous doses are taken, there are, in addition, muscular tremors and abolition of reflex action, slow pulse and respiration, miosis and motor paralysis, and death from respiratory failure.

It depresses and finally paralyzes the *reflex and motor centers of the spinal cord*, having but slight effect upon the nerves themselves. It slows the heart (by greatly lengthening the diastolic pause) and increases its power (acting either on the cardiac motor-ganglia or muscle). The *blood pressure* at first falls, but soon rises, through contraction of the arteries, and remains high until death approaches. It stimulates *intestinal peristalsis* and increases the secretions of the part. In the eye it lowers intra-ocular tension and contracts the pupil, probably by paralyzing the peripheral sympathetic nerve-fibers in the iris and at the same time stimulating the end-organs of the third pair of nerves. It is probably *eliminated* by the urine.

How should poisoning by this drug be treated?

(1) Give emetics and cathartics, and use a catheter to prevent further absorption of poison; (2) use atropine hypodermically as a physiologic antagonist, and (3) give other cardiac and respiratory stimulants, as digitalis, ammonia, and alcohol.

For what purpose is it employed medicinally?

As a *depressomotor* it is used in *tetanus, trismus neonatorum, epilepsy,* and *chorea,* though with poor success. It has also been given as a physiologic antagonist in *strychnine poisoning,* but is probably inferior to chloral for this purpose.

From its influence over *intestinal peristalsis* it is advantageously used in *habitual constipation,* especially when associated with chronic intestinal dyspepsia and dry, hard stools. The *alkaloid* in one-half to one per cent. solution is used in ocular therapeutics, to prevent or overcome adhesions of the iris, lessen intra-ocular tension, and contract the pupil.

What are its preparations and doses?

EXTRACTUM PHYSOSTIGMATIS (*extract of physostigma*), dose, gr. $\frac{1}{12}$–$\frac{1}{2}$ (0.005–0.03 gm.).

TINCTURA PHYSOSTIGMATIS (*tincture of physostigma*), dose, ♏ v–xxx (0.3–2.0 c.c.).

PHYSOSTIGMINÆ SULPHAS (*physostigmine sulphate*), a very deliquescent salt; dose, $\frac{1}{60}$–$\frac{1}{12}$ (0.001–0.005).

Physostigminæ Salicylas (*physostigmine salicylate*), preferred to the sulphate because of its greater permanency; dose, gr. $\frac{1}{60}$–$\frac{1}{12}$ (0.001–0.005 gm.).

Chloral and The Bromids have been discussed under the head of *Hypnotics* (*vid.* pp. 95 and 97).

THE NITRITES.

What are the nitrites?

The *nitrites* are salts formed by the union of *nitrous acid*[1] with a base.

Amylis nitris (*amyl nitrite*) is the only official organic nitrite (except the sweet spirits of niter, which contains ethyl nitrite, and will be considered elsewhere). It is a yellowish, oily, very volatile liquid, with a pleasant, fruity odor. *Nitroglycerin* (*glyceryl trinitrate, trinitrin, trininitroglycerin*, or *glonoin*) is a colorless, oily liquid, without odor, soluble in ether and alcohol. It forms the basis of various explosives. It is really a *trinitrate* (not a *nitrite*) of glyceryl or propenyl [$C_3H_5(NO_3)_3$]. *Erythrol tetranitrate*, another explosive, and *potassium and sodium nitrites* are also used.

What is the physiologic action of the nitrites?

They cause flushing of the face, headache, fulness and throbbing of the head, excited cardiac action, great dilatation of the arterioles and capillaries (from paralysis of their muscular coats), and consequently greatly diminished blood pressure, rapid respiration, lowered temperature, and diminished reflexes. After toxic doses the pupils dilate, the muscular system relaxes, the blood becomes darker (probably from the formation of methemoglobin), the respiration and circulation become slow and irregular, and finally death occurs from respiratory failure, sensation and consciousness being preserved to the last. They depress both the *motor and reflex spinal* centers without influencing either the sensory nerves or centers. At first the heart is faster through vagus depression, later it is slow and weak by direct action on the muscle. The *temperature* is lowered, owing to lessened oxidation. The nitrites are all *muscle poisons*. They are *elim-*

[1] See footnote on page 72.

inated by the urine, increasing greatly the amount of water and the uric acid and urea. The action of *amyl nitrite* is the most rapid but most transient; *nitroglycerin* is slower, but its effects are more lasting; *erythrol tetranitrate* is still slower and its effects last several hours.

What are the therapeutic uses of the nitrites?

The nitrites are used—(1) as *depressomotors* to relax spasm in *angina pectoris, asthma, tetanus,* puerperal and other forms of *convulsions, strychnine poisoning,* congestive and nervous *dysmenorrhea,* and in all cases of very *high arterial tension* from spasm of the arterioles; thus, in *renal asthma* the inhalation of a few drops of amyl nitrite quickly relieves the spasm, and *migraine* with capillary spasm is frequently benefited by it. Given just before the expected chill of *malarial fevers,* it will abort it, and sometimes avert the paroxysm. If amyl nitrite is inhaled when the "aura epileptica" is experienced, it will often prevent the *epileptic* attack. Nitroglycerin has proved of value in *chronic interstitial nephritis,* lessening the albuminuria and relieving the arterial spasm. Obstinate *hiccup* has been benefited by nitroglycerin.

(2) The nitrites are also employed in *syncope, cardiac dyspnea,* and in *threatened cardiac failure* during the administration of anesthetics, especially chloroform.

(3) They have also been found useful in the *nausea and vomiting* of sea-sickness and pregnancy.

What are the doses of the nitrites, and how are they administered?

AMYLIS NITRIS (*amyl nitrite*), given internally or by inhalation; dose, ℳij–v (0.1–0.3 c.c.).

SODII NITRIS (*sodium nitrite*), dose, gr. ij–iij (0.1–0.2 gm.).

Potassium nitrite is not official. It may be used in the same doses as the sodium salt.

SPIRITUS GLYCERYLIS NITRATIS (*spirit of glyceryl trinitrate; spirit of nitroglycerin*) is a 1 per cent. alcoholic solution of nitroglycerin, the dose of which is ℳss (0.03 c.c.), cautiously increased.

Triturates of the nitroglycerin, each containing gr. $\frac{1}{100}$ (0.0006 gm.), are also employed.

Erythrol tetranitrate (not official) is a solid, dose, gr. j (0.06 gm.).

Amyl nitrite is usually given by *inhalation*, but may be administered internally on sugar or even hypodermically. The other preparations are given by the mouth. If a speedy action is required, amyl nitrite should be used, and after the immediate danger is over, if it is desired to maintain the effect, the other nitrites or nitroglycerin may be given.

GELSEMIUM.

What is gelsemium, and what chemic principles does it contain?

Gelsemium is the *rhizome* and *roots* of *G. sempervirens*, the yellow or Carolina jasmine (*Fam.* Loganiaceæ), a climbing plant of the Southern States. It contains two alkaloids, *gelsemine* and *gelseminine*, combined with *gelseminic acid*, a volatile oil, resin, etc.

What are its physiologic effects?

Small doses produce languor, dizziness, and perhaps slight lowering of the pulse-rate; *large doses* diminish the force and frequency of the pulse and lower arterial pressure, depress respiration, cause frontal headache, and disordered, usually double, vision; *toxic doses* depress the central nervous system and cause extreme muscular weakness, partial blindness, dilated pupil, often internal strabismus, ptosis, incoördination, the jaw drops, articulation is impaired, general sensibility is much diminished, respiration is slowed, the pulse is very feeble, the temperature declines, a profuse cold sweat breaks out, and death occurs from respiratory failure. The mind remains clear until the end approaches. The *respiratory center* is depressed and finally paralyzed. The poison appears in toxic doses to depress the *heart* directly. It paralyzes the end-organs of the motor oculi, thus causing mydriasis with paralysis of accommodation and ptosis, and must also act on the sixth nerve, as the action of the external rectus muscle is much enfeebled.

What are its therapeutic uses?

It has been used as a *motor depressant* in *asthma*, *laryn-*

gismus stridulus, pertussis, nervous cough, and *tic douloureux;* as a *sensor-depressant* in *trigeminal neuralgia,* especially when associated with spasm, and in various other *neuralgic affections;* as a *calmative* in *mania* (full doses); as a *cardiac sedative* in *sthenic fevers* and *inflammations,* and in *ocular therapeutics.* Its chief use is in neuralgia, especially of the fifth nerve.

What are its preparations and their doses?

FLUIDEXTRACTUM GELSEMII (*fluid extract of gelsemium*), dose, ♏v–x (0.3–0.6 c.c.), repeated every two or three hours until constitutional effects are produced—ʒj (4 c.c.) has proved fatal.

TINCTURA GELSEMII (*tincture of gelsemium*), dose, ♏xx–ʒj (1.3–4.0 c.c.),

ACIDUM HYDROCYANICUM DILUTUM (DILUTED HYDROCYANIC ACID).

What are the sources of hydrocyanic acid?

Hydrocyanic or prussic acid develops in the presence of water in bitter almonds, peach kernels and leaves, wild cherry, etc., but is used in medicine only in a very diluted solution. The *diluted acid* is formed by the reaction of sulphuric acid and water upon potassium ferrocyanid or of hydrochloric acid on silver cyanid, and is a colorless, volatile liquid, with an odor resembling that of bitter almonds. It contains 2 per cent. of the absolute acid.

How may the presence of prussic acid be detected?

1. The addition of a solution of silver nitrate produces a white precipitate entirely soluble in boiling concentrated nitric acid. 2. The addition of a small amount of a mixed solution of ferrous and ferric sulphate, and afterward a little liquor potassæ, gives a dirty, greenish-blue precipitate, which changes to Prussian blue when slighty acidulated with hydrochloric acid.

What are its physiologic effects?

Locally applied it passes through the cuticle and paralyzes the end-organs of the sensitive nerves beneath. When its vapor is inhaled or when the acid is taken in sufficient doses it kills almost immediately, from arrest of circulation. If the toxic dose has not been large enough to arrest the circulation instantly, vomiting, dyspnea, and depression of the heart occur, followed by dilated pupils, convulsions, unconsciousness, and collapse and death from asphyxia. The convulsions are of *cerebral* origin.

Prussic acid is a direct nerve and muscle poison. In large doses it causes diastolic arrest by direct action either on the *heart muscle* or on its contained ganglia; in small doses it slows the heart by stimulation of the inhibitory centers. It stimulates at first the vasomotor system, and for a short time raises arterial tension, but it soon depresses and finally paralyzes the vasomotor apparatus, and the blood-pressure falls. The venous blood at first becomes of an arterial hue, as the tissues are prevented from taking up the oxygen, but after death even the arterial blood has lost its bright color. Asphyxia is due to paralysis of the respiratory center. It is rapidly eliminated by the lungs and kidneys, appearing in the urine as sulphocyanids.

How should poisoning by prussic acid be treated?

The best chemical antidotes are the hydrated oxid of iron, and nitrate of cobalt.

Evacuate, if possible, the contents of the stomach; give atropine hypodermically as a respiratory stimulant; give ammonia freely by inhalation, by the mouth, and by intravenous injection; practice artificial respiration assiduously, and use alternate hot and cold douches. Death usually results so rapidly that nothing is of much service.

What are the medicinal uses of diluted hydrocyanic acid?

It is used—1. as a *depressomotor* and *nerve sedative* in various forms of *cough*, as that of phthisis, also in *asthma* and in *whooping*-cough. In obstinate *vomiting* it is sometimes successful. In *gastrodynia* and in *enteralgia* it has proved beneficial, probably by a local action on the nerves of the parts. When successful in these cases, it is so speedily.

2. *Locally* (ʒj–iij to Oj—4–12 to 480 c.c.) it is used as an *anodyne* in neuralgia and in many cutaneous affections at-

tended with pruritus. Great caution should be used when it is thus applied, as fatal results have attended its absorption through an abraded surface.

How is it administered?

ACIDUM HYDROCYANICUM DILUTUM (*diluted hydrocyanic acid*), dose, ℞j–iij (0.06–2.0 c.c.) diluted.

THE CYANIDS.

What are the effects, uses, and doses of the cyanids?

POTASSII CYANIDUM (*Potassium Cyanid*).—*Locally*, it is an irritant. It may be absorbed through the skin when the application is prolonged, and cause poisoning. When administered *internally*, it reacts with the acids of the gastric juice and prussic acid is set free, consequently the systemic effects are identical with those of that acid, as a substitute for which it is used. Dose, gr. $\frac{1}{12}$–$\frac{1}{8}$ (0.005–0.008 gm.).

ARGENTI CYANIDUM (*silver cyanid*) is used in medicine in making prussic acid extemporaneously.

OLEUM AMYGDALÆ AMARÆ (OIL OF BITTER ALMOND).

What are the effects, uses, and dose of this oil?

Oil of bitter almond is a volatile oil obtained from bitter almond by maceration with water, and subsequent distillation. It contains *benzoic aldehyd* and *hydrocyanic acid* (due to the reaction of *amygdalin* with water, in the presence of an albuminous ferment called *emulsin*). Its effects and uses are the same as those of prussic acid. Dose, ℞¼–ss (0.015–0.03 c.c.), in emulsion.

AQUA AMYGDALÆ AMARÆ (*bitter almond water*) contains $\frac{1}{10}$ of 1 per cent. of the oil, and is used as a vehicle; dose, ʒj–iv (4–15 c.c.).

SPIRITUS AMYGDALÆ AMARÆ (*spirit of bitter almond; essence of bitter almond*) contains 1 per cent. of the oil; dose, ♏j–xx (0.06–1.2 c.c.).

SYRUPUS AMYGDALE (*syrup of almonds*), made from the spirit of bitter almond and orange-flower water, is used as a vehicle.

EMULSUM AMYGDALÆ (*almond emulsion; milk of almonds*), made from the sweet almonds alone, is also used as a vehicle.

LOBELIA.

What is lobelia and what are its active ingredients?

Lobelia is the *leaves* and *tops* of *L. inflata*, or Indian tobacco (*Fam.* Lobeliaceæ), an indigenous plant. It contains an *alkaloid, lobeline*; also *lobelic acid*, fixed and volatile oils, etc.

What are its effects and uses?

In *large doses* it causes nausea, violent vomiting with great depression, sometimes purging, feeble pulse, almost complete muscular relaxation, and, if a *lethal dose* has been taken, collapse, coma, sometimes preceded by convulsions, and death from paralysis of the respiratory center.

Large doses appear to paralyze the motor nerves, the vasomotor center, and the peripheral vagi. Its action has not been fully studied.

The *treatment of lobelia poisoning* consists in emetics, tannic acid, morphine, alcohol, ammonia, and counterirritation to the surface.

It is *used* as a *depressomotor* and *expectorant* in *asthma* and in *acute bronchitis* with spasmodic dyspnea. In other spasmodic diseases it has been superseded by more reliable and less dangerous remedies. It is too depressing in its action to be used as an emetic.

Locally, in infusion (℥j to Oj—30–480 c.c.), it is highly recommended as an application to *poison-oak dermatitis*.

What are the preparations of lobelia and their doses?

Fluidextractum Lobeliæ (*fluid extract of lobelia*), dose, as an *expectorant*, ♏j–v (0.06–0.3 c.c.); as an *emetic*, ♏xv–xx (1.0–1.2 c.c.).

Tinctura Lobeliæ (*tincture of lobelia*) contains 10 per cent. of lobelia; dose, as an *expectorant*, ♏v–xxv (0.3–1.5 c.c.); as a *motordepressant* in asthma, ʒj (4 c.c.).

CONIUM.

What is conium and what active principles does it contain?

Conium is the *full-grown but unripe fruit* of *C. maculatum*, or poison-hemlock (*Fam.* Umbelliferæ), and yields not less than 0.5 per cent. of coniine. The *active principle* is *coniine*, a volatile *liquid alkaloid.* It also contains *conydrine, methyl-coniine,* and *pseudoconydrine.* It is found in the temperate regions of the old world.

What are its physiologic effects?

Full medicinal doses cause great muscular weakness, first felt in the lower extremities, difficulty in keeping the eyelids raised, and disordered vision from paralysis of accommodation. Sometimes the pupils dilate, and sometimes there are nausea and vomiting. After a *poisonous amount* has been taken these symptoms are intensified, and difficulty of speech, delirium or coma, ascending paralysis, and death from asphyxia, preceded by convulsions of cerebral origin, occur. Conium has little, if any, action on the *cerebral hemispheres,* and but little is known of its influence on the *spinal cord.* It paralyzes the peripheral ends of *nerves,* acting much more powerfully on the motor than on sensory fibers. The effects on the *ocular apparatus* are due to peripheral oculomotor paralysis. The *pulse* is at first accelerated (paralysis of the vagi), but afterward slowed (depression of cardiac motor nerves), and the blood-pressure, which was primarily lowered, is raised when symptoms of asphyxia take place. It is eliminated by the urine. The *treatment of poisoning* consists in evacuating the contents of the stomach, giving tannic acid as an antidote, maintaining artificial respiration, and administering, as antagonists, atropine, strychnine, or picrotoxin.

What are the medicinal uses of conium?

Conium has been used as a *depressomotor* in *whooping-cough, paralysis agitans, chorea, blepharospasm, asthma,* and other spasmodic affections. It has been used as a *calmative* and *relaxant* in *maniacal* and *hysterical excitement,* and also in *melancholia,* and as an *anodyne* in *neuralgia,* especially *sciatica.*

What are the preparations and doses of conium?

FLUIDEXTRACTUM CONII (*fluid extract of conium*), dose, ♏j–v (0.06–0.3 c.c.).

As different samples of the drug vary much in the amount of coniine contained, it is safer to begin with a small dose, to be gradually increased until some effect is obtained.

WOORARA.

What is woorara?

Woorara (not official), called also woorali and curare, is an extract prepared by the South American Indians from *Strychnos toxifera* and other species of Strychnos (*Nat. Ord.* Loganiaceæ), and is used by them as an arrow-poison. It *contains* an alkaloid called *curarine.*

What are its effects and uses?

It is eliminated so rapidly that usually when administered internally no symptoms result. When it enters the system through a wound or by hypodermic injection, it paralyzes the peripheral endings of the *motor nerves,* and if the dose be sufficiently large, the *vagus* and the ends of the *sensory nerves* are also paralyzed. After a time the *nerve-trunks* and the *spinal cord* are also affected. The *voluntary muscles* are uninfluenced. Large amounts lower the *blood-pressure* and finally depress the *heart.* Death results from paralysis of the motor respiratory nerves. Small doses increase all the secretions. It is *eliminated* chiefly by the urine.

The *treatment of woorara-poisoning* consists in frequent catheterization to prevent resorption, artificial respiration, and atropine and strychnine hypodermically as antagonists. They can scarcely be relied on.

Woorara is *used* as a *depressomotor* in *tetanus* and in *hydrophobia,* and has also been employed in *epilepsy* and in *chorea.* It is given in doses of gr. $\frac{1}{10}$ (0.006 gm.), or its alkaloid, curarine, may be used in doses of gr. $\frac{1}{200}$–$\frac{1}{100}$ (0.0003–0.0006 gm.). It is an unsafe drug.

TABACUM (TOBACCO).

What is tobacco, and what does it contain?

Tobacco (not official) is the commercial *dried leaves* of *Nicotiana Tabacum* (*Fam.* Solanaceæ). It contains *nicotine,* a volatile *liquid alkaloid, nicotianin* (tobacco-camphor), and an empyreumatic oil. The smoke from tobacco contains pyridin derivatives with nature and action like nicotine.

What are its effects and uses?

To persons unaccustomed to its use, tobacco or nicotine is a depressant, nauseant, and emetic, and causes dizziness and weakness. When a toxic dose is taken, purgation, diuresis, cramps, or convulsions, followed by great muscular weakness, and, finally, paralysis, a rapid, feeble, and compressible pulse, collapse, and death from paralysis of the respiratory muscles.

It first stimulates the *spinal* centers (thus causing convulsions), but probably finally paralyzes them. It at first excites and then abolishes the functions of the peripheral endings of motor nerves, the nerve-trunks being afterward affected, but has no influence on voluntary muscles. The *cardiac* action is first depressed from some unexplained cause, afterward much increased, probably from paralysis of the peripheral inhibitory nerves, and the blood-pressure, which at first falls, is afterward elevated. Nicotine contracts the pupil, whether applied locally or administered internally.

Tobacco increases intestinal peristalsis, and is probably eliminated chiefly by the urine, which it greatly increases.

The *treatment of nicotine poisoning* consists in emetics or washing out the stomach, tannic acid, and strychnine with artificial respiration.

Tobacco is not much *used* at present as a *depressomotor*, but may be employed for this purpose in *tetanus* and in *strychnine poisoning*. In persons unaccustomed to its use, smoking a strong cigar may relieve an attack of *spasmodic asthma*. As a *local anodyne*, it has been used as a poultice to *painful ulcers*, as an ointment to inflamed *hemorrhoids*, and as a lotion to relieve *pruritus*. Great caution should be observed, as its local use has resulted in poisoning and death. There are no *official preparations*. Dose, gr. j–iij (0.06–0.19 gm.), in infusion, which in poisoning by strychnine or in tetanus must be frequently repeated until some results are obtained.

ON THE ORGANS OF CIRCULATION.

CARDIAC STIMULANTS.

What are cardiac stimulants?

They are medicines which are administered with a view to increasing the power of the heart or the force of the circulation.

Mention the remedies of this order.

Alcohol, ether, the ammonium preparations, atropine, digitalis, caffeine, adonidine, strophanthus, strychnine, cimicifuga.

ALCOHOL.

What is alcohol?

Alcohol (ethyl hydroxid) results from the fermentation of saccharine liquids. It is a colorless, inflammable liquid, uniting in all proportions with water. *Alcohol* contains 94.9 per cent. by volume of absolute alcohol, which is not used in medicine.

What are the physiologic effects of alcohol?

Locally applied it is an astringent. It evaporates rapidly and produces a feeling of cold, but if evaporation is prevented, it acts as an irritant. Taken *internally in small doses* it promotes absorption, stimulates secretions, and stimulates the movements of the stomach. As a result of this it increases appetite and digestion and temporarily stimulates the heart and respiration. It dilates the cutaneous vessels, thus causing a sensation of warmth, and diminishes the amount of urea eliminated. The *continued use* of small doses disorders the digestion and the hepatic functions, produces gastric catarrh and hyperplasia of the connective tissues, resulting in sclerosis of different viscera, and tends to the production of fatty degeneration of the walls of the vessels and various organs. In fevers where carbohydrates and fats are unavailable, alcohol may serve as a *food*, preventing proteid destruction.

Large doses disorder digestion, depress the nervous system, and cause the well-known alcoholic intoxication with muscular incoördination and weakness, hallucinations, lowered temperature, depression of the heart-muscle and reflexes, and stupor.

After toxic doses death from respiratory or cardiac failure may rapidly result, preceded by insensibility, stertorous breathing and coma, and occasionally by convulsions.

Small doses slightly increase the *temperature* of the body, but large doses reduce it by interfering with the oxygen-carrying function of the red corpuscles and with the nutritive process, and by dilating the cutaneous vessels. *Respiration* is first quickened, then slowed, and after fatal doses, paralyzed.

It appears to act as a *cerebral* stimulant, because it depresses the higher inhibitory powers of judgment, will, etc., setting free the lower functions, emotional, self-indulgent, etc. One seems to think more quickly, and in company is free from embarrassment. In toxic doses it depresses the cerebrum and cerebellum, the *spinal* reflex centers, the conductivity of both motor and sensory nerves, and finally the reflex functions of the medulla. It diminishes the *excretion* of nitrogenized waste, and is *eliminated* principally by the kidneys, and also lungs and skin, although a large proportion (more in proportion to the smallness of the dose) disappears in the system.

How should acute alcohol-narcosis be treated?

The contents of the stomach should be evacuated, ammonia or strychnine should be given, and the hot and cold douche alternately used.

What are the medicinal uses of alcohol?

As a stimulant through reflex from the stomach and by lessening the power of the inhibitory centers, alcohol is much used in shock, collapse, syncope from exhaustion, and wasting fevers. Though its prolonged use lessens the power of resistance to germs, it is useful in conditions of suppuration, pyemia, septicemia, typhoid fever, etc., acting not only to support and nourish the body, but to calm the nervous system, and, by dilating the cutaneous vessels and lessening oxidation, to reduce the fever.

In poisoning by snake-bite it is given in frequently repeated doses almost *ad libitum*, conjoined with intravenous, or, at least, hypodermic injection of ammonia.

To *improve digestion* and *nutrition* it is useful in many chronic diseases, but the danger of forming the alcohol habit should always be borne in mind when it is thus prescribed.

Locally, alcohol is used as an *antiseptic* and *stimulant* dressing for wounds, to harden the cuticle when *bed-sores* are imminent, and as a *tonic* and *cooling lotion*.

What are the official preparations of alcohol?

ALCOHOL ABSOLUTUM (*absolute alcohol*) is ethyl alcohol containing not more than 1 per cent., by weight, of water. It is not used medicinally.

ALCOHOL is commercial alcohol with the fusel oil removed, and is used in making various medicinal preparations into which alcohol enters. It contains 94.9 per cent. by volume of absolute alcohol; specific gravity, 0.816.

ALCOHOL DILUTUM (*diluted alcohol*) contains 48.9 per cent. by volume of absolute alcohol; specific gravity, 0.936.

SPIRITUS FRUMENTI (*whisky*), an alcoholic liquid obtained by the distillation of the mash of fermented grain (usually of mixtures of corn, wheat, and rye), and at least four years old; it contains 44 to 55 per cent. by volume of alcohol; specific gravity, 0.924–0.945.

SPIRITUS VINI GALLICI (*brandy*), an alcoholic liquid obtained by the distillation of fermented, unmodified juice of fresh grapes, and at least four years old; it contains from 46 to 55 per cent. by volume of alcohol; specific gravity, 0.925–0.941. It is astringent, and is, therefore, preferable to whisky if there is looseness of the bowels. It is also a stomachic sedative, and, next to champagne, tends to check vomiting more than any other alcoholic liquid.

VINUM ALBUM (*white wine*), an alcoholic liquid, made by fermenting the juice of fresh grapes, the fruit of *Vitis vinifera* (*Fam.* Vitaceæ), freed from seeds, stems, and skins, contains 8.5 to 15 per cent. by volume of absolute alcohol.

VINUM RUBRUM (*red wine*), an alcoholic liquid made by fermenting the juice of fresh red-colored grapes, the fruit of *Vitis vinifera* (*Fam.* Vitaceæ), in the presence of their skins, and contains from 8.5 to 15 per cent. by volume of absolute alcohol. It is somewhat astringent.

How is alcohol administered?

Wines may be given pure or mixed with water. Brandy and whisky are given pure or diluted with water, or in the form of milk-punch or egg-nog.

They may also be injected into the rectum, and, if cardiac failure is imminent, brandy may be used hypodermically.

ÆTHER—ETHER.

Is this substance ever used as a cardiac stimulant?

The use of *ether* as a cardiac stimulant has already been

mentioned. It acts rapidly but transiently, and may be used internally, or, better still, hypodermically in cases of sudden cardiac failure.

AMMONIUM.

What are the sources of ammonium?

Ammonium is abundantly present in nature as the result of animal and vegetable decay, but is chiefly obtained for commercial purposes from the ammoniacal liquor of gas works.

What are the general physiologic actions of ammonium preparations?

AMMONIA GAS in solution is an irritant. Kept in contact with the skin it reddens and finally vesicates. When the gas is *inhaled* it irritates and reflexly stimulates the heart and respiration. If very strong, it produces a sense of suffocation, spasm, and, if continued, inflammation of the air-passages. When *injected* into the veins of animals in sufficient quantities, it damages the blood and causes convulsions, rapid respiration, and death.

Ammonia temporarily stimulates the accelerator nerves of the *heart*, thus increasing the rapidity of its action. After intravenous injection, the *blood-pressure* at first falls, but rapidly rises as the pulse becomes quicker. It stimulates the bronchial, skin, and salivary glands. Intravenous injections of ammonia quicken *respiration* by powerfully stimulating the respiratory centers. The convulsions are due to stimulation of the *motor and reflex spinal centers*. It is *eliminated* chiefly by the urine as urea, and tends to increase the acidity of the urine and to lessen the alkalinity of the blood. Its salts are also eliminated by the bronchopulmonary mucous membrane, stimulating it and tending to liquefy the mucus. When taken internally in medicinal doses, it is antacid and carminative, but if continued for too long a poriod, it disorders digestion and causes emaciation.

What are the symptoms and treatment of poisoning by ammonia?

When a strong solution is swallowed, it causes inflammation

of the lips, mouth, fauces, pharynx, esophagus, and stomach. Edema of the glottis may occur, and secondary strictures of the esophagus or even of the pylorus may result. Death may be due to asphyxia or to collapse preceded by symptoms of corrosive poisoning. The *treatment* consists in neutralizing the alkali by mild vegetable acids (vinegar or lemonade); protecting the injured surfaces by oils and demulcents; and the occasional passage of an esophageal bougie, for at least a year, to prevent secondary stricture. The occurrence of edema of the glottis demands immediate tracheotomy or intubation.

What are the therapeutic uses of the ammonium preparations?

Ammonia is a rapid and powerful *cardiac stimulant,* but its effects are of brief duration. It is used for this purpose both internally and by inhalation in all cases of acute *cardiac failure,* and may be used to antagonize the action of *snake poison* and *prussic acid* on the heart, but should here be employed as an adjuvant to alcohol.

For *sudden cardiac failure* during *anesthesia* or from *surgical shock* it may be given hypodermically.

It has been used by intravenous injection to *maintain the fluidity of the blood* in cases of threatened *cardiac thrombosis;* and as a *stimulating expectorant* in *pneumonia,* especially when typhoid symptoms are present, It is given *as an alkali* in *acidity, flatulence,* and in *nervous headache.*

Externally it is an ingredient of stimulating and irritating liniments, and may be used as a vesicant.

What preparations of ammonium are used?

AQUA AMMONIÆ FORTIOR (*stronger ammonia water*) contains 28 per cent. by weight of gaseous ammonia. It is a powerful corrosive poison. It is best adapted for hypodermic use in doses of ♏x–xxv (0.6–1.5 c.c.), diluted with four times its volume of water, and repeated in fifteen minutes if necessary, and may be used externally as a rapid (but painful) vesicant by inverting a watch-crystal full of it on the skin.

AQUA AMMONIÆ (*ammonia-water*) contains 10 per cent.

by weight of ammonia-gas; *dose*, for internal use, gtt. x–xxx (0.6–2.0 min.), freely diluted.

SPIRITUS AMMONIÆ (*spirit of ammonia*) contains 10 per cent. by weight of the gas in solution in alcohol; dose, ♏x–xxx (0.6–2.0 c.c.), freely diluted.

SPIRITUS AMMONIÆ AROMATICUS (*aromatic spirit of ammonia*) contains also ammonium carbonate and aromatics; dose, ʒss–j (2–4 c.c.), freely diluted.

AMMONII CARBONAS (*ammonium carbonate*) is used as a cardiac stimulant, and also in threatened thrombosis. It is very valuable as a stimulating expectorant in capillary bronchitis, typhoid pneumonia, and other low forms of chronic pulmonary disease where an expectorant is required; dose, gr. v–x (0.3–0.6 gm.).

AMMONII SALICYLAS (*ammonium salicylate*) has been sometimes employed in rheumatism, but the dose is much smaller than that of the other salicylates; dose, gr. ij–v (0.12–0.3 gm.).

The *iodid, bromid*, and the *acetate, tartrate*, and *citrate of iron* and *ammonium*, and *valerianate of ammonium* have already been noticed; the *acetate, benzoate*, and *chlorid* will be discussed hereafter. The *nitrate of ammonium* is used only in making other official preparations.

The *acetate* is especially stimulating to the sweat-glands, producing diaphoresis.

ATROPINÆ (ATROPIN).

Is atropine used as a cardiac stimulant?

Atropine (*vid.* Belladonna, p. 107) is used as a cardiac stimulant in cases of sudden or threatened heart-failure; dose, gr. $\frac{1}{120}$–$\frac{1}{60}$ (0.0005–0.001 gm.), given hypodermically.

DIGITALIS.

What is digitalis?

Digitalis is the *leaves* of *D. purpurea*, or purple foxglove (*Fam.* Scrophulariaceæ), obtained *from plants of the second year's growth.* It is a European plant, cultivated in this country.

What are its chemic constituents?

The constituents of digitalis are *digitalin, digitoxin, digi-*

tonin, *digitophyllin*, and *digitalein*, with digitaleic acid, resin, gum, etc. Digitalin and digitoxin are insoluble in water and soluble in alcohol; digitonin is soluble in water and (as in infusion of digitalis) has the peculiar property of holding digitalin and digitoxin in watery solution.

What are the physiologic effects of digitalis?

Its effects are much more slowly produced, but are much more lasting than those of the medicines previously considered; and it is, therefore, more of a tonic than a stimulant to the heart. In *moderate doses* it slows and strengthens the cardiac beat, elevates the blood-pressure, and causes diuresis. It sometimes interferes with the appetite and digestion. After very *large doses*, or when too long continued, nausea and vomiting may occur; the pulse becomes dicrotic, weak, and sometimes rapid, and diaphoresis, more or less profuse, takes place. *Toxic doses* cause the same symptoms, and in addition vertigo, disordered vision, lowered reflexes, muscular tremors, lassitude, reduced temperature, delirium, stupor, usually convulsions, and death from cardiac paralysis.

In moderate doses it stimulates the vagus center and the peripheral cardioinhibitory fibers of the vagi (thus slowing the *heart* by increasing the length of the diastole), the cardiac muscle and its contained motor ganglia (thus increasing the strength and force of the systole), and the vasomotor centers (thus raising the arterial tension). It also acts directly on the muscular walls of the vessels, and thus also lessens their caliber.

When full medicinal doses are taken or when the pulse has been greatly slowed by it, a sudden change from the recumbent to the erect posture may give rise to a small, weak, rapid pulse, with lowered arterial tension, owing to over-stimulation and exhaustion of the heart.

When *fatal doses* are taken, the heart is arrested in systole.

In poisonous doses it lowers *reflex action* by stimulating Setschenow's inhibitory reflex centers and, later, by paralyzing directly the spinal cord. It also lowers the contractility of *muscles*. It usually proves *diuretic*, probably by improving the renal circulation. It is *eliminated* chiefly by the urine, and very slowly, so that its effects are cumulative. It stimulates the uterus.

How should poisoning by digitalis be treated?

(1) Give emetics and cathartics to remove the poison from the alimentary canal; (2) tannic acid as a chemic antidote; alcohol, ammonium carbonate, and opium, or saponin, as physiologic antagonists; (3) absolute recumbency must be maintained.

What are the medicinal uses of digitalis?

As a *cardiac tonic* digitalis is used in all cases of loss of cardiac power, as in *dilatation* or in *weakness of the cardiac muscle. It should never be prescribed* in simple hypertrophy, nor when hypertrophy is sufficient to compensate for valvular lesion. In advanced cases of fatty heart it should be used very cautiously, if at all, as the increased systolic power which it induces may lead to rupture of the friable cardiac walls. In *valvular diseases*, when the hypertrophy is not compensatory or when dilatation is taking place, it is invaluable. In "*irritable heart*," *functional palpitation*, and *venous engorgements* (by lengthening the diastole it allows the veins more time to empty their contents into the auricles), it is much used. The tincture (♏x–xx 0.6–1.2 c.c.) may be employed hypodermically in cases of *sudden cardiac failure.* To sustain the action of a depressed heart in various acute diseases, particularly in *pneumonia*, it is often administered.

In *delirium tremens*, when the pulse is soft and compressible, digitalis is often given in large doses with benefit.

It is also used as a *physiologic antidote* to poisoning by *aconite, delphinine*, and *muscarine*, all of which arrest the heart in diastole.

To *contract the blood-vessels* it has been used in *acute inflammations* and in *hemorrhages*, and as it is supposed to stimulate involuntary muscle-fibers generally, it is given in *menorrhagia* and in *spermatorrhea.*

As a *cardiac tonic* and *diuretic* it is used in all forms of *cardiac* and of *renal dropsy*, in acute *suppression of urine*, and in *acute desquamative nephritis.*

What are the preparations of digitalis, and how are they administered?

Digitalis leaves are sometimes given in powder or pill;

dose, gr. j (0.06 gm.) t. i. d., gradually increased. The official preparations are—

EXTRACTUM DIGITALIS (*extract of digitalis*); dose, gr. ¼ (0.016 gm.), gradually increased.

FLUIDEXTRACTUM DIGITALIS (*fluid extract of digitalis*); dose, ♏j (0.06 c.c.).

TINCTURA DIGITALIS (*tincture of digitalis*); dose, ♏v–x (0.3–0.6 c.c.), gradually increased.

INFUSUM DIGITALIS (*infusion of digitalis*)—one of the best preparations; dose, ʒss-jv (2–15 c.c.).

Digitalin (not official); dose, gr. $\frac{1}{100}$–$\frac{1}{10}$ (0.006–0.06 gm.). There are several mixtures on the market under the name of "digitalin."

Occasionally after digitalis has been taken for some time continuously, especially when free diuresis has not taken place, its action becomes suddenly manifested by the pulse rapidly falling and the supervention of other effects characteristic of the drug. This is due to delay in the elimination of the medicine, and when it occurs, the remedy should be promptly discontinued.

GLANDULÆ SUPRARENALES SICCÆ.

What are dessicated suprarenal glands?

Dessicated suprarenal glands are the suprarenal glands of the sheep (*Ovis aries*) or ox (*Bos taurus*), freed from fat and cleaned, dried, and powdered. They contain a complex body, *adrenalin*, to which their medicinal activity is due, also *neurine, choline, lecithin, jecorin,* and *pyrocatechin.*

What is the physiologic action of adrenalin?

Locally applied it is not absorbed by the skin, but is slightly anesthetic and causes a marked anemia of mucous membranes by direct stimulation of the muscles in the walls of the arterioles. Applied to the conjunctiva it causes anemia, retraction of the eyelids, dilatation of the pupil (stimulates radial muscle-fibers), and reduces intra-ocular tension. It is partly destroyed in the stomach, so to obtain a full systemic effect it must be given hypodermically. Thus administered, it stops peristalsis, increases the saliva, tears, and bile, and has a digitalis effect on the circulation. Its action, however, is very rapid, manifesting itself quickly after the injection, and lasting only an hour or two. It slows the heart by stimulating the vagus center, increases the force of its systole by stimulating the cardiac muscle, and contracts the arterioles by combined action on the vasomotor center and the arterial muscles. Blood-pressure is raised. *Large doses* cause slowing and irregularity of the heart; *poisonous doses*, rapid weak heart, dilatation of the vessels, and collapse.

The drug is destroyed in the system, but through interference with the functions of the liver and pancreas causes an increase in the sugar of the blood and glycosuria. It also causes anemia and contraction of the uterus. Its local ischemic effects are not obtained from its systemic use.

What are the therapeutic uses of adrenalin or the suprarenal gland?

Locally, it is employed to reduce the hyperemia of a mucous membrane. In the nose it shrinks the tissues and permits a clearer view and the easier manipulation of instruments. It may be added to cocaine for use in the eye or nose and for small operations. For *epistaxis* it may be used as a spray or on a pledget of cotton. It gives great relief in *hay-fever*. It has been applied locally with prompt success in *hemorrhage* from *stomach, rectum, bladder*, and *uterus*, and in *postpartum hemorrhage*.

Systemically, it has been employed as a rapid heart stimulant, especially in collapse. It has also been used with slight success in Addison's disease.

What preparations are used?

Glandulæ Suprarenales Siccæ (*dessicated suprarenal glands*); dose, gr. j–v (0.06–0.3 gm.).

Suprarenal Extract (unofficial); dose, gr. j–v (0 06–0.3 gm.), in tablet or capsule.

Adrenalin Chlorid Solution (1 : 1000); dose, ♏j–v (0.06–0.3 c.c.). For hay-fever it is best diluted with equal parts of normal salt solution and used in spray.

CAFFEINA (CAFFEINE).

What is caffeine?

Caffeine (*theine*) is a feebly basic substance, obtained from the *dried leaves* of *Thea sinensis*, or tea plant (*Fam.* Ternstrœmiaceæ), or from the *dried seeds* of *Coffea arabica*, or coffee plant (*Fam.* Rubiaceæ). It also occurs in *guarana*, a paste prepared from the crushed or ground seeds of *Paulinia cupana* (*Fam.* Sapindaceæ), *kola*, *Paraguay tea*, etc.

What are its physiologic actions?

In *medicinal doses*, caffeine is a cerebral stimulant, causing nervous restlessness, increased mental activity, and wakefulness; it also increases the cardiac force, raises the arterial pressure, and acts as a decided diuretic. After *poisonous amounts* there is also confusion of thought, with delirium, muscular tremblings, cardiac oppression, quickened respiration, cold extremities, symptoms of collapse, rise of temperature, and, in animals, tonic and clonic convulsions, muscular weakness, general paresis, and death from paralysis of respiration. It slightly increases the power and rate of the *heart*, probably by a direct stimulant effect upon the heart-muscle, and raises arterial tension by stimulating the vasomotor center. It increases the power and activity of the voluntary muscles and lessens fatigue. It is *diuretic*, not only indirectly by increasing the blood-pressure, but also by some direct action on the secreting cells of the kidney itself. The *convulsions* are due to spinal stimulation and resemble those from strychnine. In moderate doses caffeine is said to be entirely destroyed in the system; in toxic doses it is partly destroyed and partly eliminated by the kidneys. Its effect on the elimination of waste-products is at present uncertain.

What are its medicinal uses?

As a *cardiac stimulant* (more rapid in action, but not so enduring or powerful as digitalis) it is used to meet the same indications as digitalis. In cases of *sudden heart failure* it may be used hypodermically combined with equal parts of sodium salicylate, which renders it more soluble in water. Its most important function, however, is as a respiratory and cerebral stimulant.

As a combined *cardiac stimulant* and *diuretic* it is very useful in the latter stages of *chronic Bright's disease* with weak heart.

As a *diuretic* in all *renal* and *cardiac dropsies* it is very serviceable. It is also employed as a *cerebral stimulant* in nervous and neuralgic *headaches*, and combined with other antagonists in opium poisoning. The prolonged use of tea and coffee tends to produce digestive troubles, nervousness, and mental depression.

From a single large dose wakefulness, tremors, and cardiac palpitation may result.

How is caffeine administered?

CAFFEINA (*caffeine*) may be given in pill, capsule, or solution; dose, gr. ss–ij (0.03–0.12).

CAFFEINA CITRATA (*citrated caffeine*), dose, gr. ss–iij (0.03–0.2 gm.).

CAFFEINA CITRATA EFFERVESCENS (*effervescent citrated caffeine*), dose, ʒj–iij (4.0–12 c.c.).

GUARANA (*guarana*) contains *tannic acid* as well as *caffeine* in considerable quantities, and is principally used in *neuralgia* and in *sick headache*. In Brazil, whence it comes, it is also used as an astringent in diarrheal affections; dose, ʒj (4 c.c.).

FLUIDEXTRACTUM GUARANÆ (*fluid extract of guarana*); dose, ♏x–xx (0.6–1.2 c.c.).

Theobromine, the active principle of cocoa, and *theophylline* (theocin), an alkaloid occurring in tea leaves and now made synthetically, are closely allied to caffeine, but are less stimulating to the cerebrum and more diuretic; dose of either, gr. x (0.6.).

ADONIDIN.

What is adonidin?

Adonidin (not official) is a glucosid, obtained from the root of *Adonis vernalis* (*Nat. Ord.* Ranunculaceæ), a plant of northern and central Europe.

What are its effects, uses, and modes of administration?

The *effects* of adonidin are almost identical with those of digitalis, but it is expensive and unstable and is little used.

It may be alternated with digitalis for a few weeks during a course of the latter; dose, gr. ⅛–½ (0.008–0.03) every three or four hours, in pill or capsule.

STROPHANTHUS.

What is strophanthus?

Strophanthus is the *ripe seed* of *S. Kombé (Fam.* Apocynaceæ), an African plant which has been used by the natives as an arrow-poison, and called by them Kombé or Ineé. It contains a crystalline glucosid, called *strophanthin*, an alkaloid *ineine*, and *kombic acid.*

What are its effects, uses, and modes of administration?

The effects of *strophanthus* are more rapid in action, but much more evanescent, than those of digitalis. It appears to act upon the muscles directly, and to have less effect than digitalis upon the nervous system.

In *moderate doses* it greatly increases the strength of the cardiac systole, and prolongs the diastole. It has little, if any, effect in contracting the arteries. In *large doses* it increases the contractility of all the striated muscles and finally arrests the heart in systole.

It proves diuretic by increasing the arterial tension, and has no cumulative effects. It is *used* as a substitute for digitalis in *cardiac diseases* when a temporary effect or a temporary change of medicine is desirable or when the vessels are contracted. From its *diuretic* action it has been successfully employed in various forms of *edema* depending on a weak circulation, and general *cardiac* and *renal dropsies.*

What are the preparations of strophanthus and their doses?

TINCTURA STROPHANTHI (*tincture of strophanthus*); dose, ♏v–xv (0.3–1 c.c.).

STROPHANTHINUM (*strophanthin*); dose, gr. $\frac{1}{200}$ (0.0003 gm.).

SPARTEINÆ SULPHAS (SPARTEINE SULPHATE).

Is sparteine a cardiac tonic?

Sparteine has been much used as a cardiac tonic, but extensive pharmacologic investigation shows it to have no such power—see Scoparius, p. 212.

CIMICIFUGA.

What is cimicifuga?

Cimicifuga is the *rhizome* and *roots* of *C. racemosa,* black snake-root or cohosh (*Fam.* Ranunculaceæ), a common indigenous plant. It contains a *volatile oil,* to which its virtues are probably due, a crystalline principle, resin, and tannin. It is astringent and bitter, and to a slight degree stimulates cardiac and involuntary muscle. It resembles ergot in its action on the uterus, and is also diuretic and expectorant. It has been *used* as a *cardiac tonic* in fatty heart, as a *diaphoretic* in *rheumatism,* as a *diuretic* in *dropsies,* as an expectorant in *chronic bronchitis,* and as an *antispasmodic* in *chorea,* in which disease it is sometimes of value, combined with tonics and laxatives, and as an *emmenagogue.*

FLUIDEXTRACTUM CIMICIFUGÆ (*fluid extract of cimicifuga*); dose, ʒss–j (2–4 c.c.).

TINCTURA CIMICIFUGÆ (*tincture of cimicifuga*); dose, ʒss–ij (2–8 c.c.).

EXTRACTUM CIMICIFUGÆ (*extract of cimicifuga*); dose, gr. iij–v (0.2–0.3 gm.).

CONVALLARIA.

What is convallaria?

Convallaria is the *rhizome* and *roots* of *C. majalis,* or lily of the valley (*Fam.* Liliaceæ), a European plant naturalized in this country.

It contains two glucosids, *convallamarin* and *convallarin,* to the former of which it probably owes its action on the heart, while the latter appears to cause nausea, diarrhea, and gastric pain.

The results of the investigations regarding the *physiologic action* of this plant are very contradictory, but it seems to slow the heart and increase the blood-pressure in small doses. In toxic doses the cardiac action becomes rapid, the arterial pressure gradually falls, and death occurs from heart-failure.

It is *used* in all cases of *cardiac weakness* whether accompanied by valvular lesion or not, as in *dilatation* or *fatty heart.* It is also used in *palpitation.*

FLUIDEXTRACTUM CONVALLARIÆ (*fluid extract of convallaria*); dose, ♏v–xv (0.3–1.0 c.c.).

CARDIAC SEDATIVES.

What are cardiac sedatives?

Cardiac sedatives are medicines which are used to diminish the force and frequency of the cardiac contractions when they are morbidly increased, and thus to depress the circulation.

Name the principal cardiac sedatives.

Antimonials, aconite and its alkaloid, veratrum viride and its alkaloids, veratrine, gelsemium, pulsatilla, arnica, the vegetable acids.

ANTIMONIUM (ANTIMONY).

What are the sources of antimony?

Antimony is a metallic element found native in the form of black antimonious sulphid.

Mention some of the tests for antimony.

Sulphuretted hydrogen in solution forms with solution of antimonial salts an orange-colored precipitate. The metal should also be reduced by Marsh's test, and chemically and microscopically distinguished from arsenic.

What are the general physiologic effects of antimonials?

When applied *locally* to the skin, the salts of antimony produce an eruption of papules, which become pustules, somewhat resembling the eruption of small-pox. After prolonged use, the fauces sometimes present a similar eruption. *Internally*, in *small doses*, they are diaphoretic. In somewhat *larger doses* they cause nausea, depressed circulation, weakness, and increase of the mucous and cutaneous secretions. In *larger doses* they prove emetic, with very weak pulse, great general depression, and relaxation of the muscular system. In *poisonous doses* they are gastro-intestinal irritants, causing emesis, catharsis with cramps in the extremities, and collapse, often resembling Asiatic cholera, and death from asthenia, sometimes preceded by tonic and clonic spasms.

Antimonials slow the *heart*, increase the duration of its diastole, and diminish the force of its systole by direct depression of the cardiac functions; they lower the blood-pressure partly by cardiac depression and partly by paralyzing the peripheral vasomotor system. The pulse finally becomes rapid and very feeble, the pressure sinks almost to *nil*, and the heart is arrested in diastole. They depress and paralyze the reflex, sensory, and, to a less extent, the motor functions of the *spinal cord*. The *temperature* is reduced by poisonous doses. The *emesis* is probably partly from local and partly from centric irritation.

When *given for a length of time*, they cause fatty degeneration of various viscera.

Antimony is *eliminated* by the mucous membranes, especially of the stomach, by the liver, kidneys, and skin.

What is the treatment of poisoning by antimony?

Wash out the stomach to remove any poison present; give tannic acid as a chemic antidote, and opium and stimulants to overcome the resulting depression.

What are the medicinal uses of antimonials?

They are used as *cardiac sedatives* in the early stages of *acute sthenic inflammations*, but are probably inferior to aconite or veratum viride for this purpose. They are very useful in the early stages of *acute bronchitis* and in *acute laryngitis*, from their combined sedative, diaphoretic, and expectorant qualities. As *diaphoretics* they are used in minute doses, frequently repeated, in fever mixtures, or combined with minute amounts of morphine or ipecac, which increase their action. The depression which they produce should always be remembered.

As *nauseants* and *emetics* they are rarely resorted to, because of the great depression which they produce.

Sulphurated antimony, or the old Kermes mineral, is sometimes used as a nauseant in membranous croup.

Locally, as a *counterirritant* it is rarely employed.

What are the antimonial preparations?

ANTIMONII ET POTASSII TARTRAS (*antimonium and potassium tartrate; tartar emetic; tartarated antimony*); dose, *as a sedative*, gr. $\frac{1}{4}$–$\frac{1}{2}$ (0.01–0.03 gm.), increased to gr. j–ij (0.06–0.12 gm.), as tolerance to its action is established;

as a *diaphoretic* and *expectorant*, gr. $\frac{1}{16}$–$\frac{1}{4}$ (0.004–0.016 gm.), in solution, repeated every two or three hours until the desired results are produced; as an *emetic*, gr. j–ij (0.06–0.13 gm.).

VINUM ANTIMONII (*wine of antimony*) contains 4 parts of tartar emetic in 1000 of the preparation (about gr. ij–℥j). Dose, as a *diaphoretic* and *expectorant*, ♏x–xxx (0.6–2.0 c.c.); as an emetic, ʒj–iv (4–15 c.c.). It is an ingredient of Mistura Glycyrrhizæ Composita (Brown Mixture).

SYRUPUS SCILLÆ COMPOSITUS (*compound syrup of squill; Coxe's hive syrup*) contains tartar emetic, 2 parts in 1000 of the preparation (about gr. j to the ounce). It is used in croup as an *emetic* and also as an *expectorant;* dose, ♏v–ʒj (0.3–4.0 c.c.).

ACONITUM (ACONITE).

What is aconite, and what is its chemic composition?

Aconite is the *tuberous root* of *Aconitum Napellus*, aconite, monkshood, or wolfsbane (*Fam.* Ranunculaceæ), a native of the mountains of Europe and Asia, and containing not less than 0.5 per cent. of aconitine. The active principle is an alkaloid called *aconitine.* Other alkoloids have been discovered in it, viz.: *aconine, isaconitine,* and *picraconitine.*

What are its physiologic effects?

Locally applied, aconite or aconitine benumbs the sensory nerves and causes a sensation of tingling. *Internally* in *small doses* it lessens the force and frequency of the cardiac contractions, diminishes the blood-pressure, causes tingling and numbness in the lips, tongue, and extremities, and produces a feeling of weakness. When *large doses* are taken, these symptoms are more marked, the pulse becomes irregular, weak, and slow (sometimes rapid), a tendency to fainting is manifested on assuming the erect posture or on any exertion, and the respirations are reduced in number. After *poisonous* doses these symptoms are much intensified; the countenance is anxious, a cold sweat covers the body, the pulse and respiration are very slow, weak, and irregular, general anesthesia is present, and collapse and death from syncope, sometimes preceded by convulsions, occur.

Aconite affects the *heart* by directly depressing the cardiac muscle and its contained motor ganglia, and stimulating the cardio-inhibitory apparatus. It slightly stimulates the vaso-motor center, later paralyzes it. It paralyzes the peripheral end organs of both *motor* and *sensory nerves*, the latter being first affected by it, and the nerve-trunks and centers being only involved as the poisoning deepens. The loss of reflex function is probably due to interference with conduction. It depresses and finally paralyzes the *respiratory center*. It is excreted mainly by the kidneys.

What is the treatment of poisoning by aconite?

Evacuate the contents of the stomach and wash it out by means of the stomach-pump; keep the sufferer perfectly quiet, with his head low; give cardiac stimulants, as alcohol, ether, or ammonia, and administer digitalis hypodermically.

What are the medicinal uses of aconite?

As a *cardiac sedative* aconite is of great value in the early stages of all *acute inflammations* and all *fevers*, in which the patient is vigorous and young and the pulse tense, full, bounding, and strong, and is only *contraindicated* when the heart is weak, when there is gastro-enteric inflammation, or where a typhoid condition is present. Thus it is used to diminish the circulation, arterial tension, and temperature, and to promote diaphoresis and diuresis in *acute coryza*, acute *broncho-pulmonary* catarrhs, *acute pleuritis* and *acute peritonitis*, in *acute meningitis*, either cerebral or spinal, and in the *essential fevers*, when not of the asthenic type. In *scarlet fever* and in *measles* (when the temperature is high) it is of great value, and is often used during the exacerbations of remittent malarial fevers.

In *cardiac hypertrophy* uncomplicated by valvular lesion, or even if the latter is present provided the hypertrophy be in excess of the requirements of the system, or an overacting heart, it is an invaluable medicine.

As a *local anesthetic* it has been advantageously given internally and applied externally in *neuralgia*, particularly of the face and head, and in *chronic muscular rheumatism* and *rheumatic neuralgia*. It is applied to the gums by dentists as an anodyne.

What are the preparations of aconite and their doses?

FLUIDEXTRACTUM ACONITI (*fluid extract of aconite*); dose, ♏ss–ij (0.03–0.12 c.c.).

TINCTURA ACONITI (*tincture of aconite*), now of 10 per cent. strength; but in the Pharmacopœia of 1890 it was of 35 per cent. strength; dose, ♏iij–x (0.2–0.7 c.c.), frequently combined with other medicines in fever mixtures.

In fevers and inflammations aconite is preferably given in small doses, repeated every few hours, and carefully watched until its effects on the pulse are obtained.

ACONITINA (*aconitine*) should be used internally with great caution, as it is a powerful poison. It has been given in *tic douloureux* with success, and, combined with digitalin, is sometimes employed to slow and steady a rapid heart in *pneumonia*. Dose, gr. $\frac{1}{610}$–$\frac{1}{200}$ (0.0001–0.0003 gm.).

VERATRUM.

What is veratrum, and what does it contain?

It is the *rhizome* and *roots* of *Veratrum viride*, American or swamp hellebore or Indian poke, or *Veratrum album*, white hellebore (*Fam.* Liliaceæ), a plant indigenous to swampy places in the eastern part of the United States. It contains two alkaloids, *veratrine* and *jervine*, to which its effects are due; also *rubijervine*, *pseudojervine*, resin, etc.

What is its physiologic action?

Both veratrine and jervine are related chemically and physiologically to aconitine, but in addition they markedly prolong the relaxation of cardiac and voluntary muscle, while increasing the power of the individual contraction. The heart is slowed by the prolonged diastole due to the muscle action and to stimulation of the vagus endings and center. Blood-pressure is lessened, and the respiratory center is at first stimulated. The sensory nerve-endings are first irritated and then anesthetized. Veratrine causes violent sneezing and cough from the irritation; it also induces vomiting and diarrhea. It is excreted by the urine.

In poisonous doses there are great irritation of the alimentary tract, burning in the mouth, salivation, vomiting, purging, slow, feeble pulse, muscular weakness, twitching, headache, and dilated pupils. Consciousness is not lost. Death results from paralysis of the heart or respiration. Poisoning rarely occurs, as an overdose causes emesis. Should dangerous symptoms arise, they should be treated with alcoholic and other stimulants, as in aconite-poisoning.

What are the medicinal uses of veratrum viride?

It is given as a *cardiac sedative* in the same *inflammatory* and *cardiac affections* in which aconite is administered, and its *contraindications* are identical with those of the latter drug, with the addition that in peritonitis it is not a safe remedy, because of its liability to cause vomiting. In *acute lobar pneumonia* it is considered much safer than aconite. It has been highly recommended in *puerperal eclampsia*, in doses of ♏x–xx (0.6–1.2 c.c.) of the tincture, given hypodermically, partly as an arterial sedative and partly as a reflex depressant.

What are its preparations and their doses?

FLUIDEXTRACTUM VERATRI (*fluid extract of veratrum viride*); dose, ♏j–iv (0.06–0.25 c.c.).

TINCTURA VERATRI (*tincture of veratrum viride*), formerly of 40 per cent. strength, now 10 per cent.; dose, ♏v–xx (0.3–1.3 c.c.).

Its effects are better obtained by giving small and increasing doses at intervals of an hour, being careful not to cause vomiting, and closely watching the pulse.

VERATRINA (VERATRINE).

What is veratrine?

Veratrine is a *mixture of alkaloids* obtained from the seed of *Asagræa officinalis* (*Nat. Ord.* Liliaceæ), a Mexican plant, known as *Sabadilla.*

How may its presence be detected?

When warmed in concentrated hydrochloric acid, a persistent dark-red color is produced, resembling a strong solution of potassium permanganate. This is *Trapp's test for veratrine.*

What are its actions and uses?

The mixture of alkaloids known commercially as "veratrine" consists of *cevadine, veratridine, cevadilline, sabadine,* and *sabadinine.* The action of these alkaloids is similar to that of veratrine and jervine (see Veratrum Viride), but they are so powerful and irritating that their use is entirely confined to external application in *neuralgia, rheumatism,* etc., as a counterirritant.

UNGUENTUM VERATRINÆ (*ointment of veratrine*) contains 4 per cent. of veratrine.

OLEATUM VERATRINÆ (*oleate of veratrine*) contains 2 per cent. of veratrine.

GELSEMIUM.

Is gelsemium used as a cardiac sedative?

It has been employed for this purpose in sthenic inflammation and fevers. Its medicinal uses have been described among the depressomotors.

ARNICA.

What is arnica?

It is the *flower-heads* of *Arnica montana,* leopard's bane (*Fam.* Compositæ). It contains *arnicin,* a *volatile oil, resins,* etc.

What are its effects and uses?

Locally applied arnica is a stimulant and often a decided irritant. *Internally* it slows the heart, but seems to raise the arterial pressure slightly. In large doses it is emetic and cathartic, causes great muscular weakness, a rapid pulse, and if the dose be excessive, collapse. It seems to be eliminated by the skin and kidneys. Arnica is not much *used* in this country except as an *external* application to sprains and contusions. When thus employed, its irritant qualities should be borne in mind. The preparations are:

TINCTURA ARNICÆ (*tincture of arnica*); dose, ♏x–xxx (0.6–2.0 c.c.).

THE VEGETABLE ACIDS.

Name the vegetable acids.

The official vegetable acids are acetic, citric, and tartaric acids.

What are their general effects and uses.

When applied to an abraded surface, they are irritant (tartaric acid being most, and citric the least, powerful). Given *internally* they increase the saliva and thus diminish thirst in fever. In *large doses* they are gastro-intestinal irritants and cardiac sedatives. They are probably oxidized in the blood and converted into carbonic acid, which abstracts part of the base of the alkaline phosphates and converts them into acid phosphates, thus increasing the acidity of the urine. When taken in large quantities they cause flatulence, tormina, and diarrhea. Their long-continued use disorders the digestion, and causes emaciation and an anemic condition. They are eliminated, chiefly as carbonates, by the intestines and kidneys.

The vegetable acids are *used* as *refrigerants* and perhaps cardiac sedatives in *fevers* (citric acid), as *antiscorbutic agents* (citric or acetic acid), in *acute rheumatism* (lemon-juice is, however, inferior to the alkaline treatment), and as *diuretic* to increase the amount of urine and render it acid in reaction (tartaric or citric acid).

They are also used as *chemic antidotes* to poisoning by the alkalis.

Glacial acetic acid is used as a *caustic* to remove corns and warts, and as an inhalant to irritate the nasal mucous membrane and reflexly stimulate heart and respiration in fainting. A 2 per cent. solution of acetic acid is much used as a uterine injection in postpartum hemorrhage and as a vaginal injection in leukorrhea. The acid is added to liniments and cooling lotions. The preparations are:

ACIDUM ACETICUM GLACIALE (*glacial acetic acid*) (nearly or quite absolute acetic acid) and ACIDUM ACETICUM (*acetic acid*) (containing 36 per cent. by weight of absolute acetic acid) are used externally as caustics.

ACIDUM TRICHLORACETICUM (*trichloracetic acid*), obtained by the oxidation of hydrated chloral with nitric acid, occurs in crystals which are soluble in water and alcohol. It is used externally as a caustic.

ACIDUM ACETICUM DILUTUM (*diluted acetic acid*) may be used internally; dose, ʒj–ij (4–8 c.c.) diluted. It is a pure form of vinegar.

Acidum Citricum (*citric acid*), ℥j (30 c.c.) to water Oj (480 c.c.), may be used as a substitute for lemonade.

Syrupus Acidi Citrici (*syrup of citric acid*) contains 10 parts of the acid in 1000 of the preparation, and is used in making "solution of citrate of magnesia."

Limonis Succus (*lemon-juice*), Oleum Limonis (*oil of lemon*), and Tinctura Limonis Corticis (*tincture of lemon peel*) are also official.

Acidum Tartaricum (*tartaric acid*) is rarely used in medicine, except as an ingredient of Seidlitz powders.

ON THE SEXUAL ORGANS.

APHRODISIACS.

What are aphrodisiacs?

Aphrodisiacs are medicines used to excite the functions of the genital organs when they are morbidly depressed.

What medicines are used for this purpose?

When the *nutritive functions are not properly performed*, the tonics or alteratives, especially phosphorus, zinc phosphid, the phosphates and hypophosphites, the salts of iron, gold, or arsenic, and cod-liver oil are used. When there is *an absence of sexual desire*, small doses of opium, very minute amounts of alcohol, cannabis indica, musk, or small doses of camphor may be useful by stimulating the cerebral centers. If impotence be due to *want of erectile power*, the tonics and alteratives are of use, as are also agents acting on the genital center in the lumbar portion of the spinal cord and agents which either determine a flow of blood to the part by increasing the general or local circulation or which, by contracting the veins, aid in producing and maintaining erection. Thus, nux vomica or its alkaloid, the cardiac stimulants, hamamelis, ergot, cantharides, and myrrh are useful in this condition. Good hygiene, cold baths, proper food, sea air and bathing, electricity, and moral means are important. The above medicines have either been considered already or will be found in their appropriate places.

ANAPHRODISIACS.

What are anaphrodisiacs?

Anaphrodisiacs are medicines which are used to depress the sexual functions when they are morbidly excited

What medicines are employed for this purpose?

Morbid excitation of the sexual organs is treated by medicines which depress the functions of the body generally, as nauseants and purgatives, or those which, by depressing the brain or spinal cord, will prove sedative to centers governing these organs: thus full doses of opium or of camphor will depress the cerebral center, while potassium or ammonium bromid (very useful), monobromated camphor, iodin and the iodids, potassium nitrate, ammonium chlorid, belladonna, tobacco, and conium act more especially on the spinal center and nerves. Medicines diminishing the circulation of the parts will also prove advantageous, as the cardiac sedatives or full doses of digitalis and the bromids. Cocaine locally applied acts by contracting the vessels and diminishing the irritability of the sensory nerves.

Other agents used for this purpose are the local use of cold, general blood-letting, a low diet, avoidance of stimulation, and the withdrawal of blood to other parts of the body, as by hard mental work or exercise with the upper extremities.

SABAL.

What is sabal?

Sabal (*saw palmetto*) is the partially dried ripe fruit of *Serenoa serrulata* (*Fam.* Palmæ). It contains resin, fixed and volatile oils, and a trace of an alkaloid. It is said to have nutritive and aphrodisiac properties; dose, gr. xv (1 gm.).

OXYTOCICS.

What are oxytocics?

Oxytocics are medicines which are employed to increase the power of a contracting uterus, thus aiding in the expulsion of its contents.

Name the medicines belonging to this order.

Ergot; hydrastis; hydrastinine hydrochloride; gossypii radicis cortex; and quinine.

ERGOTA (ERGOT).

What is ergot?

Ergot is the *sclerotium* of *Claviceps purpurea* (*Fam.* Hypocreaceæ), replacing the grain of *Secale sereale* (*Fam.* Gramineæ), or, in other words, it is a fungus growing from the diseased ovary of rye. "When more than a year old it is unfit for use."

What does it contain?

Its essential constituents are *cornutin*, *ergotinic acid*, and *sphacelotoxin* (sphacelic acid). It also contains about 30 per cent. of fixed oil. *Ergochrysin* and *chrysotoxin* are new products recently described by Jacoby, and it is thought may represent the true active principles of the drug.

What are its physiologic effects?

The effects of ergot are chiefly manifested on the uterus of the pregnant female and on the circulation. In the *non-pregnant, small doses* produce no perceptible effect; *moderate doses* slow and strengthen the heart by stimulating the vagi and the heart muscle, and enormously increase the blood-pressure by stimulating the vasomotor centers and the muscles in the vessel-walls. *Large doses* cause nausea and vomiting, increased peristalsis, and purging. *Toxic doses* depress the heart by acting directly on its muscle or contained ganglia, and lower the blood-pressure, partly by its action on the heart and partly from depression of the vasomotor centers.

When *poisonous doses are given to animals* there are salivation, vomiting, and sometimes diarrhea, rapid pulse and respiration, dilated pupil, trembling, great thirst, prostration, paraplegia, convulsions, and death. The nervous symptoms appear to be due to action on the nerve-centers.

Ergot possesses the property of causing contraction of all non-striated muscular fibers: thus it contracts the arterioles, increases intestinal peristalsis, and increases the power as well as the duration of the uterine contractions during labor, but does not always originate them during pregnancy or at other times, except immediately prior to and after parturition. The uterine contraction is continuous and not intermittent.

What is ergotism?

When ergot is used continuously in large amounts as an article of diet it produces a condition of chronic poisoning which manifests itself either by gangrene (usually dry, but occasionally moist and attended with septicemia) or by tetanic spasms.

What are the medicinal uses of ergot?

Ergot is used *as an oxytocic* in *small doses* in *uterine inertia* during the second stage of labor, when there is no resistance either on the part of the bony canal or the soft parts of the mother. When thus administered, it energizes the uterine contractions, but if given in large doses it renders them tetanic and continuous, thus greatly increasing the danger both to the mother and child.

To prevent *postpartum hemorrhage* by contracting the uterus, and thus compressing the uterine sinuses, it is invaluable. To affect the uterus it takes fifteen to thirty minutes if given by mouth, and five to ten minutes when given hypodermically. It is valuable in subinvolution.

It has been used to *induce premature labor*, but is at best an uncertain remedy for this purpose. To arrest hemorrhage in cases of *threatened abortion* ergot is worse than useless unless the uterus is emptied. In these cases, by contracting the cervix, it imprisons the ovum, and thus, by preventing its escape, keeps the uterus distended. If given at all in these cases, its administration should be conjoined with the application of vaginal tampons. It is also given to aid the expulsion of *uterine polypi*.

As a hemostatic, it is used in all *hemorrhages* where surgical means of arrest cannot be employed, but may increase the bleeding by raising the blood-pressure. In *menorrhagia*, *epistaxis*, *hemorrhage from the gums*, and in *bronchopulmonary*, *intestinal*, or *renal hemorrhage* it is said to be efficient. In *hema-*

temesis it is not so serviceable. In *purpura* it acts benficially. From its influence in contracting blood-vessels it has been used in the early stages of *pneumonia* and other *inflammatory affections*, in *spinal congestions*, in *cerebrospinal meningitis*, and for the cure of *internal aneurysms*. It has been injected hypodermically near the seat of disease for the cure of *varices*, *hemorrhoids*, and *impotence* due to dilatation of the dorsal vein of the penis. In *glycosuria* and in *polyuria* it does good, as also in *malaria*, and, from its influence on unstriped muscular fibers generally, it is useful in *relaxation of the sphincters*, *diarrhea*, *dysentery*, *spermatorrhea*, *uterine subinvolution*, and to diminish the size of *subperitoneal uterine fibroids*.

What are the preparations of ergot and their doses?

EXTRACTUM ERGOTÆ (*extract of ergot*) is five times as strong as the fluid extract; dose, gr. v–xv (0.3–1.0 gm.). It may be used hypodermically, dissolved in water and filtered.

FLUIDEXTRACTUM ERGOTÆ (*fluid extract of ergot*); dose, ♏v–xxx (0.3–2 c.c.), or at the end of labor ʒj–ij (4–8 c.c.).

VINUM ERGOTÆ (*wine of ergot*) represents 20 per cent. of ergot; dose, ʒj–iv (4–15 c.c.).

HYDRASTIS.

What is hydrastis?

Hydrastis is the *rhizome and roots* of *H. canadensis*, yellow root or golden seal (*Fam.* Ranunculaceæ). It has been already considered under the Bitter Tonics (*q. v.*).

HYDRASTININÆ HYDROCHLORIDUM (HYDRASTININE HYDROCHLORIDE).

What is this substance?

It is the hydrochloride of an artificial alkaloid produced by the oxidation of hydrastine, and has been found to produce uterine contractions, stimulating also the muscular fibers of the heart, arterioles, and intestines. It probably stimulates the voluntary muscles, but in a lesser degree.

In fatal doses it depresses powerfully the entire motor nervous tract and causes death by respiratory failure.

It has been used with success in menorrhagia and metrorrhagia and other uterine hemorrhages, but is less useful than ergot in postpartum hemorrhage or subinvolution. Dose, gr. ¼–j (0.016–0.06 gm.).

STYPTICIN.

What is stypticin?

It is cotarnine hydrochlorid, a substance closely related to hydrastinine. It is very efficient in uterine hemorrhage, especially in menorrhagia and fibroids. Dose, gr. ⅛ (0.008 gm.) several times a day.

GOSSYPII CORTEX (COTTON-ROOT BARK).

What is gossypii cortex?

It is the *bark of the root* of *Gossypium herbaceum* or of other cultivated species of Gossypium (*Fam.* Malvaceæ).

Given to animals, it first slows and then quickens the cardiac action, which is always enfeebled by first stimulating and then paralyzing the cardioinhibitory apparatus and depressing the cardiomotor ganglia. It stimulates and then depresses the vasomotor centers, causing a rise, but subsequently a fall, in the blood-pressure. It stimulates non-striated muscular fibers, and appears to excite rhythmic contractions of the gravid uterus and to increase their power when present. It depresses the reflex centers of the cord, and causes death by respiratory paralysis, generally preceded by convulsions, which are not of cerebral origin.

It has been *recommended* as a substitute for ergot in *uterine inertia, postpartum hemorrhage,* and to aid the expulsion of *uterine myomata.* It has been used in *chronic metritis,* and, although not so efficient as ergot, is useful in *menorrhagia.*

The fresh drug is probably the most efficient, according to reports from the South.

QUININA (QUININE).

Is quinine oxytocic?

Although quinine is used for this purpose, it probably possesses no action on the uterus *per se,* though it may strengthen the muscular contractions in uterine inertia.

UTERINE SEDATIVES.

What are uterine sedatives?

They are medicines which are employed to depress the uterine muscular or nervous apparatus and restrain violent, irregular, or untimely uterine contractions.

What medicines are used for this purpose, and when are they employed?

They are principally useful during pregnancy, to prevent abortion which is threatening but not inevitable. They are also of service in arresting the irregular uterine contractions which sometimes occur prior to labor, and are called "false labor pains." For the former purpose opium, cannabis indica, and the motor depressants, as chloral, the bromids, tartar emetic, and viburnum, especially the first- and last-named remedies, are used, while for the latter opium and chloral are employed. To moderate too-violent contractions during labor ether is the best remedy. Of these medicines, all have been described except

VIBURNUM PRUNIFOLIUM.

What is viburnum prunifolium?

It is the *bark* of the root of *V. prunifolium*, sloe or black haw, or of *V. Lentago* (*Fam.* Caprifoliaceæ), a small indigenous tree. It *contains valerianic acid*, a bitter principle (*viburnin*), resin, tannin, etc. Its *physiologic effects* are not understood. It appears to diminish reflex irritability and to have a sedative effect on involuntary muscular fiber and possibly lowers blood-pressure. Toxic effects are seen only after enormous doses have been administered, and consist of headache, dryness of the mouth and throat, and disordered vision.

It has been employed as a *uterine sedative* in *habitual* and in *threatened abortion*, in congestive and neuralgic *dysmenorrhea*, in *menorrhagias*, in *nervous disturbances occurring at the climacteric* period, and in *false labor-pains* and *after-pains*. It has also been used in *colicky diarrhea and dysentery*, and is even recommended for *cramps occurring in the voluntary muscles*.

FLUIDEXTRACTUM VIBURNI PRUNIFOLII (*fluid extract of*

viburnum prunifolium); dose, ʒss–ij (2–8 c.c.) in elixir of orange.

VIBURNUM OPULUS.

What is viburnum opulus?

It is the bark of *V. opulus*, cramp bark (*Fam.* Caprifoliaceæ), a small indigenous tree. It is similar in composition and uses to viburnum prunifolium, but has less effect on the uterus, and more in relieving colic and cramps.

FLUIDEXTRACTUM VIBURNI OPULI (*fluid extract of viburnum opulus*); dose, ʒss–ij (2–8 c.c.).

EMMENAGOGUES.

What are emmenagogues?

Emmenagogues are medicines employed to increase or reëstablish the menstrual flow when it is scanty or suppressed from other causes than pregnancy or the climacteric period.

When the catamenia are arrested from pregnancy, medicines used to bring them on cannot but be injurious to the woman, as the doses necessary are sufficient to cause poisoning, one of the symptoms of which may be uterine hemorrhage. This is especially true of cantharides and of the volatile oils.

What medicines are used as emmenagogues?

When amenorrhea depends upon anemia or chlorosis, the best emmenagogues are iron (combined with aloes or myrrh), arsenic, or manganese. When local anemia or an atonic condition of the uterus is present, aloes (*q. v.*) is very useful. If, on the other hand, pelvic plethora exists with constipation and a scanty flow often of a thick black discharge accompanied with pelvic pain and fulness, the saline cathartics are employed.

In suppression of the menses from cold, aloes and potassium permanganate are usually more successful. In amenorrhea due to an atonic condition of the uterus the more stimulating emmenagogues are given, generally with aloetic purgatives.

STIMULATING EMMENAGOGUES.

Name the stimulating emmenagogues.

Savine, tansy, apiol, cantharides, and guaiac.

SABINA (SAVINE).

What is savine?

Savine is the *tops* of *Juniperus Sabina* (*Fam.* Coniferæ), a small evergreen shrub of southern Europe. It contains a *volatile oil* and a resin. When applied *locally*, savine is irritant. In *medicinal doses* it increases the circulation, is a gastric, uterine, and renal irritant, and proves diuretic. In overdoses it is a gastro-intestinal irritant, with great depression, unconsciousness, convulsions, hemorrhages from the uterus and kidneys, suppression of urine, and, in pregnant females, abortion. Death occurs from collapse. Savine is *used* in relaxed states of the uterus and uterine vessels, and has proved successful in the treatment both of *amenorrhea* and *menorrhagia* when due to atonic condition of this organ. It is a dangerous drug.

FLUIDEXTRACTUM SABINÆ (*fluid extract of savine*); dose, ♏v–x (0.3–0.6 c.c.).

OLEUM SABINÆ (*oil of savine*), the best preparation for internal use; dose, ♏j–v (0.06–0.3 c.c.). In capsules or emulsion every three or four hours.

TANACETUM (TANSY).

What is tansy?

Tansy (not official) is the *leaves* and *tops* of *Tanacetun vulgare* (*Fam.* Compositæ). It contains a volatile oil and a bitter principle (*tanacetin*). It is a gastro-intestinal irritant and diuretic, and in large doses causes death from respiratory paralysis, preceded by epileptiform convulsions of cerebral origin and unconsciousness. It is used as a stimulating emmenagogue, but is a very dangerous remedy. The minimum fatal quantity is unknown. Dose, gr. x–xxv (0.6–1.5 gm.), in infusion; of the oil, ♏j (0.06 c.c.) may be given. It is much used in domestic practice.

APIOL.

What is apiol?

Apiol (not official), or parsley-camphor, is obtained from the volatile oil of the root of *Petroselinum sativum* (*Fam.* Umbelliferæ). It is very efficacious as a stimulating emmenagogue in *functional* and *anemic amenorrhea* and in *neuralgic dysmenorrhea*, but is contraindicated in any condition of plethora. Dose, ♏iij–x (0.2–0.6 c.c.) in gelatin capsules given morning and evening for four or five days before the expected menstrual period.

The French capsules or pearls usually contain gr. iv. (0.25 gm.) of apiol.

CANTHARIDES—GUAIAC.

What are these substances?

Cantharides will be considered under Irritants. The tincture is used as a stimulating emmenagogue; dose, ♏iij–v (0.2–0.3 c.c.), t. i. d., great care being taken to avoid strangury.

Guaiac has been considered with the Alteratives.

ON THE ALIMENTARY CANAL.

EMETICS.

What are emetics, and how do they act?

Emetics are medicines which are given to induce vomiting. They may act either by directly irritating the stomach, thus causing expulsion of its contents in a reflex manner, when they are called *local emetics*, or by acting, after absorption, on the center of the medulla which governs emesis, when they are called *systemic emetics*. It does not always follow that a remedy is a systemic emetic because it causes vomiting when given hypodermically or per rectum, for it may be eliminated by, and produce irritation of, the gastric mucous membrane, thus exciting reflex vomiting.

For what purposes are emetics used?

Emetics are used—(1) To unload the stomach; (2) to depress the circulatory system by inducing nausea (as in the early stages of bronchitis or of tonsillitis, in which emetics, frequently repeated in small doses, will sometimes arrest the inflammation); (3) to relax the muscular system and relieve spasm (as in spasmodic croup); (4) to promote secretion and excretion; (5) to expel foreign bodies or secretions from the air-passages; (6) as revulsives.

What are the contraindications to their employment?

They should never be employed in cases of cerebral or gastric inflammation, and should be used cautiously, if at all, in the later stages of pregnancy, in hernia, or where great depression exists, as in the later stages of capillary bronchitis or of croup.

Name the medicines employed as emetics?

The vegetable emetics are ipecac, apomorphine, and mustard. The *mineral emetics* are zinc sulphate, copper sulphate, alum, turpeth mineral, and tartar emetic.

IPECACUANHA (IPECAC).

What is ipecac, and what chemic principles does it contain?

Ipecac is the *root* of *Cephaëlis Ipecacuanha*, Rio, Brazilian or Para ipecac, or of *C. acuminata*, Carthagena ipecac (*Fam.* Rubiaceæ), yielding not less than 2 per cent. of ipecac alkaloids. They are plants of Brazil. Its effects depend upon an alkaloid, *emetine;* it also contains cephaeline, psychotrine, and ipecacuanhic acid.

What are its physiologic actions?

Locally applied, ipecac is an irritant, either to the skin or mucous membranes. Given *internally* in *small doses*, repeated, it increases the perspiration, saliva, bile, the secretions from the bronchopulmonary and gastro-intestinal mucous membranes, and causes nausea. In sufficient amounts it greatly augments the secretions and induces vomiting, without much nausea or depression, no matter how exhibited, emesis being more rapid when it is taken by the mouth. In minute doses it is sedative to the stomach.

Toxic doses in animals depress the *respiration* and paralyze the *heart* directly. Postmortem examination shows the mucous membranes of the stomach, intestines, and lungs to be intensely congested. Sometimes, however, the lungs are almost exsanguine.

What are the medicinal uses of ipecac?

Ipecac is employed as an *emetic*, and is the safest remedy

which can be given for this purpose, especially to children. It is particularly of service when it is desired to evacuate the contents of an overloaded stomach without producing much depression, as an adjunct to other remedies in *croup* and in the earlier stages of *capillary bronchitis.* In narcotic poisoning it is not so efficient as the mineral emetics.

As an *expectorant* it is added to cough medicines in the dry stage of bronchitis. As a *cholagogue* it is a valuable addition to purgative pills. As a *hemostatic* it is highly recommended in *hemoptysis* and *postpartum hemorrhage.*

In the treatment of *dysentery,* especially when epidemic, it is of great service, given in large dose (gr. xx–ʒij (1.2–8.0 gm.), every few hours). When thus administered, a tolerance is soon established, and no nausea or vomiting is produced. It is also useful in various kinds of *diarrhea,* especially of choleriform and tuberculous diarrhea. *Reflex vomiting,* as the vomiting of pregnancy, has sometimes been arrested by minute doses of the wine of ipecac.

What are the preparations of ipecac and their doses?

Ipecac may be given in powder; dose, as an *emetic,* gr. x–xx (0.6–1.2 gm.); as a *nauseant,* gr. ss–ij (0.03–0.12 gm.); as an *expectorant* and *diaphoretic,* gr. $\frac{1}{4}$–$\frac{1}{2}$ (0.016–0.03 gm.); as a *stomachic tonic* and *hepatic stimulant,* gr. $\frac{1}{12}$–$\frac{1}{8}$ (0.005–0.008 gm.).

FLUIDEXTRACTUM IPECACUANHÆ (*fluid extract of ipecac*); dose, as an emetic, ♏xx–xxx (1.2–2.0 c.c.), repeated until vomiting occurs.

VINUM IPECACUANHÆ (*wine of ipecac*) contains 10 per cent. of the fluid extract; dose, as emetic, ʒj–iv (4–16 c.c.).

SYRUPUS IPECACUANHÆ (*syrup of ipecac*) contains 7 per cent. of the fluid extract; as an emetic, ʒj–ij (4–8 c.c.) may be given to a child, or as an expectorant, ♏v–x (0.3–0.6 c.c.).

Powder of ipecac and opium (Dover's powder) and *tincture of ipecac and opium* have been considered under Opium.

APOMORPHINÆ HYDROCHLORIDUM (APOMORPHINE HYDROCHLORIDE).

What is apomorphine hydrochloride?

It is the *hydrochloride* of an *artificial alkaloid* obtained from morphine or codeine.

What are its physiologic actions?

Given to warm-blooded animals in *small doses* it causes vomiting; after *large doses* there is salivation, violent vomiting, and muscular tremors; *toxic doses* induce great restlessness, paresis, convulsions, hurried respiration, and death from asphyxia, without the occurrence of emesis.

It is a systemic emetic, probably in medicinal doses stimulating the reflex center for *vomiting*, but in large doses depressing and paralyzing it. No matter how administered, emesis takes place promptly, with but little nausea and rarely accompanied by much depression. Large doses appear to stimulate and finally paralyze the respiratory center. It increases the *pulse-rate* by stimulating the accelerator fibers (?), and in large doses, by stimulating the vasomotor center, it raises the arterial pressure. In toxic doses it depresses the cardiac muscle and thus reduces the blood-pressure. In large doses it is at first a *cerebral* stimulant, but later depresses and paralyzes the brain. The cause of the convulsion is not understood. It is a *muscle* poison.

What are the uses and doses of apomorphine hydrochloride?

It may be employed *as an emetic* whenever prompt evacuation of the stomach is required, and may be administered either hypodermically or by the mouth. In *narcotic poisoning* it is highly recommended.

As an expectorant in the early stages of *acute bronchitis* or in *chronic bronchitis* without much expectoration, it is very serviceable, and can be advantageously employed in *capillary bronchitis* of children, both as an expectorant and emetic. The adult dose as an *emetic* is gr. $\frac{1}{16}$ (0.004 gm.) hypodermically, or gr. $\frac{1}{10}$–$\frac{1}{8}$ (0.005–0.008 gm.) by the mouth. As an *expectorant* smaller doses are required. It has recently been employed as a hypnotic, but its other effects are so disagreeable that it is no longer so used.

SINAPIS (MUSTARD).

What is mustard, and how is it used as an emetic?

Mustard is the *seed* of *Brassica nigra* and of *Sinapis alba* (*Fam.* Cruciferæ). Mustard flour is irritant to the mucous membranes as well as to the skin, and is a prompt and efficient local emetic, especially useful when torpor of the stomach is present. It will be more fully considered hereafter. Dose, as an emetic, from a teaspoonful to a tablespoonful (4–16 c.c.) of the flour, in a glass of tepid water, repeated, if necessary, in fifteen or twenty minutes.

What mineral emetics are employed?

ZINCI SULPHAS (*zinc sulphate*) is a prompt and efficient local emetic. Dose, gr. x–xx (0.6–1.2 gm.), or even gr. xxx (2 gm.) in narcotic poisoning.

CUPRI SULPHAS (*copper sulphate*) is a prompt local emetic, but more irritating than the zinc salt. Dose, gr. iij–v (0.2–0.3 gm.) or even gr. x (0.6 gm.) in narcotic poisoning. It is the best emetic in poisoning by phosphorus, (*q. v.*).

ALUMEN (*alum*) is also a local emetic of value, especially useful in *membranous croup*, and useful also in *capillary bronchitis;* dose, a teaspoonful (4 c.c.) of the powdered drug in molasses, or, better, in syrup of ipecac.

HYDRARGYRI SUBSULPHAS FLAVUS (not official) (*yellow mercurial subsulphate; Turpeth mineral*), used as an emetic in *croup;* dose, gr. j–v (0.06–0.3 gm.) repeated every ten or fifteen minutes until free vomiting occurs.

ANTIMONII ET POTASSII TARTRAS (*antimonium and potassium tartrate; tartar emetic*) is rarely used as an emetic because of the great depression which it induces; dose, gr. j–ij (0.06–0.13 gm.).

Of these substances the first three will be found under the head of astringents, while the last two have already been considered.

GASTRIC SEDATIVES.

What are gastric sedatives?

They are medicines employed to diminish gastric irritability and thus allay nausea and vomiting.

What medicines are used for this purpose?

When vomiting is due to *acute irritation*, as from an overloaded stomach, the ingestion of acrid substances, or cholera morbus, it is best treated, after the contents have been evacuated, by minute doses of calomel (gr. $\frac{1}{10}$—0.005 gm.) with sodium bicarbonate (gr. j—0.06 gm.); pellets of ice dissolved in the mouth; lime-water and rest. A small dose of brandy or champagne will sometimes "settle the stomach." If *irritability persists*, small doses of morphine or of diluted hydrocyanic acid or creosote, or bismuth and sodium bicarbonate, answer better. When due to the formation of gases from *fermentation*, creosote, resorcin, carbolic acid, thymol, sulphurous acid, the sulphites, or charcoal are given.

Ether-vomiting is best met with teaspoonful (4 c.c.) doses of very hot water given every ten or fifteen minutes. *Reflex vomiting*, as of sea-sickness or of pregnancy, usually requires a medicine which will depress the center in the medulla presiding over the act, as opium, the bromids, or diluted hydrocyanic acid. Among other remedies used for the latter variety of vomiting may be mentioned tincture of nux vomica (gtt. ¼-j—0.015-0.06 c.c.); cerium oxalate (gr. ¼-v—0.015-0.3 gm.); wine of ipecac (gtt. ¼-ij—0.015-0.12 c.c.), and Fowler's solution (♏ ¼-j—0.015-0.06 c.c.). Counterirritation over the epigastrium often aids the action of gastric sedatives. The above remedies have already been noticed or will be discussed in their appropriate places.

CARMINATIVES.

What are carminatives?

Carminatives are medicines employed to aid the expulsion of gases from the stomach and intestines.

What medicines are used as carminatives?

The *aromatics*, which owe their virtues principally to the volatile oil which they contain, are especially used for this purpose. Other drugs containing volatile oils, as asafetida, eucalyptus, etc., are also carminative; and ether is sometimes employed for the same object.

What are the general effects of the aromatics?

Locally they are irritant and rubefacient. The oils are also local anesthetics. *Internally* in *medicinal doses* they are gastric and intestinal stimulants, increasing peristalsis and temporarily increasing to a slight extent the force and frequency of the pulse. In *larger doses* they stimulate the brain and cause a species of intoxication. In *very large doses* they are irritant and narcotic poisons.

What are their medicinal uses?

The aromatics are used internally as *carminatives;* to prevent the *griping* of purgatives; to *correct* the unpleasant *taste* or *smell* of other medicines, and as *gastric stimulants.*

Locally they are employed as *rubefacients, antiseptics,* and *anodynes.* They should *never be used* when inflammation of the stomach or bowels is present, but in diarrhea due to relaxation they are often of service.

Name the aromatics, their chemic constituents, preparations, and doses.

CAPSICUM, or red pepper, is the *fruit* of *C. fastigiatum* (*Fam.* Solanaceæ). It contains a *resin,* a *fixed* and a *volatile oil.* It is *used* as a *condiment,* as a *gastric stimulant,* particularly in the case of drunkards, as an addendum to tonic pills, as a *carminative* in cases of feeble digestion, as a *gargle* in tonsillitis, and externally as a *rubefacient.*

FLUIDEXTRACTUM CAPSICI (*fluid extract of capsicum*); dose, ♏v–x (0.3–0.6 c.c.).

TINCTURA CAPSICI (*tincture of capsicum*); dose, ♏v–ʒj (0.3–4.0 c.c.).

OLEORESINA CAPSICI (*oleoresin of capsicum*); dose, gr. ss–j (0.03–0.06 gm.).

EMPLASTRUM CAPSICI (*plaster of capsicum*), for external use.

PIPER (*pepper*) is the *unripe fruit* of *Piper nigrum* (*Nat. Ord.* Piperaceæ). It contains a *volatile oil,* an acrid *resin,* and a neutral principle, *piperin,* which increases the respiration and circulation, dilates the pupil, and finally paralyzes the heart in systole. It has been used as an *antiperiodic.* Pepper is used as a *condiment* and sometimes as a *stomachic stimulant,* combined with other medicines, in atonic dyspepsia, and as a *carminative.*

Oleoresina Piperis (*oleoresin of pepper*); dose, gr. ss–ij (0.03–0.13 gm.).

Piperinum (*piperin*); dose, gr. j–v (0.06–0.3 gm.).

Cinnamomum Saigonicum (*Saigon cinnamon*), *the bark* of an undetermined species of cinnamomum (*Fam.* Lauraceæ) (which comes from Cochin-China); and **Cinnamomum Zeylanicum** (*Ceylon cinnamon*), *the inner bark of the shoots of Cinnamomum Zeylanicum* (*Fam.* Lauraceæ), are recognized by the Pharmacopeia. They contain *volatile oil, tannic acid,* etc., are slightly astringent, and are used as *carminatives, flavoring ingredients,* and *vehicles.*

Tinctura Cinnamomi (*tincture of cinnamon*) represents 20 per cent. of Saigon cinnamon; dose, ʒj–ij (4–8 c.c.).

Aqua Cinnamomi (*cinnamon water*) contains 0.2 per cent. of the oil of cinnamon, and is used as a vehicle.

Oleum Cinnamomi (*oil of cinnamon*) is a volatile oil distilled from Cassia cinnamon, and yields not less than 75 per cent. by volume of cinnamic aldehyde; dose, ♏j–iij (0.06–0.18 c.c.).

Cinnaldehydum (*cinnamic aldehyde*) is often employed instead of the oil of cinnamon; dose, ♏j–ij (0.06–0.12).

Spiritus Cinnamomi (*spirit of cinnamon*) contains 10 per cent. of the oil; dose, ♏x–xxx (0.6–2.0 c.c.).

Pulvis Aromaticus (*aromatic powder*) contains 35 per cent. of Saigon cinnamon; dose, gr. v–xxx (0.3–2.0 gm.).

Myristica (*nutmeg*); **Macis** (*mace*).—These are parts of the *fruit* of *Myristica fragrans* (*Fam.* Myristicaceæ), the *arillode of the seed* being mace, and *the kernel,* nutmegs. Mace is not official. Both contain volatile oils. They are aromatic stimulants, carminatives, and in large doses narcotics. The oil of mace is used as a stimulant to the growth of the hair.

Oleum Myristicæ (*oil of nutmeg*); dose, ♏j–v (0.06–0.3 c.c.).

Caryophyllus (*cloves*) is the *dried flower buds* of *Eugenia aromatica* (*Fam.* Myrtaceæ). They contain *volatile oil, tan-*

nic acid, caryophyllin, and *eugenol.* They are gastric stimulants and carminatives, but are principally employed as a condiment. The oil is used as a local anodyne to carious teeth.

OLEUM CARYOPHYLLI (*oil of cloves*); dose, ♏iij–v (0.2–0.3 c.c.).

EUGENOL (*eugenol*); dose, ♏j–v (0.06–0.3).

PIMENTA, or allspice, is the *nearly ripe fruit* of *Pimenta officinalis* (*Fam.* Myrtaceæ). It contains a *volatile oil* and is carminative.

OLEUM PIMENTÆ (*oil of pimenta*); dose, ♏iij–v (0.18–0.3 c.c.).

ZINGIBER (*ginger*) is the *rhizome* of *Z. officinale* (*Fam.* Zingiberaceæ). It contains a *volatile oil* and an acrid *resin.* It is a *gastric stimulant* and *carminative,* much employed in flatulency and colic and as an addition to other stomachics.

FLUIDEXTRACTUM ZINGIBERIS (*fluid extract of ginger*); dose, ♏x–xxx (0.6–2.0 c.c.).

TINCTURA ZINGIBERIS (*tincture of ginger*); dose, ʒss–j (2–4 c.c.).

SYRUPUS ZINGIBERIS (*syrup of ginger*), used as a vehicle for other medicines.

OLEORESINA ZINGIBERIS (*oleoresin of ginger*), used as a corrective in purgative pills to prevent griping; dose, ♏ss–ij (0.03–0.12 c.c.).

CARDAMOMUM (*cardamom*) is the *nearly ripe fruit of Elettaria repens* (*Fam.* Zingiberaceæ), and contains a *volatile oil.* It is used as a gastric stimulant and carminative, and as an adjuvant and corrective of other medicines.

TINCTURA CARDAMOMI (*tincture of cardamom*); dose, ʒj–ij (4–8 c.c.).

TINCTURA CARDAMOMI COMPOSITA (*compound tincture of cardamom*) contains also caraway, cassia, cinnamon, and cochineal; dose, ʒj–ij (4–8 c.c.).

PULVIS AROMATICUS (*aromatic powder*) consists of Saigon cinnamon and ginger (35 per cent. each), with cardamom and nutmeg (15 per cent. each). An excellent carminative preparation. Dose, gr. v–xxx (0.3–2.0 gm.).

FLUIDEXTRACTUM AROMATICUM (*aromatic fluid extract*) is a fluid extract of aromatic powder. Dose, ♏v–xxx (0.3–2.0 c.c.).

OLEUM CAJUPUTI (*oil of cajuput*) is the *volatile oil* distilled from the *leaves* of *Melaleuca Leucadendron* (*Fam.* Myrtaceæ), and is very destructive to low organisms. It has been employed as a remedy against ascarides, and, locally, in parasitic skin-diseases, but is chiefly used as a gastric stimulant and carminative in flatulent colic and to prevent the griping of cathartics. Dose, ♏j–v (0.06–0.3 c.c.).

CALAMUS is the *unpeeled, dried rhizome* of *Acorus Calamus* (*Fam.* Araceæ). It contains a *volatile oil* and a glucosid, *acorin*. It is an aromatic stimulant and is somewhat tonic.

FLUIDEXTRACTUM CALAMI (*fluid extract of calamus*); dose, ♏x–xxx (0.6–2.0 c.c.).

OLEUM GAULTHERIÆ (*oil of gaultheria; oil of wintergreen*) is a *volatile oil* distilled from the leaves of *G. procumbens*, or wintergeen (*Fam.* Ericaceæ), and has been considered under the head of Salicylic Acid. It consists almost entirely of methyl salicylate, and is nearly identical with volatile oil of Betula (*vid.* Salicylates); dose in rheumatism, ♏v–xv (0.3–1 c.c.).

SPIRITUS GAULTHERIÆ (*spirit of gaultheria*) contains 5 per cent. of the oil; dose, ♏x–xxx (0.6–2.0 c.c.).

The following herbs, belonging to the *Fam.* Labiatæ, contain volatile oils, and are used as carminatives, gastric stimulants, and flavoring ingredients:

OLEUM LAVANDULÆ FLORUM (*oil of lavender flowers*) is a *volatile oil* distilled from the *fresh flowering tops* of *L. officinalis*. Dose, ♏j–v (0.06–0.3 c.c.). *Spiritus lavandulæ* (*spirit of lavender*) and *Tinctura Lavandulæ Composita* (*compound tincture of lavender*) are also official; dose of either, ʒss–j (2–4 c.c.).

MENTHA PIPERITA (*peppermint*) and MENTHA VIRIDIS (*spearmint*).—The *leaves* and *tops* are official. The *oils* (*oleum menthæ piperitæ* and *oleum menthæ viridis*, dose,

♏j–v—0.06–0.3 c.c.) are usually given in the form of *spirit* (*spiritus menthæ piperitæ and spiritus menthæ viridis*), dose, ♏v–xxx (0.3–2.0 c.c.). The *waters* (*aqua menthæ piperitæ* and *aqua menthæ viridis*) are used as vehicles. *Troches of peppermint* (*not official*) are sometimes used in flatulent colic.

OLEUM ROSMARINI (*oil of rosemary*) is a *volatile oil* distilled from the *fresh flowering tops* of *Rosmarinus officinalis.* It is carminative, but is chiefly used as an ingredient of rubefacient liniments. It enters into "soap liniment."

HEDEOMA (*pennyroyal*).—The *leaves* and *flowering tops* of *H. pulegioides* are official. The *volatile oil* (*oleum hedeomæ*) may be given in doses of ♏j–v (0.06–0.3 c.c.). It is said to be emmenagogue.

MARRUBIUM (*horehound*).—The *leaves* and *flowering tops* of *M. vulgare* are used as a gastric stimulant and expectorant.

SALVIA (*sage*).—The *leaves* of *S. officinalis* are slightly astringent as well as aromatic. An infusion is sometimes used as a gargle in sore throat.

OLEUM THYMI (*oil of thyme*), a *volatile oil distilled* from the *leaves* and *flowering tops* of *Thymus vulgaris*, contains much *thymol* (*q. v.*), and is therefore not only aromatic and carminative, but antiseptic and antifermentative.

The following *fruits* resembling *seeds* are derived from plants belonging to the *Fam.* Umbelliferæ:

FŒNICULUM (*fennel*), from *F. vulgare.* Of the *oil* (*oleum fœniculi*) the dose is ♏v–x (0.3–0.6 c.c.). A *water* (*aqua fœniculi*) is also official.

CARUM (*caraway*), from *C. Carvi.* Dose of the *oil* (*oleum cari*) ♏j–x (0.06–0.6 c.c.).

ANISUM (*anise*), from *Pimpinella Anisum.* Dose of the *oil* (*oleum anisi*) ♏v–xv (0.3–1.0 c.c.). A *spirit* (*spiritus anisi*) and a *water* (*aqua anisi*) are also official.

CORIANDRUM (*coriander*), from *C. sativum.* The *oil* (*oleum coriandri*) is official.

The following preparations are used only as flavors and vehicles:

AURANTII AMARI CORTEX (*bitter orange peel*); AURANTII DULCIS CORTEX (*sweet orange peel*). These are respectively the *rind* of the *fruits* of *Citrus vulgaris* (bitter orange) and of *C. aurantium* (sweet orange) (*Fam.* Rutaceæ). The following preparations are official:

Stronger orange-flower water (*aqua aurantii florum fortior; triple orange-flower water*), water saturated with the volatile oil of fresh orange flowers, obtained as a by-product in the distillation of the oil of orange-flowers; *orange-flower water* (*aqua aurantii florum*), equal volumes of stronger orange-flower water and distilled water freshly mixed; *syrup of orange-flowers* (*syrupus aurantii florum; syrup of orange peel* (*syrupus aurantii*); *oil of orange peel* (*oleum aurantii corticis*); *compound spirit of orange* (*spiritus aurantii compositus*) contains oil of orange peel (200), oil of lemon (50), oil of coriander (20), and oil of anise (5) in 1000 parts of the preparation. It is used in making *elixir aromaticum* (*aromatic elixir*), which contains 12 parts of the compound spirit in 1000 parts of the preparation; *fluid extract of bitter orange peel* (*fluidextractum aurantii amari*); *tinctures of bitter* and *of sweet orange peel* (*tinctura aurantii amari; tinctura aurantii dulcis*)—dose of either tincture, ʒj–ij (4–8 c.c.).

VANILLA, the *cured, full-grown,* but *immature fruit* of *V. planifolia* (*Fam.* Orchidaceæ), contains *vanillin.* The *tincture* (*tinctura vanillæ*) and *vanillinum* (*vanillin*) are official.

The *oil of turpentine* is an excellent carminative and will be considered hereafter.

CATHARTICS.

What are cathartics?

Cathartics are medicines employed to produce an evacuation from the bowels either by increasing intestinal peristalsis or by increasing the secretions of the canal and its appendages.

For what purposes are they used?

They are used—(1) To unload the bowels; (2) to deplete the blood-vessels by abstracting water from the blood; (3) to promote absorption; (4) to stimulate secretion; (5) to eliminate noxious material from the blood (as the poison of uremia); (6) to act as revulsives, and (7) to influence the pelvic circulation.

How may cathartics be classified?

Cathartics are divided into laxatives, simple purgatives, salines, and drastics.

Laxatives.

What are laxatives?

Laxatives are such substances as unload the bowels, acting without irritation and not causing active purgation.

Name the laxatives.

Tamarind, manna, cassia fistula, frangula, cascara sagrada, castor oil, sulphur.

TAMARINDUS (TAMARIND). MANNA.

What are these substances?

TAMARINDUS (*tamarind*) is the *preserved pulp of the fruit* of *T. indica (Fam.* Leguminosæ), a tree of India, and naturalized in the West Indies. Eaten as a preserve (℥ss–j; 15–30 c.c.) it is laxative. An infusion makes a pleasant refrigerant drink. It enters into *confection of senna.*

MANNA is the *concrete saccharine exudation* of *Fraxinus Ornus* (*Fam.* Oleaceæ). It contains *mannit, fraxin,* and *resin,* and is usually combined with other cathartics. Dose for an adult, ʒj–ij (30–60 c.c.); for children, ʒj–iv (4–15 c.c.). It enters into *compound infusion of senna.*

CASSIA FISTULA. FRANGULA. RHAMNUS PURSHIANA.

What are these substances?

CASSIA FISTULA is the *fruit* of *C. Fistula* or purging cassia (*Fam.* Leguminosæ). It is an ingredient of the *confection of senna.* Dose, ʒj–℥j (4–30 c.c.).

FRANGULA is the *bark* of *Rhamnus Frangula* or alder buckthorn (*Fam.* Rhamnaceæ). It contains *frangulin* and *emodin,* and as it is an active emetic and hydragogue when fresh, it should be kept a year at least before being used; dose of the *fluid extract* (*fluidextractum frangulæ*), ʒss–j (2–4 c.c.).

RHAMNUS PURSHIANA (*cascara sagrada* or *chittem bark*) is the *bark* of *R. Purshiana* (*Fam.* Rhamnaceæ), a tree of California. It contains several resins and is an efficient laxative, very useful in habitual constipation; dose of the *fluid extract* (*fluidextractum rhamni purshianæ*), or of the *aromatic fluid extract* (*fluidextractum rhamni purshianæ aromaticum*), ♏x–ʒj (0.6–4.0 c.c.); of the *extract* (*extractum rhamni purshianæ*), gr. ij–v (0.12–0.3 gm.).

OLEUM RICINI (CASTOR OIL).

What is castor oil?

It is a *fixed oil* expressed from the *seed* of *Ricinus communis,* or Palmi Christi (*Fam.* Euphorbiaceæ).

What are its effects and uses?

In *small doses* it is a mild laxative, in *larger amounts* a simple purgative. Its action is sometimes followed by constipation. Applied with friction to the abdomen of children it frequently purges. It is very useful whenever it is desired to evacuate the bowels and remove any irritant materials, as undigested food. For this purpose it is often used in acute dysenteries and diarrheas, especially of children; dose, ʒj–℥j (4–30 c.c.), best given floating on whisky, lemon juice, or peppermint water; or in sarsaparilla soda-water, or mixed with glycerin and an aromatic oil. As an alterative in chronic dysentery it is given in doses of ♏x (0.6 c.c.) three times a day.

SULPHUR.

What is sulphur?

Sulphur is a chemic element obtained by purifying native sulphur or by decomposing native sulphids.

What are its effects, uses, and preparations?

It acts as a mild laxative and is eliminated in all the

excretions. Its continued use causes flatulence from the formation of sulphureted hydrogen. It is used as a *laxative*, especially in cases of *hemorrhoids*, and as an *alterative* both internally and externally in *chronic rheumatism*, *muscular rheumatism*, *sciatica*, and in various forms of *skin disease*, especially those of parasitic origin. As sulphur is excreted largely by the hair, it has been used locally and internally in the treatment of *alopecia*. It is also used as an *expectorant*. It is official as SULPHUR SUBLIMATUM (*sublimed sulphur*, sometimes called "flowers of sulphur"), SULPHUR LOTUM (*washed sulphur*), and SULPHUR PRÆCIPITATUM (*precipitated sulphur*); dose of either preparation, ʒj–iv (4–15 c.c.) in syrup. UNGUENTUM SULPHURIS (*sulphur ointment*, containing 15 per cent. of washed sulphur) is used externally.

SIMPLE PURGATIVES.

What are the simple purgatives?

They are medicines employed to produce active purgation, but which do not produce sufficient irritation to cause inflammation or depression, even when large doses are given.

Name the agents of this group.

Castor oil, rhubarb, juglans, aloes, senna, leptandra, euonymus, and mercurials.

Castor oil has been described with the *Laxatives*.

RHEUM (RHUBARB). JUGLANS.

What are these medicines?

RHUBARB is the rhizome of *Rheum officinale*, *Rheum palmatum*, and the variety *tanguticum*, and probably *other species* of *Rheum* (*Fam.* Polygonaceæ). It contains *chrysophan*, *chrysophanic acid*, four resins (*erythroretin*, *emodin*, *phæoretin*, and *aporetin*), *rheotannic* and *rheumic acids*. It is a tonic and mild purgative, and, owing to the rheotannic acid, is astringent, and hence after purging it has a tendency to cause constipation. It tinges the milk and urine yellow, and stimulates the flow of bile. It is much used in *diarrhea*, from relaxation, in the early stages of *summer complaint* of children, and in *dyspepsia* with constipation. The official preparations and their doses are: the *extract* (*extractum rhei*), gr. v–xx (0.3–1.3 gm.); *compound pills* (*pilulæ rhei compositæ*), each contains gr. ij (0.13 gm.) of rhubarb, gr. iss (0.1 gm.) of aloes, with myrrh and oil of peppermint, dose, 1 to 4; *compound powder* (*pulvis rhei compositus*), contains rhubarb and magnesia, dose, ʒss–j (2–4 c.c.); *fluid extract* (*fluidextractum rhei*), ♏xx–xxx (1.2–2.0 c.c.); *mixture of rhubarb and soda* (*mistura rhei et sodæ*), for a child, ʒss–j (2–4 c.c.), for an adult, ʒj–iv (4–16 c.c.); *syrup* (*syrupus rhei*), ♏x–xx (0.6–1.2 c.c.), for an infant; *aromatic* or *spiced syrup*, (*syrupus rhei aromaticus*), for an infant, ʒss–j (2–4 c.c.); *tincture* (*tinctura rhei*), ʒj–ij (4–8 c.c.); *aromatic tincture* (*tinctura rhei aromaticus*), ʒss–j (2–4 c.c.).

JUGLANS (not official) is the *bark* of the *root* of *Juglans cinerea*, butternut or white walnut (*Fam.* Juglandaceæ), collected in autumn. It is used as a substitute for rhubarb, and especially stimulates the flow of bile. The *extract* (*extractum juglandis*) may be given in doses of gr. x–xxx (0.6–2.0 gm.).

ALOE—ALOES.

What is aloes?

Aloes is the *inspissated juice* of the *leaves* of *Aloë Perryi*, socotrine aloes, of *Aloë vera*, Barbadoes aloes, of *Aloë Chinensis*, and of *other species* of *Aloë* (*Fam.* Liliaceæ). Each variety contains a neutral crystalline principle, *aloin*. It is a tonic to the mucous membrane and a purgative, being slow in its action and affecting principally the large intestine, and apparently causing a determination of blood to the pelvic viscera. It is also a hepatic stimulant. It is *used* in habitual constipation especially when torpor of the large bowel exists; in *hemorrhoids* from relaxation of the veins and congestion of the portal circle; in *amenorrhea* and in *menorrhagia* due to want of tone of the uterine vessels. It is contraindicated in threatened abortion. The official preparations are made of *purified* (socotrine) *aloes* (*aloë purificata*), and are, *pills* (*pilulæ aloes*), each containing gr. ij (0.13 gm.) of aloes; *pills* of *aloes and mastiche* (*pilulæ aloes et mastiches*), called also

Lady Webster's dinner-pill, each containing gr. ij (0.13 gm.) of aloes; *pills of aloes and myrrh* (*pilulæ aloes et myrrhæ*) or *Rufus' pill*, each containing gr. ij (0.13 gm.) of aloes; *pill of aloes and iron* (*pilulæ aloes et ferri*), each containing gr. j (0.07 gm.) of aloes, of dried ferrous sulphate, and of aromatic powder (the two last-named pills are useful in amenorrhea); *extract* (*extractum aloes*), dose, gr. j–v (0.06–0.3 gm.); *tincture* (*tinctura aloes*), dose, ʒj–iv (4–16 c.c.); *tincture of aloes and myrrh* (*tinctura aloes et myrrhæ*), dose, ʒj–ij (4–8 c.c.).

ALOINUM (*aloin*) is official, dose, gr. $\frac{1}{10}$–j (0.006–0.06 gm.), and enters into *pilulæ laxativæ compositæ* (compound laxative pills; pills of aloin, belladonna, ipecac, and strychnine). Each pill contains gr. $\frac{1}{5}$ (0.013 gm.) of aloin, gr. $\frac{1}{8}$ (0.008 gm.) of extract of belladonna leaves, gr. $\frac{1}{16}$ (0.004 gm.) of ipecac, and gr. $\frac{1}{128}$ (0.0008 gm.) of strychnine.

SENNA. LEPTANDRA. EUONYMUS.

What are these medicines?

SENNA is the *leaflets* of *Cassia acutifolia* (Alexandria senna) and of *C. angustifolia* (Indian senna) (*Fam.* Leguminosæ). It contains *cathartic acid, chrysophanic acid, sennit,* and *sennacrol.* It is a prompt and efficient purgative, and probably acts on the entire length of the intestine, causing some griping. It is a mild hepatic stimulant. It is used where a prompt and decided cathartic effect is desired, usually in combination to prevent griping. Its preparations are: the *fluid extract* (*fluidextractum sennæ*), dose, ʒj–iv (4–15 c.c.); *confection* (*confectio sennæ*), an excellent purgative during pregnancy, ʒj–ij (4–8 gm.); *compound infusion* (*infusum sennæ compositum*), also called *black draft*, ℥ss–iv (15–120 c.c.); *syrup* (*syrupus sennæ*), ʒj–ij (4–8 c.c.); *compound powder of glycyrrhiza* (or of *licorice*) (*pulvis glycyrrhizæ compositus*), an excellent purgative; dose, a teaspoonful (4 gm.) at bedtime.

LEPTANDRA is the *rhizome* and *roots* of *Veronica virginica,* Culver's root or physic (*Fam.* Scrophulariaceæ). It contains *leptandrin,* and is a feeble stimulant to the liver and intestinal glands. Dose of the *extract* (*extractum leptandræ*), gr. j–iv (0.06–0.25 gm.); of the *fluid extract* (*fluidextractum leptandræ*), ℥ss–j (2–4 c.c.).

EUONYMUS, or wahoo, the bark of the root of *E. atropurpureus* (*Fam.* Celastraceæ), contains a bitter principle, *euonymin, resin, euonic acid,* etc. It is a powerful hepatic stimulant, increases the intestinal secretion, and is *used* as a purgative in torpidity of the liver and intestine. Dose of the *extract* (*extractum euonymi*), gr. ij–iv (0.13–0.25 gm.) in pill, and of the *fluid extract* (*fluidextractum euonymi*) ♏v–xv (0.3–1 c.c.).

MERCURIAL CATHARTICS.

What mercurials are used as simple purgatives?

HYDRARGYRI CHLORIDUM MITE (*mercurous chlorid* or *calomel*); dose, gr. ss–j to x (0.03–0.6 gm.), at bedtime given in a single dose or in small divided doses of gr. $\frac{1}{20}$–$\frac{1}{4}$ (0.003–0.015 gm.); and MASSA HYDRARGYRI (*mercurial* or *blue mass*), dose, gr. v–xv (0.3–1.0 gm.). They will be found under the head of *Alteratives*.

SALINE CATHARTICS.

What are saline cathartics?

The saline cathartics are certain *salts* which produce an evacuation of the bowel not only by increasing peristalsis from their irritant effect, but also by preventing absorption from the alimentary tract and promoting outward osmosis from the blood, thus rendering the stool liquid, depleting the blood-vessels, and consequently favoring removal of effused fluids.

Name the medicines of this group.

The magnesium salts, some of the sodium and some of the potassium salts, and manganese sulphate.

Describe the effects, uses, preparations, and doses of the magnesium salts.

MAGNESII OXIDUM (*magnesia; calcined magnesia*) and MAGNESII OXIDUM PONDEROSUM (*heavy magnesia*; is similar to *Henry's*, *Husband's*, and *Ellis'* magnesias) are antacid and cathartic, are mild in their action, and are excellent preparations for children; dose as an antacid, gr. xx (1.2 gm.), as a cathartic, ʒj (4 gm.) or more.

MAGNESII CARBONAS (*magnesium carbonate; magnesia alba*), not much used; dose as an antacid, gr. x–xx (0.6–1.2 gm.); as a cathartic, ʒj–ij (4–8 gm.).

MAGNESII SULPHAS (*magnesium sulphate; Epsom salt*) is much more powerful than the preceding preparations, and produces free, watery purgation with very little irritation. It is used as a *purgative* to remove *fecal accumulation;* as a *depletant* in *enterocolitis* and *acute dysentery* (with opium); to *aid absorption* (given in very concentrated solutions) in *dropsical effusions*, especially hydrothorax; and for the relief of *colica pictonum* and other forms of lead-poisoning; dose, ℥ss–j (15–30 gm.). Its taste is bitter.

MAGNESII SULPHAS EFFERVESCENS (*effervescent magnesium sulphate*); dose, ʒiv (15 gm.), taken in water while effervescing.

LIQUOR MAGNESII CITRATIS (*solution of magnesium citrate*). The citrates are similar in effect to the sulphate, but are more apt to irritate; this preparation, however, is well borne by the stomach; dose, half to a whole bottleful (180–360 c.c.).

What salts of sodium are used as cathartics?

SODII SULPHAS (*sodium sulphate; Glauber's salt*) is similar in its effects to Epsom salt, but more irritant and disagreeable. It is a mild hepatic stimulant. It is not much used; dose, ʒj–iv (4–15 gm.).

SODII PHOSPHAS (*sodium phosphate*) is a mild cathartic and hepatic stimulant. It is an excellant purgative in *catarrhal conditions of the bowel*, in *catarrhal jaundice*, and in *chronic infantile diarrhea* with pasty stools; dose, ʒj–℥j (4–30 gm.).

SODII PHOSPHAS EXSICCATUS (*dried sodium phosphate*); dose, gr. xv (1 gm.)

SODII PHOSPHAS EFFERVESCENS (*effervescent sodium phosphate*); dose, ʒij (8 gm.), taken in water while effervescing.

LIQUOR SODII PHOSPHATIS COMPOSITUS (*compound solu-*

tion of sodium phosphate); dose, ʒj–iij (4–12 c.c.), well diluted.

Sodii Pyrophosphas (*sodium pyrophosphate*) resembles the preceding salt in action and uses; dose, ʒss–iv (2–15 gm.).

What potassium salts are used as cathartics?

Potassii Sulphas (*potassium sulphate*) was formerly, but is not at present, much used; dose, gr. xv–ʒj (1–4 gm.).

Potassii Bitartras (*potassium bitartrate; cream of tartar; cremor tartar*) is a diuretic, refrigerant, and cathartic. In overdoses it causes gastro-enteritis. Dose as *diuretic*, gr. x–ʒj (0.6–4.0 gm.); as a *mild laxative*, ʒss–j (2–4 gm.); as a saline cathartic, ℥ss (15 gm.).

Potassii et Sodii Tartras (*potassium and sodium tartrate; Rochelle salt*) resembles Epsom salt, but is not so powerful; dose, ℥ss–j (15–30 gm.).

Pulvis Effervescens Compositus (*compound effervescing powder; Seidlitz powder*) consists of Rochelle salt ʒij (7.75 gm.), with sodium bicarbonate gr. xl (2.59 gm.) in a blue, and tartaric acid gr. xxxv (2.25 gm.) in a white, paper, their contents to be dissolved separately, the solutions mixed and taken on an empty stomach while effervescing.

What is manganese sulphate?

Mangani Sulphas (*manganese sulphate*) has been discussed with the tonics. It is a hepatic stimulant and cathartic also, resembling Epsom salt, but is a dangerous remedy, and is not much employed; dose, gr. j–v (0.06–0.3 gm.).

DRASTIC CATHARTICS.

What are drastic cathartics?

Cathartics which cause much irritation and act very powerfully are so called. Most of them in overdoses cause irritant poisoning. When they produce very free, watery evacuations they are sometimes spoken of as "hydragogues." The more powerful drastics are used as revulsives in cerebral affections.

Describe the medicines employed as drastics?

Jalapa (*jalap*), the *tuberous root* of *Exogonium Purga*

(*Fam.* Convolvulaceæ), a Mexican plant, contains a *resin,* to which its purgative properties are due. It is required to yield not less than 8 per cent. of total resin, and not more than 1.5 per cent. of resin soluble in ether.

It is a prompt and powerful hydragogue and cholagogue, in overdoses causing gastro-intestinal irritation and even death. It is *used* as a hydragogue in *dropsies* of cardiac or renal origin, as in ascites or anasarca, and sometimes as a cerebral revulsant. Its preparations are *compound powder* (*pulvis jalapæ compositus*), containing 35 per cent. of jalap with cream of tartar, dose, gr. x–ʒj (0.6–4.0 gm.); and the *resin* (*resina jalapæ*), dose, gr. j–v (0.06–0.3 gm.), which enters into the *compound cathartic* and the *vegetable cathartic pills.*

Bryonia (*bryony*) (not official), the *root* of *B. alba* and *B. dioica* (*Fam.* Cucurbitaceæ), European climbing vines, contains a glucosid, *bryonin,* probably the active principle. It is a violent hydragogue cathartic, resembling jalap in its *effects,* and also proving *diuretic* and emmenagogue. It is *used* as a hydragogue in dropsies, especially in hydrothorax and hydropericardium. The *tincture* (*tinctura bryoniæ*) may be used in doses of ʒss–j (2–4 c.c.).

Podophyllum, the *rhizome* of *P. peltatum,* Mayapple or mandrake (*Fam.* Berberidaceæ), a common indigenous plant, containing a resinous substance which yields *podophyllotoxin,* consisting of picropodophyllin, the purgative principle, and podophyllinic acid, which is inert.

It is an active hydragogue and cholagogue, acting slowly and especially on the upper part of the small intestine, and causing much irritation. In overdoses it is a gastro-intestinal irritant capable of causing death.

It is *used* as a purgative and cholagogue in acute and chronic *constipation, bilious attacks,* and in *torpor of the liver.* The dose of the *fluid extract* (*fluidextractum podophylli*) is ♏x–xx (0.6–1.2 c.c.); of the *resin,* gr. $\frac{1}{10}$–$\frac{1}{2}$ (0.006–0.03 gm.); the latter preparation is the only one in common use, and enters into the *Pills of Podophyllum, Belladonna and Capsicum.*

Podophyllotoxin (not official) may be used in the form of a

1 per cent. alcoholic solution, the dose of which is ℞ x–xxx (0.6–2.0 c.c.). It is used hypodermically; dose, gr. ¼ (0.016 gm.).

IRIS (not official), the *rhizome* and *roots* of *I. versicolor*, or blue-flag (*Fam.* Iridaceæ), contains a purgative *resin.* It is a powerful stimulant to the liver and intestinal glands, *acting* like podophyllum, but with less irritation. It is *diuretic*, and in overdoses irritant and depressant. It is *used* in *dropsies, jaundice of malarial origin*, and *torpor of the liver.* Dose of the *extract* (*extractum iridis*), gr. ij–iv (0.1–0.25 gm.); of the *fluid extract* (*fluidextractum iridis*), ℞ x–ʒj (0.6–4.0 c.c.).

SCAMMONIUM (*scammony*) is a *gum-resin* obtained by incising the living *root* of *Convolvulus Scammonia* (*Fam.* Convolvulaceæ), a Syrian plant. The resin *scammonin* is the active portion. It is a *violent hydragogue*, resembling jalap in its action, but much more irritating. It is never given except in combination with other cathartics. The dose of the *resin* (*resina scammonii*) is gr. ij–viij (0.13–0.5 gm.). It is one of the ingredients of *compound extract of colocynth.*

COLOCYNTHIS (*colocynth*), the *peeled, dried fruit* of *Citrullus colocynthis*, or bitter apple (*Fam.* Cucurbitaceæ), contains a glucosid (the purgative principle) called *colocynthin;* also a *resin, colocynthitin*, etc.

It is a *hepatic stimulant* and *violent hydragogue*, and in overdoses causes death from gastro-enteritis. It is never given alone, but is *used* in small doses to increase the effects of milder cathartics. The *extract* (*extractum colocynthidis*) is used in combination with other purgatives; dose, gr. ij–v (0.13–0.3 gm.); *compound extract* (*extractum colocynthidis compositum*), containing also aloes, resin of scammony, cardamom, and soap; dose, gr. iij–x (0.2–0.6 gm.).

CAMBOGIA (*gamboge*) is a *gum-resin* obtained from *Garcinia Hanburii* (*Fam.* Guttiferæ), a tree of Siam. The resin is the purgative principle, and is called *cambogic acid.* It is a very powerful *hydragogue cathartic*, and in overdoses has caused death. It is rarely *used* alone, and enters into *compound cathartic pills;* dose, gr. ij–v (0.13–03 gm.).

Pilulæ Catharticæ Compositæ (*compound cathartic pills*). Each pill contains of compound extract of colocynth gr. j⅕ (0.08 gm.); of calomel, gr. j (0.06 gm.); of resin of jalap, gr. ⅓ (0.02 gm.); and of gamboge, gr. ¼ (0.015 gm.).

Pilulæ Catharticæ Vegetabiles (*vegetable cathartic pills*). Each pill contains of compound extract of colocynth gr. j (0.06 gm.); of extract of hyoscyamus gr. ½ (0.03 gm.); of resin of jalap, gr. ⅓ (0.02 gm.); of extract of leptandra and of resin of podophyllum, each, gr. ¼ (0.015 gm.), with oil of peppermint.

Elaterinum (*elaterin*) is a *neutral principle* extracted from elaterium, a substance deposited by the juice of the fruit of *Ecballium Elaterium*, or squirting cucumber (*Fam.* Cucurbitaceæ). It is one of the most powerful of the *hydragogues*, also proving *diuretic*, and in excessive doses often causing death. It is much *used* in *dropsies*, in *uremia*, and as a cerebral *revulsive*. The dose is gr. $\frac{1}{20}$ (0.003 gm.); of the *trituration* (*trituratio elaterini*), which is *10 per cent.*, gr. ¼–ss (0.016–0.03 gm.).

Oleum Tiglii (*croton oil*) is a *fixed oil* expressed from the *seeds* of *Croton Tiglium* (*Fam.* Euphorbiaceæ), a tree of India. It contains crotonic acid and crotonoleic acid, the latter of which is irritant.

When applied to the skin, croton oil is an intense irritant, causing a papular eruption which soon becomes pustular. Given internally, it is a powerful and rapid hydragogue cathartic, causing severe griping pains and to some extent depressing the circulation. In overdoses it produces great depression and often proves fatal. In *obstinate constipation* it is very serviceable, and as a *revulsive* in cerebral affections, as apoplexy, it is the best hydragogue. It has been used externally as a *counterirritant* (*q. v.*), and with sulphur ointment for ring-worm. Dose, ♏j–ij (0.06–0.12 c.c.), which may be given in pill or emulsion, or mixed with a few drops of glycerin or olive oil and placed on the patient's tongue when he cannot or will not swallow.

ENEMATA.

What are enemata?

Enemata are liquids injected into the rectum. They may be *nutritive, cathartic*, or *forced enemata*.

Nutritive enemata are used to nourish the patient when the stomach cannot retain or digest food. They should be small in amount, not exceeding ℥iij–vj (90–180 c.c.) at a time, nor should they be too frequently repeated, else they will cause irritability of the rectum. They should be combined with some digestant, as pepsin or pancreatin.

Cathartic enemata are used to unload the bowels when irritation or inflammation of the stomach is present; to aid the action of cathartics taken by the mouth; to remove fecal accumulations or retained and irritating secretions from the large intestine; to relieve tympanites; to remove ascarides; or to act as revulsives. The fluid used may be cold or warm water, either simple or medicated, and the quantity will depend on the case. The injection should be made slowly and carefully, and the introduction of air is to be avoided.

Forced enemata are made slowly and gradually, the fluid, either warm water or warmed oil, being poured into a large funnel or rubber bag (fountain syringe) to which a long rubber tube is attached, armed with an injection pipe. By elevating the funnel or bag the fluid flows in a steady stream, the force being regulated by the height at which the bag is held. Forced enemata are employed principally to reduce intussusception of the bowels.

ANTHELMINTICS.

What are anthelmintics?

Anthelmintics are medicines used to kill (*vermicides*) or cause the expulsion of (*vermifuges*) intestinal worms.

How are they administered?

They should be given fasting, and should be followed in four to six hours by a purgative, as calomel or castor oil.

Describe the medicines used as anthelmintics.

SPIGELIA, or pinkroot, the *rhizome* and *roots* of *S. marilandica* or Carolina pink (*Fam.* Loganiaceæ), contains a *bitter principle, volatile oil, resin, tannic acid,* etc. It slows the heart by stimulating the inhibiting centers, reduces arterial pressure by depressing the heart, and in overdoses quickens the pulse, increases the blood-pressure, dilates the pupil, causes delirium, and, in fatal cases, death from respiratory paralysis. It is very efficient in causing the expulsion of *lumbrici*, but should be followed by a purge. Dose of the *fluid extract* (*fluidextractum spigeliæ*), ʒj–ij (4–8 c.c.), or to a child, ♏x (0.6 c.c.) on sugar. It is often given with senna.

CHENOPODIUM (not official), or American wormseed, the *fruit* of *C. ambrosioides* or Jerusalem oak (*Fam.* Chenopodiaceæ), contains a *volatile oil*, to which its effects are due. It is a very efficient remedy for the expulsion of *lumbrici*, and should be followed by a brisk cathartic. The *oil* (not official) is given in doses of ♏v–x (0.25–0.5 c.c.) on sugar, to a child three years old, before meals.

SANTONICA, or Levant wormseed, is the *unexpanded flowerheads* of *Artemisia pauciflora* (*Fam.* Compositæ). The active principle is *santonin*. *Large doses* cause salivation, rapid breathing, slow, labored pulse, trembling, yellow vision and yellow urine, unconsciousness, convulsions, dilated pupils, and death. It is used almost exclusively as a remedy for *lumbrici*. Dose of *santonin* (*santoninum*) for an adult, gr. ss–v (0.03–0.3 gm.); for a child two years old, gr. ¼ (0.016 gm.). *Troches of santonin* (*trochisi santonini*), each contains gr. ss (0.03 gm.) of santonin; dose, 1 to 6 troches.

ASPIDIUM, the *rhizome* of *Dryopteris filix-mas*, or malefern, and *D. marginalis* (*Fam.* Filices), contains *filicic acid, volatile* and *fixed oils, resin,* etc., and is used as a *teniacide*. Like all remedies employed for this purpose, its administration should be preceded by a fast of twenty-four hours and followed by a brisk cathartic. In overdoses it has caused death from enteritis. Dose of the *oleoresin* (*oleoresina aspidii*), ʒss–j (2–4 c.c.).

GRANATUM (*pomegranate*), the *bark* of the *stem* and *root* of *Punica Granatum* (*Fam.* Punicaceæ), contains four alkaloids, *pelletierine* and three allied alkaloids, which are powerful *teniacides*, as is also granatum itself. In overdoses they are said to act on the muscles like woorara. Dose of pomegranate in decoction ℥ij (60 c.c.) to water Oij (1000 c.c.), boiled to Oj (500 c.c); ℥ij (60 c.c.), repeated three times at an hour's interval before breakfast; of the *fluid extract* (*fluid-extractum granati*), ʒj–iij (4–12 c.c.); of *pelletierine tannate*, gr. v–x (0.3–0.6 gm.).

CUSSO (*Kousso; Brayera*, the panicles of the pistillate flowers of *Hagenia abyssinica* (*Fam.* Rosaceæ), contains tannic acid, resin, volatile oil, and *kosotoxin* (an amorphous, highly active resin), and is used as a *teniacide;* dose of the *fluid extract* (not official), ʒij–iv (8–15 c.c.).

KAMALA (not official), the *glands* and *hairs* from the capsules of *Mallotus philippinensis* (*Fam.* Euphorbiaceæ), contains *rottlerin* and *isorottlerin*, resinoid substances, and is used as a *teniacide;* dose, ʒj–ij (4–8 c.c.) of the powder in syrup.

PEPO (*pumpkin-seed*), the *ripe seed* of *Cucurbita pepo* or pumpkin (*Fam.* Cucurbitaceæ), contains a *resin*, and is one of the most powerful *teniacides* in the materia medica and perfectly harmless; dose of the fresh seed (powdered with sugar, or made into an infusion), ℥j–ij (30–60 c.c.).

OLEUM TEREBINTHINÆ (*oil of turpentine*) is an efficient but not a harmless remedy for *tenia* and *lumbrici*. It will be found under the head of Diuretics. Dose, ℥ss–j (15–30 c.c.), combined with castor oil.

HYDRARGYRI CHLORIDUM MITE (*mercurous chlorid or calomel*) is used alone or combined with other anthelmintics for the expulsion of *lumbrici* and (rarely) *tenia*. It should be given in full purgative doses (*v.* Alteratives).

THYMOL, a phenol occurring in the volatile oil of *Thymus vulgaris* (*Fam.* Labiatæ) and in some other volatile oils, is a very efficient remedy for the *hook-worm*, *Uncinaria* (or *Anchylostomum*) *duodenalis* or *Americana*. Dose, gr. v–xv (0.3–1 gm.).

What remedies are used for the destruction of ascarides?

Mild purgatives, as *calomel* or *sulphur*, may be used to dislodge them from the small intestine, but *injections of quassia infusion, common salt, naphthol, tannin, alum*, or *lime-water* must be employed to get rid of those in the colon. *Injections of sweet oil* at bedtime are useful to kill any which may be in the rectum and prevent the excessive itching which they cause. The child should be prevented from scratching the anus, as the ova are very tenacious, and, adhering to the finger-nails, may be conveyed to the mouth and reproduce the trouble.

What are useful adjuncts to the anthelmintics?

Iron and *bitter tonics*, by restoring tone to the mucous membranes, prevent the excessive secretion of mucus which forms a suitable nidus for the development of parasites.

Medicines Acting on the Body by their Effect on the Various Secretions and Excretions.

DIURETICS.

What are diuretics?

Diuretics are medicines used to increase the excretion of urine, acting either *directly* on the secreting cells of the kidney or *indirectly* by their influence on the blood-pressure in the glomeruli.

For what purposes are they used?

They are used—(1) To maintain the *function of the kidneys* in suppression of urine independent of the cause; (2) to promote the excretion of *urinary solids* (injurious waste-products) or of poisons from the blood, as in uremia, gout, rheumatism, fevers, and in cases of various metallic and vegetable poisons; (3) to promote the excretion of *water*, thus tending to dilute highly concentrated urine or to aid in the removal of effused (dropsical) fluids; and (4) to alter the *chemic reaction* of the urine and render that fluid more bland, thus lessening vesical and urethral irritation and any tendency which may exist to the formation of calculi.

A certain relation exists between the functions of the skin, kidneys, and bowels, so that free catharsis or free diaphoresis will diminish the urinary secretion, and vice versâ.

How may diuretics be classified?

They may be divided into alkaline, hydragogue, and alterative diuretics.

Alkaline Diuretics.

What are the alkaline diuretics?

They are those salts which, without materially increasing

the amount of water, usually increase the elimination of its solid ingredients and modify or alter its chemic reaction.

Name the alkaline diuretics.

The potassium and lithium salts and strontium lactate.

POTASSIUM.

What is the source of potassium ?

Potassium is obtained from the ashes of plants, from native *niter*, and from *tartar* or *argols*, deposited from wine during fermentation.

What are the general physiologic actions of its salts ?

Locally applied, *caustic potash* destroys tissues by abstracting water, dissolving albumin, and saponifying fats. *Internally*, in *small doses* before meals, they increase the acidity of the gastric juice ; in *large doses*, or after meals, they neutralize the acid present in the stomach.

When there is hydrochloric acid present, it is neutralized and the chlorid formed. The *bicarbonates* are sedative to the stomach, neutralizing excessive acidity and preventing acid fermentation. Given before meals they tend to increase the production of hydrochloric acid in the gastric juice. These and the *salts formed with the vegetable acids* increase the alkalinity of the blood and diminish the acidity of the urine. The potassium salts depress brain, spinal cord, and muscle, and in large doses paralyze the heart. The organic salts are diuretic. The strong alkalis promote tissue-waste. Caustic potash is a corrosive poison, eating the esophagus and stomach-wall, and often followed long after by cicatricial stenoses. The *treatment* of potassium poisoning consists in neutralizing the alkali by a vegetable acid, giving demulcents and fixed oils as protectives, and stimulating if requisite.

What are the therapeutic uses of the potassium salts ?

The potassium salts are used as *diuretics*, increasing both the water and salts of the urine, and rendering the urine alkaline in *acute rheumatism*, *uric-acid diathesis*, in *desquamative nephritis*, and to alkalinize the urine in *cystic* and *urethral irritation*.

What are the potassium preparations, their uses and doses?

LIQUOR POTASSII HYDROXIDI (*solution of potassium hydroxide*) contains 6 per cent. of potassium hydroxid, and is *antacid* and *diuretic*. It is used to render the urine alkaline in cystic irritability and in gonorrhea; dose, ♏x–xx (0.6–1.2 c.c.), freely diluted.

POTASSII CARBONAS (*potassium carbonate; salts of tartar*) is *antacid* and *diuretic*, but is more irritating to the stomach than the bicarbonate; dose, gr. x–xx (0.6–1.2 gm.).

POTASSII BICARBONAS (*potassium bicarbonate; saleratus*) is *antacid* and *diuretic*; dose, gr. xx–ʒj (1.2–4.0 gm.). It is much used in the treatment of *acute rheumatism*, especially in plethoric persons, ℥ss–iss (15–45 gm.) are given in the first twenty-four hours, half as much during the second day, and afterward enough to keep the urine alkaline.

POTASSII CITRAS (*potassium citrate*) is used as a *diuretic* in acute rheumatism, and as a refrigerant diaphoretic in fevers and acute inflammations; dose, gr. xx (1.2 gm.) in solution every hour or two.

LIQUOR POTASSII CITRATIS (*solution of potassium citrate*) contains 8 per cent. of the bicarbonate and 6 per cent. of citric acid. It is often prescribed with sweet spirits of niter, in fever mixtures; dose, ℥ss (15 c.c.)

POTASSII CITRAS EFFERVESCENS (*effervescent potassium citrate*) is made by mixing thoroughly, drying, and powdering citric acid (63), potassium bicarbonate (90), and sugar (47). Dose, ʒss–j (2–4 gm.).

Neutral mixture (not official) is made by neutralizing fresh lemon-juice with the bicarbonate. The official *solution of potassium citrate* has superseded it, as being the more exact and more elegant method of prescribing the same medicine; dose, ℥ss–j (15–30 c.c.).

Effervescing draft (not official) is made by adding ℥j (30 c.c.) of a solution of the bicarbonate (ʒj–℥iij—4 gm.–90 c.c.) to ℥j (30 c.c.) of lemon-juice and water (equal parts). It is particularly acceptable to febrile patients with irritable stomachs.

POTASSII ACETAS (*potassium acetate*) is *antacid, diuretic*, and in large doses a *mild cathartic*. It is chiefly used as a *diuretic* in acute rheumatism, and to some extent in dropsies and in uric-acid diathesis; dose, gr. xx–ʒj (1.2–4.0 gm.)

POTASSII BITARTRAS (*potassium bitartrate; cream of tartar*) is a *diuretic* and *saline cathartic* (*q. v.*) much employed in dropsies.

POTASSII NITRAS (*potassium nitrate; saltpeter; niter*) *locally* applied is a powerful irritant to the mucous membranes and to raw surfaces. It passes through the system unchanged, and is eliminated chiefly by the urine, increasing the amount passed, but not affecting its reaction to the same extent as the other salts. *Poisoning* occurs more frequently from the nitrate than from any other potassium salt, the symptoms being burning pain in the throat and epigastrium, hematemesis and bloody stools, muscular weakness, syncope, collapse, sometimes preceded by convulsions or paralysis, suppression of urine, and death. The *treatment* consists in evacuating the contents of the stomach and administering opiates, demulcents, and stimulants.

It is *used* in *acute rheumatism* as a *diuretic*, but is probably inferior to the salts formed with the vegetable acids. It is used in *fevers* for the same purpose, and has been given in small doses combined with Dover's powder as a *diaphoretic* in *acute muscular rheumatism*. Dose of potassium nitrate, gr. x–xxx (0.6–2.0 gm.). *Papers of potassium nitrate* (not official), made by immersing strips of unsized paper in a solution of the salt, are burned, and the fumes inhaled with success in spasmodic asthma. It is probable that the *nitrite* is formed by the combustion, and is the active agent in these cases.

POTASSII CHLORAS (*potassium chlorate*) is a *local* irritant. *Internally* in large doses it causes gastro-enteritis, affects the circulation as do the other potassium salts, damages the blood-corpuscles, and interferes with oxygenation by the formation of methemoglobin, and produces a condition of acute tubal nephritis. Cases of poisoning are not infrequent, and death is usually preceded by profuse salivation, great dyspnea, cyanosis, delirium, coma, tonic and clonic spasms, and sometimes ecchymoses and jaundice. It increases the excretion of urine, but does not affect its chemic reaction.

It has been *used* as a diuretic in dropsies, but is dangerous and inferior to other preparations. As an *alterative* in the exanthemata it is now little employed. In *mercurial, follicular*, or *aphthous stomatitis* it is of unquestionable value, given internally with sugar or used as a gargle. In ordinary *sore throat* and in *tonsillitis* it is useful as a local application; dose, gr. v–xxx (0.3–2.0 gm.). It must be given freely diluted. It should not be prescribed in powder with readily oxidizable or combustible substances, as when triturated with them it forms explosive compounds. As a gargle, ʒss–iv (2–15 gm.) in water Oj (500 c.c.) may be used.

The *troches* (*trochisci potassii chloratis*) each contain gr. v (0.3 gm.) of the salt.

The other potassium preparations have been or will be considered in their appropriate places.

LITHIUM.

What are the sources of lithium?

Lithium is a chemic element found native in the form of silicates, phosphates, etc.

What are the physiologic effects and uses of the lithium salts?

The lithium salts appear to resemble those of potassium. They are eliminated by the urine as urates, increasing the urine and rendering it less acid. As the urate of lithium is much more soluble than the urate either of sodium or of potassium, the lithium preparations are advantageously *used* in the treatment of *chronic gout* and *lithemia*, and as a *local application* to gouty deposits either before or after the skin has broken. They have also been employed internally in *glycosuria*.

What are the preparations of lithium and their doses?

Lithii Carbonas (*lithium carbonate*), dose, gr. v–x (0.3–0.6 gm.) freely diluted. As a local sorbefacient for gouty deposits a solution (gr. v–℥j—0.3 gm.–30 c.c.) should be kept constantly applied.

Lithii Citras (*lithium citrate*); dose, gr. v–xx (0.3–1.2 gm.).

Lithii Citras Effervescens (*effervescent lithium citrate*) is made by triturating and thoroughly drying citric acid (370) with sugar (about 200); then triturating the mixture with lithium carbonate (70), sodium bicarbonate (280), and sugar (enough to make the product weigh 1000); dose, ʒj–ij (4–8 c.c.)

LITHII BENZOAS (*lithium benzoate*); dose, gr. v–xx (0.3–1.2 gm.).

Lithium bromid and *lithium salicylate* have been *previously* mentioned.

What sodium salt has been used as a diuretic?

SODII ACETAS (*sodium acetate*) is supposed to possess properties similar to those of potassium acetate, and has been used for the same purposes and in the same doses.

What preparation of strontium is used as a diuretic?

STRONTIUM LACTATE (not official) has been used as a diuretic, especially in *acute desquamative nephritis*, with scanty urine, where it has been found to increase the amount of urine and diminish the albumin present in that excretion. It has also been used in *other forms of kidney disease*, but is much less efficient in chronic than in acute cases. It has been used as an *intestinal antiseptic*, but is of little value for this purpose. Dose, gr. v–xv (0.3–1.0 gm.) in solution.

Hydragogue Diuretics.

What are hydragogue diuretics?

The medicines of this group greatly increase the flow of the *watery* element of the urine, and are hence used in the treatment of dropsies.

Name the hydragogue diuretics.

Squill, digitalis, caffeine, sodiotheobromine salicylate, apocynum, broom, dandelion, sweet spirit of niter, and mercurials.

SCILLA (SQUILL).

What is squill?

Squill is the *bulb* of *Urginea maritima* (*Fam.* Liliaceæ) deprived of its dry, membranaceous outer scales, and cut into thin slices, the central portions being rejected. It contains *scillipicrin*, *scillitoxin*, and *scillin*. In *small doses* squill increases the mucous secretions and is a stimulating expectorant, while it markedly increases the urinary secretion. In *large doses* it causes nausea, vomiting, and sometimes purging, and in *excessive doses* produces in addition great abdominal pain, with scanty, bloody, or even suppressed urine, great depression, collapse, convulsions, and death.

Scillipicrin appears to be the diuretic principle. *Scillitoxin* slows the pulse, and in overdoses causes diastolic cardiac arrest by stimulating the peripheral vagi; after large doses the vagi are finally paralyzed and the pulse becomes rapid. *Scillin* is devoid of diuretic effects, but appears to be the emetic principle.

The *treatment of poisoning* consists in evacuating the contents of the stomach and the use of opiates and demulcents. If collapse occurs, alcohol must be employed.

Squill is *used* as a *diuretic* in *dropsy*, but should not be employed if kidney disease or cystitis is present. It is frequently combined with digitalis in cardiac dropsies, and in chronic pleurisy or pericarditis is often given with calomel. As an *expectorant* it is much used in *bronchial* affections. As an *emetic* it is too dangerous a remedy to employ.

As a *diuretic* or *expectorant* squill may be given in doses of gr. j–ij (0.06–0.13 c.c.) repeated every two hours and gradually increased until nausea occurs. Doses of gr. vj–xij (0.4–0.8 gm.) generally prove emetic. The dose of the *fluid extract* (*fluidextractum scillæ*) is ♏j–ij (0.06–0.12 c.c.); of the *tincture* (*tinctura scillæ*), ♏x–xxx (0.6–2.0 c.c.); of the *vinegar* (*acetum scillæ*), ♏x–xxx (0.6–2.0 c.c.); of the *syrup* (*syrupus scillæ*), ʒss–j (2–4 c.c.); of the *compound syrup* (*syrupus scillæ compositus; Coxe's hive syrup*), containing squill and senega and gr. j (0.06 gm.) of tartar emetic in each ounce (30 c.c.), ♏v–ʒj (0.3–4.0 c.c.).

DIGITALIS; CAFFEINE; THEOBROMINE; THEOPHYLLINE.

Are these drugs used as diuretics?

The uses of these remedies as diuretics have already been discussed under the head of Cardiac Stimulants. For this purpose the best preparations of digitalis are the *infusion*, the *powdered leaves*, and the *tincture*.

SODIOTHEOBROMINE SALICYLATE.

What is sodiotheobromine salicylate?

Sodiotheobromine salicylate, or *diuretin* (*the proprietary name*), is a non-official preparation "obtained by mixing aqueous solutions of equal molecules of sodium theobromine and salicylic acid, and evaporating to dryness; a definite compound appears to be formed, containing theoretically 49.7 per cent. of theobromine and 38.1 per cent. of salicylic acid. It occurs as a white powder, odorless, of a saline, alkaline taste, and soluble in one-half its weight of warm water, the solution remaining perfect on cooling."[1]

Theobromine is dimethylxanthine, a body closely related to caffeine (trimethylxanthine), but exerting a much less stimulating effect on the cerebrum and greater effect on the kidneys. As it is not readily soluble and is irritating to the stomach, it has been combined with sodium salicylate to overcome these defects. Diuretin is a powerful direct diuretic, stimulating the kidney-cells and increasing both the liquid and the solids of the urine. It occasionally irritates the stomach. It is employed as a diuretic in dropsical effusions in doses of gr. x–xv (0.6–1.0 gm.) repeated every two or three hours.

APOCYNUM.

What is apocynum?

Apocynum, Canadian hemp, or milk-weed, is the *rhizome* of *A. cannabinum* or of closely allied species of *Apocynum* (*Fam.* Apocynaceæ) and contains *apocynin* and *apocynein*, a glucosid. These substances are supposed to be cardiac tonics, acting on the heart similarly to digitalis. They are also diuretic. Apocynum is laxative in *small*, but emetic and cathartic in large, doses. It is chiefly *used* as a diuretic in dropsies, and should not be given in quantities sufficient to purge when the former effect is desired; *fluidextractum apocyni* (*fluid extract of apocynum*); dose, ♏v–xxx (0.3–2.0 c.c.).

SCOPARIUS.

What is scoparius?

Scoparius is the *tops* of *Cytisus Scoparius*, or broom (*Fam.*

[1] National Dispensatory.

Leguminosæ), and contains a volatile liquid alkaloid, *sparteine*, and a neutral principle, *scoparin*, in which the diuretic properties are supposed to reside. Broom is an efficient hydragogue diuretic, and in large doses produces free purging and sometimes vomiting. It is much *used* in the treatment of *dropsies*, and is best given in decoction, ℥ss (15 c.c.) to water Oj (500 c.c.), boiled down to Oss (250 c.c.); dose, ℥j (30 c.c.) every two or three hours until an effect is produced; or the *fluid extract* (not official) may be given in doses of ʒss–j (2–4 c.c.).

Sparteine sulphate, dose, gr. $\frac{1}{6}$–j (0.01–0.06 gm.), has been much employed as a cardiac tonic, but the consensus of opinion among pharmacologists is that it is not such, but a depressant to the nerve-centers and endings, like coniine. It is, therefore, not a cardiac stimulant.

TARAXACUM.

What is taraxacum?

It is the *root* of *Taraxacum officinale* or dandelion (*Fam.* Compositæ), gathered in the autumn, and contains a bitter principle, *taraxacin;* also *taraxacerin*, *inulin*, resin, etc.

It is *diuretic*, laxative, bitter, and slightly cholagogue, and is *used* in dropsies of hepatic origin and dyspepsia with torpor of the liver. Dose of the *extract* (*extractum taraxaci*), gr. xx–ʒj (1.2–4.0 gm.), of the *fluid extract* (*fluidextractum taraxaci*) ʒj–ij (4–8 c.c.).

SPIRITUS ÆTHERIS NITROSI (SPIRIT OF NITROUS ETHER).

Is this medicine a diuretic?

Sweet spirit of niter is diuretic in large doses if the surface of the body is kept cool. It is usually combined with other diuretics, but may be given alone where the urinary secretion is scanty from simple congestion or from purely functional causes. It will be considered more fully under Diaphoretics. Dose, ʒj–iv (4–15 c.c.) freely diluted.

MERCURIALS.

Are the mercurial preparations ever used as diuretics?

Calomel (*q. v.*) has been employed as a diuretic in cardiac dropsy; dose, gr. ¼–iss (0.016–0.1 gm.) four or five times a day. It is a useful adjunct to squill in hydrothorax and hydropericardium.

Corrosive sublimate will probably prove to be a more powerful diuretic, as by its action on the liver it increases the formation of urea, which of itself always increases the excretion of water by the urine.

ALTERATIVE DIURETICS.

What are alterative diuretics?

They are medicines which are employed not only as diuretics, but also for their effect on the mucous membrane of the urinary tract, by which they are possibly to some extent excreted, or on which they exercise an alterant and sedative effect during their passage in the urine.

Name the medicines belonging to this group.

Buchu, pareira, uva ursi, chimaphila, triticum, juniper, oil of erigeron, oil of santal, stigmata maydis, turpentine, copaiba, cubeb, matico, cantharides.

BUCHU; PAREIRA.

What are these medicines?

Buchu, the *leaves* of *Barosma betulina* and *B. crenulata* (*Fam.* Rutaceæ), natives of South Africa, contains a *volatile oil* and a *bitter principle.* It is a mild tonic and diuretic, and slightly stimulates the genito-urinary mucous membranes, having also an alterative effect upon them.

It is *used* in chronic catarrhal conditions of the genito-urinary mucous tract, as *chronic pyelitis, chronic cystitis,* and especially in irritation of the neck of the bladder; dose of the *fluid extract* (*fluidextractum buchu*), ʒss–j (2–4 c.c.).

Pareira, the *root* of *Chondodendron tomentosum* (*Fam.* Menispermaceæ), a Brazilian plant, contains a bitter alkaloid *buxine,* and has been used with success in the treatment of *chronic cystitis, gleet,* and "*irritable bladder.*" It is said to be also tonic and laxative. Dose of the *fluid extract* (*fluidextractum pareiræ*), ʒss–j (2–4 c.c.).

UVA URSI; CHIMAPHILA.

What are these medicines?

UVA URSI is the *leaves* of *Arctostaphylos Uva-ursi*, or bearberry (*Fam.* Ericaceæ), and contains *tannic* and *gallic acid*, a glucosid called *arbutin*, *ericolin* (a bitter substance), etc. It is used as a mild astringent tonic and diuretic in *chronic pyelitis* and *cystitis*, and has also been employed in *chronic bronchitis*.

Arbutin is the diuretic principle, and as it is, partially at least, eliminated as hydroquinone it is supposed to act as an antiseptic to the urogenital tract. It has been employed in the above diseases and internally in *gonorrhea*.

Dose of the *fluid extract* (*fluidextractum uvæ ursi*), ʒss–ij (3–8 c.c.), t. i. d.

CHIMAPHILA, the *leaves* of *C. umbellata*, pipsissewa, wintergreen, or ground holly (*Fam.* Ericaceæ), contains *arbutin*, *tannic acid*, *chimaphilin*, etc. It is tonic, astringent, and diuretic, resembling buchu and uva ursi in its effects and uses. Special alterative qualities have been claimed for it in scrofulous affections.

Dose of the *fluid extract* (*fluidextractum chimaphilæ*), ʒss–j (2–4 c.c.), t. i. d.

TRITICUM.

What is triticum?

Triticum, the *rhizome* of *Agropyron repens*, or couch grass (*Fam.* Gramineæ), gathered in the spring, contains *triticin* and several *sugars*, and is feebly diuretic. It is useful in cystitis and in irritation of the neck of the bladder.

Dose of the *fluid extract* (*fluidextractum tritici*), ʒss–ij (2–8 c.c.).

OLEUM JUNIPERI (OIL OF JUNIPER).

What is oil of juniper?

Oil of juniper is a *volatile oil* distilled from the *fruit* of *Juniperus communis* (*Fam.* Coniferæ); dose, ♏v–xv (0.3–1 c.c.). It is a stimulant to the kidneys, capable in overdoses of causing strangury and bloody urine, and is sometimes used as an emmenagogue. It is chiefly employed as an adjuvant to other diuretics, particularly the alkaline group. As an *alterative diuretic* it is used in *chronic pyelitis* and *chronic cystitis.* It is sometimes given in *subacute renal congestion,* but is contraindicated where active inflammation is present. It is occasionally used as a *carminative* and *stomachic.* The preparations (official) are the *spirit* (*spiritus juniperi*), containing 5 per cent. of the oil; dose, ʒj–ij (4–8 c.c.); the *compound spirit* (*spiritus juniperi compositus*) contains also the oils of caraway and fennel in alcohol and water, and is about the same strength as *gin,* which is often used as a substitute for it; dose, ʒj–iv (4–15 c.c.).

OLEUM ERIGERONTIS (OIL OF ERIGERON).

What is the oil of erigeron?

It is the *volatile oil distilled* from the fresh flowering *herb* of *Erigeron canadense,* or Canada fleabane (*Fam.* Compositæ) and yields, on distillation, a *resin* and a *terpene,* It is *diuretic, hemostatic,* and *emmenagogue,* and is useful in hemorrhages due to relaxation of the genito-urinary mucous membrane. It has been used with success in *gonorrhea.* Dose, ♏v–xxx (0.3–2.0 c.c.) on sugar or in capsule, every two or three hours.

OLEUM SANTALI (OIL OF SANTAL).

What is the oil of santal?

It is a *volatile oil* (*Sandal-wood oil*) distilled from the *wood* of *Santalum album* (*Fam.* Santalaceæ). It is an *alterative, diuretic,* and *blennorrhetic,* sometimes causing vertigo, when its use should be discontinued or the dose decreased. Occasionally it produces gastro-intestinal irritation. It is used in the second stage of *gonorrhea,* and in *chronic bronchitis.* Dose, ♏v–xx (0.3–1.2 c.c.), in emulsion or capsule, t. i. d.

ZEA.

What is this substance?

Zea, or corn-silk, the *fresh styles* and *stigmas* of *Zea Mays,* or Indian corn (*Fam.* Gramineæ), is a mild, stimulating diuretic, and is strongly recommended in *cystitis,* both acute and chronic, in *gonorrhea,* in *irritability of the bladder* depending upon a highly concentrated urine, in *nocturnal incontinence* in children, and even in *cardiac dropsy*. It is given in infusion *ad libitum*, or in the form of *fluid extract* (unofficial), of which the dose is ʒj–ij (4–8 c.c.) every hour or two.

TEREBINTHINA (TURPENTINE).

What are the official varieties of turpentine?

1. TEREBINTHINA (*turpentine* or *white turpentine*) is a *concrete oleoresin* obtained from *Pinus palustris*, yellow or pitch pine, and other varieties of Pinus (*Fam.* Pinaceæ) trees indigenous to the Southern States.

2. TEREBINTHINA CANADENSIS (*Canada turpentine; Canada balsam* or *balsam of fir*) is a *liquid oleoresin* obtained from *Abies balsamea*, the American silver-fir, or balm of Gilead tree (*Fam.* Coniferæ), found in the northern portions of North America.

What do the turpentines contain?

They contain a *resin* or rosin (*resina*) and a *volatile oil* (*oleum terebinthinæ*).

What are the effects and uses of turpentine?

The *effects* of turpentine are those of the oil which it contains. It is rarely *used* internally, but has been given as an alterative to the bronchopulmonary and genito-urinary mucous membranes in chronic catarrhal conditions, and has been used as an anthelmintic, but for all these purposes the oil is preferred.

Dose as a *diuretic* and *blennorrhetic*, gr. xx–ʒj (1.3–4.0 gm.), in pill or emulsion; as an *anthelmintic*, ℥ss–j (15–30 gm.).

RESINA (*resin*) is used only externally as a basis for plasters and ointments. It enters into *ceratum resinæ* (*rosin cerate* or *basilicon ointment*), *ceratum resinæ compositum* (*compound rosin cerate*), and *ceratum cantharidis* (*cantharides cerate*).

OLEUM TEREBINTHINÆ (OIL OF TURPENTINE).

What is the oil of turpentine?

Oil of turpentine or spirit of turpentine is a *volatile oil distilled* from turpentine.

What are its effects and uses?

Locally it is rubefacient. *Internally* it is carminative, in large doses causing mental exhilaration and increasing the force and frequency of the pulse and proving cathartic. It is eliminated by the lungs and kidneys, imparting a violet-like odor to the urine. In *excessive doses* it is capable of causing death (rare). The symptoms of poisoning are unconsciousness, bloody, often suppressed, urine, and rapid, feeble pulse. Vomiting and strangury or purging sometimes occur, and occasionally the pupils are dilated. Small doses seem to increase the pulse-rate by direct action on the *heart,* while large doses stimulate the vagi and slow the heart. Moderate doses are diuretic, but when large amounts are given renal irritation results. It is *used* as an *alterative diuretic* in *chronic cystitis, gleet,* and *chronic pyelitis.* In *impotence* and *spermatorrhea* depending on relaxation it is sometimes employed. In *typhoid pneumonia* and *bronchitis* and in *hypostatic pulmonary congestion,* as in typhoid fever, it is often used externally and internally with the happiest effect. It is very useful in *ulceration of the stomach* or *intestines,* and in *typhoid fever* when the tongue becomes brown and dry, or cracked, red, and glazed, or when the ulcers are very slow to heal; it acts not only locally, but also as a cardiac stimulant. In *hemorrhages* from the lungs, stomach, or bowels, in *postpartum hemorrhages,* and in *purpura hæmorrhagica* it is sometimes useful. As an addition to stimulating enemata to cause the expulsion of flatus or to rouse the system in shock it is much resorted to. It is also used as an *anthelmintic.*

Locally as a counterirritant, either as a liniment or fomentation, it is much used in *bronchitis* and in *muscular rheumatism,* and in the latter manner in *peritonitis, hysteria, abdominal pains,* and *flatulency.* Dose, ♏v–xv (0.3–1.0 c.c.) four or five times daily in emulsion or capsule; as a cathartic enema or anthelmintic, f℥ss–j (15–30 c.c.) may be given. Externally a *liniment* (*linimentum terebinthinæ*) is employed, or the oil may be used either full strength or diluted with sweet oil. A saturated solution of camphor in oil of turpentine is a good rubefacient liniment.

Oleum Terebinthinæ Rectificatum (*rectified oil of turpentine*; dose, ♏v–xxx (0.3–2.0 c.c.).

COPAIBA.

What is copaiba?

Copaiba is an oleoresin derived from one or more South American species of *Copaiba* (*Fam.* Leguminosæ). It is cathartic, and sometimes emetic in large doses, slightly stimulates the circulation, and acts as an alterative blennorrhetic on the mucous membranes by which it is excreted. After large doses a resinous precipitate will occur if nitric acid be added to the urine, which, however, is soluble in alcohol. When the *resin* is taken in considerable quantities, the urine responds to the copper tests for sugar. Copaiba is chiefly eliminated by the genito-urinary mucous membranes and to a slight extent by the lungs. Its use is sometimes followed by urticaria. It is *used* in *chronic genito-urinary inflammations,* especially in *gonorrhea* after the subsidence of the acute stage. In *bronchorrhea* it is sometimes employed. The *oil* has been lauded as a hydragogue diuretic in dropsies when not of renal origin. The *dose of copaiba* is ♏x–ʒj (0.6–4.0 c.c.) or more, in emulsion, pill, or capsule. Of the *oil* (*oleum copaibæ*) the dose is ♏v–xv (0.3–1 c.c.) in emulsion or capsule.

CUBEBA (CUBEB).

What is cubeb?

Cubeb is the *unripe,* but *fully grown, fruit* of *Piper Cubeba* (*Fam.* Piperaceæ), an East Indian plant. It contains a *volatile oil,* a neutral principle (*cubebin*), and *cubebic acid.* Cubeb is diuretic and carminative, slightly accelerating the pulse. In large doses it often causes vomiting and purging. It is eliminated by the mucous membranes and urine, increasing the excretion of uric acid. Its use is sometimes followed by urticaria. The addition of nitric acid to the urine after the use of cubeb produces a resinous precipitate.

It is *used* in *gonorrhea* and is less apt than copaiba to disorder the digestion. It is also used in *bronchitis,* and has been smoked in cigarettes to relieve *sore throat* and *hoarseness.* The powder, used as a snuff, is employed in *coryza.* The *dose* of powdered cubeb is ʒss–iij (2–12 gm.); of the *oil* (*oleum cubebæ*), ♏x–xv (0.6–1 gm.), gradually increased. It is not so efficacious as the *oleoresin* (*oleoresina cubebæ*);

dose, ♏v–xxx (0.3–2.0 c.c.), given in emulsion. Of the *tincture* (not official) the dose is ʒj–ij (4–8 c.c.); of the *fluid extract* (*fluidextractum cubebæ*), ʒss–j (2–4 c.c.). The troches (*trochisci cubebæ*) each contain gr. ⅓ (0.02 gm.) of the oleoresin.

MATICO.

What is matico?

Matico is the *leaves* of *Piper angustifolium* (*Fam.* Piperaceæ), a shrub of Peru. It contains a *volatile oil, resin, artanthic* and *tannic acids*, etc. It is *used* as an *alterative blennorrhetic* in *gonorrhea*, as a *hemostatic* in *internal hemorrhages*, and locally as a *styptic*. Dose of the *fluid extract* (*fluidextractum matico*), ʒss–j (2–4 c.c.).

CANTHARIS (CANTHARIDES).

Is cantharides used as an alterative diuretic?

Cantharides is an intense stimulant and irritant to the kidneys, being diuretic in small doses, and frequently causing strangury, priapism, and bloody urine. It is sometimes used in *gleet*, and in spermatorrhea and impotence from weakness. It will be noticed at length under Epispastics. Dose of the *tincture* (*tinctura cantharidis*), ♏v–x (0.3–0.6 c.c.), t. i. d.

HEXAMETHYLENAMINA (*hexamethylene*), a condensation product of formaldehyde and ammonia, known also as *aminoform, cystogen, urotropin*, occurs in readily soluble crystals. It is said to give off formaldehyde in acid urine and to markedly reduce the number of bacteria in infected urine (cystitis, typhoid fever, etc.). Dose, gr. iij–viij (0.2–0.5 gm.), dissolved in plenty of water.

METHYLTHIONINÆ HYDROCHLORIDUM (*methylthionin hydrochlorid; methylene blue*) is a dark-green crystalline powder which makes a deep-blue solution in water. It has been given for *neuralgia, sciatica*, and *ataxic* pains, and in *malaria*, with only partial success. It stains the urine greenish when taken internally, and is somewhat a *urinary disin-*

fectant. It is employed also as a general stain in bacterial and blood work. The dose is gr. ij–v (0.12–0.3 gm.) in capsule.

DIAPHORETICS.

What are diaphoretics?

Diaphoretics are medicines which increase the secretion of sweat, either—(1) by stimulating the secretory nerve-fibers in the glands; (2) by stimulating the nerve-center governing the secretion of sweat; or (3) by relaxing the skin, dilating the blood-vessels, and regulating the force of the circulation.

For what purposes are they used and how are they classified?

They are used—(1) To abort an oncoming disease (as a catarrh or inflammation of mucous or serous membranes after exposure to cold), or aid in its subsidence (as in the paroxysm of a malarial fever); (2) to aid absorption, as in dropsies; and (3) to eliminate poisons from the blood.

They are divided into nauseating, sedative, saline, and special diaphoretics.

Nauseating Diaphoretics.

What are the nauseating diaphoretics?

The act of emesis is accompanied by general relaxation and diaphoresis, and even in nausea a more or less pronounced perspiration occurs. Any of the emetics in doses just sufficient to nauseate will produce this effect, but the only one which is in general use for this purpose is IPECAC (*vid.* Emetics), which is used either alone (in doses of gr. ss–j every two hours) or combined with opium in the form of DOVER'S POWDER (*vid.* Opium) in the early stages of *inflammations*, in "*cold,*" in *muscular rheumatism*, and in acute *suppression of the menses* to break up the train of morbid symptoms.

Sedative Diaphoretics.

What are sedative diaphoretics?

When the circulation is much excited, as in fevers and inflammations generally, medicines which tend to reduce the force and rapidity of the circulation and to lower the temperature act as diaphoretics. Many of these agents (particularly *antimonials, aconite,* and *veratrum viride*) tend to nauseate or even to cause vomiting when given in full doses. In *sthenic inflammations* the ANTIMONIAL PREPARATIONS (*q. v.*), especially if combined with minute doses of morphine, are often very efficacious, and may be used in the *early stages of laryngitis* and *bronchitis* and in combination with other remedies in fever. ACONITE and VERATRUM are also sometimes resorted to in the early stages of sthenic inflammations for their combined sedative and sudorific effect. In this group also should be placed SALICYLIC ACID and other ANTIPYRETICS (*q. v.*) which produce more or less profuse perspiration.

Saline Diaphoretics.

What are the saline diaphoretics?

While some of the saline diaphoretics have a sedative effect upon the circulation, which is not, however, so marked as from the remedies of the preceding group, they have no tendency to nauseate even when given in large doses; on the contrary, they are acceptable to the stomach, and form the basis of most fever mixtures.

POTASSIUM CITRATE and its preparations have been noticed among the Diuretics.

LIQUOR AMMONII ACETATIS (SOLUTION OF AMMONIUM ACETATE).

What is the solution of ammonium acetate?

The *solution of ammonium acetate* or *spirit of Mindererus* is a mild stimulant, diaphoretic, and diuretic, often employed in febrile and inflammatory affections combined with other remedies. Dose, ℥ss–j (15–30 c.c.).

SPIRITUS ÆTHERIS NITROSI (SPIRIT OF NITROUS ETHER).

What is this substance?

Spirit of nitrous ether, or *sweet spirit of niter,* is a solution of about 4 per cent. of nitrous ether (ethyl nitrite) in alcohol. In *small doses* it is a diaphoretic and stimulant; in *larger doses* an antispasmodic, and, if the skin be kept cool, diuretic; in *excessive doses*, either internally or when inhaled, it is a depressomotor, acting similarly to the other nitrites (*q. v.*) and capable of causing death. It is much *used* as a diaphoretic in *fevers*, and occasionally as a diuretic (*q. v.*) and antispasmodic for nervous children. *Dose* for an *adult*, ʒj–iv (4–15 c.c.). It is given as a diaphoretic in minute doses, frequently repeated and largely diluted, the body being kept warm.

Special Diaphoretics.

PILOCARPUS.

What is pilocarpus?

Pilocarpus, or *jaborandi*, is the *leaflets* of *P. Jaborandi* or of *P. microphyllus* (*Fam.* Rutaceæ), a Brazilian shrub, and contains not less than 0.5 per cent. of alkaloids.

What are its chief chemic constituents?

It contains an alkaloid, *pilocarpine*, and a *volatile oil;* a second alkaloid, *jaborine*, probably a derivative of pilocarpine, has been isolated, and lately two other derivative alkaloids, *pilocarpidine* and *jaborandine*, have been described.

What are the physiologic effects of these substances?

In medicinal doses *pilocarpine*, by acting on the ends of the secretory nerves, stimulates the salivary, lachrimal, and skin-glands, the mucous glands of the mouth, nose, bronchi, etc., and probably the digestive glands. Bile, urine, and milk are not increased. The solid as well as the fluid portions of the secretions are increased. The face is flushed, respiration quickened, and the pupil contracted; the heart is strong and at first rapid, but is soon slowed. It seems to stimulate the nutrition of the hair and to increase the leukocytes in the blood. Applied to the eye it contracts the pupil (by peripheral action) and increases the tension of accommodation. *Pilocarpine* and *atropine* are antagonists as regards their action on the heart, intestine, and pupil, and on the secretions of perspiration and saliva. *Jaborine* acts upon the heart, pupil, intestine, and salivary glands like atropine.

Pilocarpidine causes profuse diaphoresis, salivation, vomiting, and purging; while *jaborandine* resembles atropine in its cardiac effects.

What are the medicinal uses of pilocarpus and its alkaloid?

Pilocarpus or pilocarpine is used as a *diaphoretic* to abort disease in incipient catarrh and at the onset of a paroxysm of malarial fever, and to aid in the removal of dropsical effusions, especially when the kidneys are impaired. Its use is limited, as it is followed by much depression. In the night-sweats of tuberculosis it is useful by stimulating the glands to normal functioning.

In 1 per cent. solution it is employed to contract the pupil in glaucoma. To stimulate the growth of hair in *alopecia*, pilocarpine may be administered internally or hypodermically, and applied locally as well, and it has been employed hypodermically with success to lessen severe and prolonged hiccup, and congestion of the labyrinth of the ear.

It should *not be given* in diseases of the gastro-intestinal mucous membrane, nor in weak heart due to cardiac disease.

What are the official preparations of pilocarpus and their doses?

FLUIDEXTRACTUM PILOCARPI (*fluid extract of pilocarpus*); dose, ʒss–j (2–4 c.c.).

PILOCARPINÆ HYDROCHLORIDUM (*pilocarpine hydrochlorid* and PILOCARPINÆ NITRAS (*pilocarpine nitrate*); dose, gr. $\frac{1}{8}$–ss (0.008–0.03 c.c.) are well adapted to hypodermic use.

EXPECTORANTS.

What are expectorants?

Expectorants are remedies which are given to modify the secretions of, and promote their expulsion from, the air-passages.

How may they be classified?

They are divided into sedative and stimulating expectorants.

Sedative Expectorants.

What are sedative expectorants?

They are remedies which increase the secretion and at the same time tend to lower the blood-pressure, cause nausea, and, if frequently repeated, vomiting.

Name the sedative expectorants.

Ipecac, apomorphine, tartar emetic, pilocarpine, lobelia, and grindelia. Of these, ipecac and apomorphine have been discussed with the Emetics, tartar emetic with the Sedatives, pilocarpine with the Diaphoretics, and lobelia with the Depressomotors.

GRINDELIA.

What is grindelia?

Grindelia is the *leaves* and *flowering tops* of *G. robusta* and *G. squarrosa* (*Fam.* Compositæ). It appears to depress the motor nerves and muscles, and in large doses to slow the heart and reduce the blood-pressure. Toxic doses produce narcosis with dilated pupils. It is eliminated by the kidneys, increasing the flow of urine, and to some extent by the bronchopulmonary mucous membrane. It has been highly recommended in *spasmodic* and *cardiac asthma*, in *hay-asthma* and *hay-fever*, in *whooping-cough*, and in *acute* and *chronic bronchitis*. In *chronic cystitis* it has been advantageously employed, and as a *local* application in *vaginitis* and in *poisoning* by rhus toxicodendron has met with some success. Dose of the *fluid extract* (*fluidextractum grindeliæ*), ♏x–ʒj (0.6–4.0 c.c.).

Stimulating Expectorants.

What are stimulating expectorants?

They are remedies which probably modify the secretion by toning up the bronchopulmonary mucous membrane through which they are eliminated. Most of them seem to exert an alterative effect in passing through the membrane, and many of them elevate the arterial tension.

Name the stimulating expectorants.

Ammonium salts, senega, quillaja, quebracho, asclepias,

eriodictyon, garlic, sanguinaria, ammoniac, benzoin, Peruvian balsam, balsam of Tolu, squill, eucalyptus, serpentaria, turpentine, tar, terpin hydrate, and terebene.

What ammonium salts are used as expectorants, and what is their action?

The carbonate and chlorid are used. The ammonium compounds are slightly stimulating to the heart and respiration, and increase the secretions of the skin and bronchial and salivary glands. They fluidify the bronchial mucus.

AMMONII CHLORIDUM (AMMONIUM CHLORID).

What is ammonium chlorid?

Ammonium chlorid, called also *ammonium muriate* or *sal ammoniac*, is a crystalline salt obtained from gas liquor.

What are its effects and uses?

Locally it is irritant. In medicinal doses it is believed to influence especially the mucous membranes, promoting very decidedly nutritive changes and hastening epithelial exfoliation. It is thus considered to be an alterative. When given continuously for a length of time, it diminishes the solids of the blood and stimulates the secretions. It is supposed to stimulate the hepatic functions. The amount of urea excreted is greatly increased, as are all the other solids of the urine except uric acid. Large doses are purgative. It is used as a *stimulating* and *alterative expectorant* in the moist stage of *acute* and in *chronic bronchitis*, in *pneumonia* and the various *catarrhs* of children. Abroad it is employed also in *gastric* and *intestinal catarrhs*, in *chronic hepatitis*, and in the early stages of *hepatic cirrhosis*. In cases of *albuminoid liver, spleen*, or *kidneys* it is very useful. In subacute *muscular rheumatism* and in *neuralgia*, especially ovarian, it is advantageous, and it has been used internally as an alterative and employed locally as a sorbefacient in scrofulous *adenitis of the cervical glands* and *uterine fibroid tumors*.

Dose, gr. x–xxx (0.6–2.0 gm.). The unpleasant taste may be partially disguised by licorice. The *troches* (*trochisci ammonii chloridi*) each contain about gr. ij (0.12 gm.) of the salt.

SENEGA.

What is senega?

Senega is the *root* of *Polygala Senega*, or senega snake-root (*Fam.* Polygalaceæ), and contains *polygalic acid* or *senegin*, a glucosid identical with *saponin*.

What are its effects and uses?

Locally it is an irritant. *Internally* it stimulates the mucous membranes, and in large doses is emetic and cathartic. It is given as a *stimulating expectorant* in the latter stages of acute and in subacute and chronic *bronchitis*, especially when the mucous membranes are wanting in tone. It has also been used as an *emmenagogue* in *amenorrhea* and as a *diuretic* in dropsies. Dose of the *fluid extract* (*fluidextractum senegæ*), ♏x–xx (0.6–1.2 c.c.); of the *syrup* (*syrupus senegæ*), ʒj–ij (4–8 c.c.). It is an ingredient of the *compound syrup of squill*.

QUILLAJA.

What is quillaja?

Quillaja, or soap-bark, is the *inner bark* of *Q. Saponaria* (*Fam.* Rosaceæ), a South American tree, containing *saponin*, which foams like soap when in infusion. *Locally*, *saponin* is an irritant and protoplasmic poison. Given *internally* in sufficient doses it is a nerve and muscle poison, and completely antagonizes the effects of digitalis on the heart, which it paralyzes in diastole. It increases the secretion of bronchial mucus. Quillaja has been *used* as an *expectorant* in *chronic bronchitis*, *emphysema*, and *dilated bronchi*. It is also used to aid in emulsifying oils. Dose of the *tincture* (*tinctura quillajæ*), ♏xv–xxx (1–2 c.c.), and of the *fluid extract* (*fluidextractum quillajæ*), ♏ij–v (0.12–0.3 c.c.).

ASPIDOSPERMA.

What is aspidosperma?

Aspidosperma, or *quebracho* (not official), is the *bark* of *A. Quebrachoblancho* (*Fam.* Apocynaceæ). It contains five alkaloids, *aspidospermatine*, *aspidospermine*, *quebrachine*, *hypoquebrachine*, and *quebrachamine*. It has been used in *dyspnea* independent of cause, but as it appears to have no action on the heart or kidney, it probably is of service only in *bronchial asthma* and *emphysema.* It has also been used as a *bitter tonic.* Dose of the *fluid extract,* ♏xv–ʒj (1–4 c.c.).

ERIODICTYON.

What is eriodictyon?

It is the *leaves* of *E. californicum,* or California tar-bush (*Fam.* Hydrophyllaceæ), and is known also as *yerba santa.* It is used as an *expectorant* in *chronic pulmonary disorders,* and, as it lessens the appreciation of bitter tastes, is used as a *vehicle,* in the form of elixir, to disguise the taste of quinine and other bitter drugs. Dose of the *fluid extract* (*fluidextractum eriodictyi*), ♏xx–ʒj (1.2–4.0 c.c.).

ALLIUM (GARLIC).

What is garlic?

Garlic (not official) is the *bulb* of *Allium sativum* (*Fam.* Liliaceæ) and contains a very volatile *oil.* *Locally* applied it is a rubefacient. Taken *internally* it is a condiment, stimulating digestion, increasing the secretions generally, especially the bronchopulmonary, and quickening the circulation. It is *used as a stimulating expectorant* in subacute and chronic *bronchitis* and in *acute bronchitis of infants,* especially when the disease begins to assume the capillary form. Externally it is used as a counterirritant in the above diseases, and in infantile convulsions, applied to the spine, legs, and feet in the form of a poultice. Dose of the *syrup* (*syrupus allii*), ʒj (4 c.c.) for a child.

SANGUINARIA.

What is sanguinaria?

Sanguinaria, or blood-root, the *rhizome* of *S. canadensis* (*Fam.* Papaveraceæ), collected after the death of the foliage, contains an alkaloid, *sanguinarine.* It is a *local* irritant. *Large doses* cause vomiting with great depression, a slow irregular pulse (from direct action on the heart), and lowered blood-pressure, dilated pupil, collapse, and death from paralysis of the respiratory center, sometimes preceded by convulsions of spinal origin and lowered reflex activity. *Moderate doses* increase the arterial pressure from stimulation of the vasomotor centers, which are paralyzed by larger doses. It stimulates the liver, the mucous membranes, and the salivary and intestinal glands. It is used chiefly as a *stimulating expectorant* in lingering cases of *bronchitis.* Dose of the *tincture* (*tinctura sanguinariæ*), ℞v–xxx (0.3–2.0 c.c.); of the *fluid extract* (*fluidextractum sanguinariæ*), ℞ij–v (0.12–0.3 c.c.). *Sanguinarine* (not official) has also been used as an expectorant in the dose of gr. $\frac{1}{12}$–$\frac{1}{8}$ (0.005–0.008 gm.).

AMMONIACUM (AMMONIAC).

What is ammoniac?

Ammoniac (not official) is a *gum-resin* obtained from *Dorema Ammoniacum* (*Fam.* Umbelliferæ). It is used internally as a *stimulating expectorant* in *chronic bronchitis* and in *bronchorrhea,* and locally as a *counterirritant.* Dose, gr. x–xxx (0.6–2.0 gm.).

BENZOINUM (BENZOIN).

What is benzoin?

Benzoin, a *balsamic resin* obtained from *Styrax Benzoin,* or Benjamin tree, and another unidentified species of *Styrax* (*Fam.* Styraceæ), contains *benzoic acid, resin, volatile oil,* and often *cinnamic acid.*

Some of the effects of benzoin are due to *benzoic acid* (*vid.* Antiseptics). *Locally* it is an irritant. Internally it stimulates the bronchopulmonary and genito-urinary mucous membrane. It is eliminated chiefly by the urine as hippuric acid, increasing the acidity of that excretion.

It is chiefly *used* by inhalation (compound tincture ʒj (4 c.c.), in a cupful (120 c.c.) of boiling water) in *laryngitis,* or to quiet spasmodic laryngeal cough, as in influenza. It has also been employed internally in *chronic bronchitis* and in *chronic cystitis with alkaline urine and phosphatic deposits,* but for the latter purpose benzoic acid or its salts are preferred. It is added to ointments to prevent rancidity, and is much employed in the form of fumigating pastilles, or added to the water in a croup-kettle, or as a wash for the complexion. It is also used locally as an *antiseptic and protective* (*compound tincture*) in *fissured nipple, chapped hands,* and *fissure of the anus,* and has even been employed as a substitute for carbolic and salicylic acids, for its antiseptic effects, in the *treatment of wounds.* Dose of the *tincture* (*tinctura benzoini*), ʒss–j (2–4 c.c.); of the *compound tincture* (*tinctura benzoini composita*), ʒss–ij (2–8 c.c.).

Benzoinated lard (*adeps benzoinatus*) contains 2 per cent. of benzoin.

BALSAMUM PERUVIANUM (BALSAM OF PERU). BALSAMUM TOLUTANUM (BALSAM OF TOLU).

What are these substances?

BALSAM OF PERU is a *balsam* obtained from *Toluifera Pereiræ* (*Fam.* Leguminosæ), and contains *cinnamein, resin, benzylic benzoate,* and *cinnamic* and *benzoic acids.*

It is a stimulant and tonic to the mucous membranes, and has been used in various catarrhs. Dose, ʒss (2 c.c.) in emulsion. In the form of "balsam gauze" it is much used as a stimulant to the formation of granulations in wounds, ulcers, etc.

BALSAM OF TOLU is a *balsam* obtained from *Toluifera Balsamum* (*Fam.* Leguminosæ), and contains *resins, benzylic benzoate,* and *cinnamate, tolene,* and *cinnamic* and *benzoic acids.* Its effects and uses are similar to those of balsam of Peru, to which it is preferred for internal use because of its more pleasant taste. Dose, gr. x–xxx (0.6–2.0 gm.) in emulsion, every few hours. It is, however, principally used as a vehicle. Dose of the *tincture* (*tinctura tolutana*) is ʒj–ij (4–8 c.c.); of the *syrup* (*syrupus tolutanus*), ʒj–iv (4–15 c.c.). It is also an ingredient of the *compound tincture of benzoin.*

PIX LIQUIDA (TAR).

What is tar?

Tar is a product obtained by destructive distillation of the wood of *Pinus palustris* and other species of Pinus (*Fam.* Pinaceæ). When distilled, it yields *pyroligneous acid, oil of tar*, and a black residuum known as *pitch*. The *oil of tar* contains *creosote*. Tar resembles turpentine in its effects on the mucous membranes, but is more *antiseptic*. *Externally* it is an *irritant*. It is used as a *stimulating expectorant* in the later stages of *acute bronchitis*, particularly where the disease does not yield readily to other treatment, and in *chronic bronchitis*. *Externally* it is employed in *chronic skin-diseases*, especially in chronic eczema.

Tar-water (not official) may be given in doses of ℥ss–j(15–30 c.c.), or the syrup (*syrupus picis liquidæ*), which is better, in doses of ℥ss (15 c.c.). *Locally*, the *oil* (*oleum picis liquidæ*) is used as a substitute for "oil of cade" (*oleum cadinum*), which is also official, or the *ointment* (*unguentum picis liquidæ*) may be applied.

TERPINI HYDRAS (TERPIN HYDRATE).

What is terpin hydrate?

It is the *hydrate* of the diatomic alcohol *terpin*. It occurs in colorless, rhombic, lustrous prisms; is odorless, but has a slightly aromatic, rather bitter taste.

It *acts* on the *nervous system* and on *mucous membranes* in a manner similar to turpentine. It is eliminated by the urine, to which it imparts a turpentine odor. When given in large doses or for a long time it may cause strangury, albuminuria, or even hematuria.

From its stimulating influence on mucous membranes it has been much *used* as an *expectorant* in *bronchitis*, either acute or chronic, especially when the secretion is very free.

It has also been used in *cystitis*, in *gonorrhea*, and in *chronic kidney disease*. Dose, gr. j–iij (0.06–0.2 gm.) every four hours, in pill or capsule.

TEREBENUM (TEREBENE).

What is terebene?

Terebene is a liquid consisting of *dipentene* and other hydrocarbons, obtained by the action of concentrated sulphuric acid in oil of turpentine. In its general effect it resembles turpentine. It is a good *stimulating expectorant*, very useful in the declining stages of *acute* and *chronic bronchitis.* It is also useful in *emphysema, phthisis,* and *pleurisy.* In *fetid bronchitis* and *bronchiectasis* it is very efficacious. It has also been employed in *flatulent dyspepsia* and *genito-urinary inflammation.* Dose, ♏v–xx (0.3–1.2 c.c.), in capsule or emulsion t. i. d., or its vapor may be inhaled diluted with steam.

What substances are often used as expectorants which have been previously considered in other medicinal groups?

Squill and turpentine (*vid.* Diuretics), eucalyptus, serpentaria, and prunus virginiana (*vid.* Aromatic Bitters).

ASTRINGENTS.

What are astringents?

Astringents are remedies employed to cause contraction of the tissues with which they come in contact and thus lessen secretion.

For what purposes are they used?

They are used to check profuse secretion (*e. g.*, ptyalism, etc.) or morbid discharges (*e. g.*, diarrhea), to overcome relaxation of the tissues, and as hemostatics and styptics.

How may the astringents be classified?

They are divided into vegetable and mineral astringents.

Vegetable Astringents.

What are the vegetable astringents?

They are tannic and gallic acids, and the various plants which are used as astringents on account of containing these principles.

Name the vegetable astringents.

Tannic acid, gallic acid, nutgalls, catechu, kino, krameria, hematoxylon, white oak, geranium, witch-hazel, red rose, sumac, chestnut leaves, and gambir.

ACIDUM TANNICUM (TANNIC ACID).

What is tannic acid?

Tannic acid (*gallotannic acid; digallic acid*) is a monobasic *organic acid* obtained from nutgall. It is widely distributed throughout the vegetable kingdom, and exists under two forms, *gallotannic acid* (which is the official variety and strikes a blue-black color with the ferric salts) and *kinotannic acid* (which produces a greenish-black color with the same salts). Gallotannic acid is a light yellowish, amorphous powder, usually cohering in the form of glistening scales or spongy masses, without smell, but having a strongly astringent taste.

It is freely soluble in water and in alcohol, and may readily be dissolved in glycerin by the aid of moderate heat.

What are its physiologic effects?

Tannic acid is a powerful astringent, coagulating albumins, contracting blood-vessels, and constringing tissues with which it comes in contact. It checks the secretions of the alimentary canal when taken internally, and restrains peristalsis, thus tending to constipate. It is converted into an alkaline tannate and into gallic acid in the *primæ viæ*, and slowly absorbed. It is eliminated by the feces and urine under its own form and as gallic and pyrogallic acids.

For what purposes is it used in medicine?

Tannic acid is employed whenever the part to be acted on is so situated that the drug can come in direct contact with it. Thus, it is given to *arrest morbid discharges* from the bowels in *diarrhea* and *dysentery*, both internally and by enema, and is used externally for the same purpose in *leukorrhea, gleet, colliquative sweating*, and as an application to *chronic ulcers*. To *counteract relaxation of tissues* it is employed in the treatment of *spongy gums, chronic pharyngitis* and *laryngitis, mercurial stomatitis*, and *hemorrhoids*. It is also used to *arrest hemorrhage* from the nose, gums, pharynx, stomach, and bowels, to *harden tissues* subjected to pressure, as in threatened bed-sores and tender feet, and as an *antidote* to *antimony* and other metallic poisons and alkaloidal poisons.

Dose, in diarrhea, gr. j–xv (0.06–1.0 gm.) in pill, in hemorrhage, gr. v–xx (0.3–1.3 gm.) in powder. The *troches* (*trochisci acidi tannici*) each contain gr. j. (0.06 gm.), and may be used for relaxed palate or sore throat.

The *ointment* (*unguentum acidi tannici*), the *collodion* (*collodium stypticum*), or the *glycerite* (*glyceritum acidi tannici*), a solution in glycerin, may be used locally.

ACIDUM GALLICUM (GALLIC ACID).

What is gallic acid?

Gallic acid is an *organic acid*, usually prepared from *tannic acid*, and is tannic acid + a molecule of water; thus $HC_{14}H_9O_9$ (tannic acid) + $3H_2O = 2(HC_7H_5O_5 + H_2O)$, gallic acid. It occurs as white or pale-fawn-colored, silky, interlaced needles or triclinic prisms; odorless, having an astringent or slightly acidulous taste. It is very soluble in boiling alcohol and boiling water, less so in cold alcohol, glycerin, ether, or cold water. It does not coagulate albumin, and hence is not so efficacious as a local astringent, but is preferred to tannic acid when it is desirable that the astringent should be absorbed and act through the blood on some remote part. It is a question whether or not an astringent action can be thus produced. It is used as a *hemostatic* in *hemoptysis*, *hematuria*, and *uterine hemorrhage*. It is also employed to *lessen secretion*, as in *colliquative sweats* and *bronchorrhea*, and to *check morbid discharges*, as in *chronic albuminuria*. Dose, gr. v–xxx (0.3–2.0 gm.), in powder, pill, or solution.

Describe the preparations, doses, and uses of the vegetable astringents which owe their virtues to tannic and gallic acids.

GALLA (*nutgall*) is an *excrescence* on *Quercus infectoria*, the gall oak (*Fam.* Cupuliferæ), caused by the punctures and deposited ova of a fly (*Cynips tinctoria*). Before the maturity of the larvæ and their escape from the gall, the galls contain *tannic acid* (50 to 60 per cent.) and *gallic acid* (3 per cent.); afterward they are much inferior and contain comparatively little of these substances.

They are but little used except as the source of tannic and gallic acids. The *tincture* (*tinctura gallæ*) is chiefly used as a chemic test. The *ointment* (*unguentum gallæ*), combined with powdered opium, is sometimes applied to hemorrhoids.

GAMBIR; CATECHU.

CATECHU, an *extract* prepared from the *wood* of *Acacia catechu* (*Fam.* Leguminosæ), is no longer official, and has been replaced by GAMBIR, an extract prepared from the leaves and twigs of *Ourouparia Gambir* (*Fam.* Rubiaceæ). *Gambir* is a powerful astringent, much used in *diarrheas* and to some extent in *hemorrhages*, and locally as an *astringent* in sore throat, as an injection in *gonorrhea* and *leukorrhea*, and as a *styptic*. Dose, gr. x–xxx (0.6–2.0 gm.), in emulsion or capsules. Of the *compound tincture* (*tinctura gambir composita*), ʒj–iij (4–12 c.c.) may be given. The *troches* (*trochisci gambir*) each contain gr. j (0.06 gm.).

KINO, the *inspissated juice of Pterocarpus Marsupium* (*Fam.* Leguminosæ), contains *kinotannic acid, kinoïn, pyrocatechin*, etc., and has similar properties and uses to catechu. Dose of the powder, gr. x–xxx (0.6–2.0 gm.); of the *tincture* (*tinctura kino*), ʒj–ij (4–8 c.c.).

KRAMERIA, the *root* of *K. triandra, K. ixina*, and *K. argentea* (*Fam.* Krameriaceæ), South American shrubs, contains *kramerotannic acid*, and is a powerful astringent, similar to kino and catechu. Dose of the *extract* (*extractum krameriæ*), gr. v–xv (0.3–1.0 gm.); of the *fluid extract* (*fluidextractum krameriæ*), ʒss–j (2–4 c.c.); of the *tincture* (*tinctura krameriæ*), ʒss–ij (2–8 c.c.); of the *syrup* (*syrupus krameriæ*), ʒj–iv (4–15 c.c.). The *troches* (*trochisci krameriæ*) each contain gr. j (0.06 gm.).

HÆMATOXLYON, logwood or Campeachy wood, is the *heartwood* of *H. campechianum* (*Fam.* Leguminosæ), containing *tannic acid, hematoxylon*, etc. It is a good astringent in diarrheas due to relaxation, especially in children, but the discharges will stain the linen blood-red. Of the *extract* (*extractum hæmatoxyli*), the dose is gr. x–xxx (0.6–2.0 gm.).

QUERCUS, or white oak (*Fam.* Cupuliferæ); the *bark* is official, and contains *quercitannic acid*. It is occasionally used in *diarrheas*, but more often as an enema in *hemorrhoids* and *prolapsus ani*, or as a vaginal wash in *leukorrhea* or relaxed conditions with tendency to cystocele or rectocele. It makes an indelible stain on linen. The dose of the *fluid extract* (*fluidextractum quercus*) is ℳx–xxx (0.7–2.0 c.c.).

GERANIUM, the *rhizome* of *G. maculatum*, crow's foot or crane's bill (*Fam.* Geraniaceæ), contains *tannic* and *gallic acids*, and is an efficient indigenous astringent. Dose of the *fluid extract* (*fluidextractum geranii*), ʒss–j (2–4 c.c.).

HAMAMELIS, the *leaves* and the *bark and twigs* of *H. virginiana*, or witch-hazel (*Fam.* Hamamelidaceæ), contains *tannic acid*, a *bitter principle*, and a volatile oil. It is an astringent and seems to contract the veins of the skin and mucous membranes. It has been used in passive hemorrhages as a hemostatic, as an astringent enema or suppository in hemorrhoids, and locally in congestions and inflammations. Dose of the *fluid extract* (*fluidextractum hamamelidis*), ʒss–j (2–4 c.c.) The colorless "extract of witch-hazel" sold in the stores is a watery and alcoholic distillate of the leaves and twigs, and is official under the name of *aqua hamamelidis* (*hamamelis water*). It contains volatile oil, but no tannic acid.

ROSA GALLICA (*red rose*) (*Fam.* Rosaceæ) is the *petals* collected before expanding. It is a very mild astringent, and is used as a flavoring ingredient. The preparations of red rose are a *fluid extract* (*fluidextractum rosæ*), a *honey* (*mel rosæ*), a *syrup* (*syrupus rosæ*), and a *confection* (*confectio rosæ*). *Stronger rose water* (*aqua rosæ fortior*), and another milder *water* (*aqua rosæ*), from which is made an *ointment* (*unguentum aquæ rosæ; cold cream*), are also official.

RHUS GLABRA (*sumach*) (*Fam.* Anacardiaceæ). The *fruit* is official. It is a good astringent in sore mouth and pharyngitis. The *fluid extract* (*fluidextractum rhoïs glabræ*) may be diluted with two or more parts of water and used as a gargle.

Mineral Astringents.

Name the mineral astringents.

Most of the metallic salts possess astringent properties, but those especially used for this purpose are the lead salts, aluminium salts, the salts of copper, of zinc, of silver, and of bismuth, and cerium oxalate.

PLUMBUM (LEAD).

What is the source of lead?

Lead is obtained by roasting *galena,* the native sulphid.

What are its physiologic actions?

Metallic lead is inert, as are probably also the *sulphid* and *sulphate,* *All other salts of lead,* when *applied locally* in solution, are astringent, or if the solution be strong, irritant. In medicinal doses they are astringent to the alimentary canal, decreasing its secretions and also the secretion of bile. They are but slowly absorbed. When taken for some time, they reduce the volume and frequency of the pulse by stimulation of the cardio-inhibitory center and the peripheral filaments of the vagi. They are *eliminated* by the liver and kidneys.

What are its toxicologic actions?

In large doses several of the lead salts are capable of causing *acute poisoning,* the symptoms being intense gastro-intestinal irritation, vomiting, coma, paralysis, and collapse.

Chronic poisoning is caused by saturation of the system with lead either by drinking pure water conveyed in lead pipes (the contained air forming a soluble oxid), constantly eating substances adulterated with lead salts, exposure in lead factories, handling paint containing white lead, etc. *Lead colic* (or painters' colic), the most common form, consists of sharp pains about the umbilicus, obstinate constipation, hard, contracted abdomen, and often nausea and vomiting. This is probably due to intense stimulation of the intestinal ganglia by the lead, causing arrest of peristalsis and spasm of the muscular coat of the bowel. It is quickly relieved by belladonna, atropine, or pilocarpine. Sometimes the poisoning takes the form of *lead arthralgia,* manifesting itself by severe pains in the joints and limbs and cramps; or *lead encephalopathy,* with severe headache and cerebral symptoms.

Lead paralysis is loss of voluntary motion in groups of

muscles, particularly the flexors of the upper extremity, causing *wrist-drop*. Electromuscular contractility is affected, the muscles waste, and often anesthesia of the affected or opposite side is present. The poison may also affect the brain, kidney, or other organs. An important symptom of lead-poisoning is a *blue line upon the gums where they join the teeth*, and in case of doubt lead may be detected in the urine by the chemic tests.

What are the tests for lead, and how should saturnine poisoning be treated?

Sulphuretted hydrogen, gives a *black*, and a solution of *potassium iodid* a *yellow, precipitate* with soluble lead salts. The *treatment* of *acute poisoning* consists in evacuating the contents of the stomach and administering diluted sulphuric acid, or sodium or magnesium sulphate as a chemic antidote. In *chronic poisoning*, discover its source and remove it (in the case of painters, insist on scrupulous cleanliness of the hands and nails, and the use of very diluted sulphuric acid as a drink); give purgatives to overcome the resulting constipation; give diluted sulphuric acid or the soluble sulphates, with baths of potassium sulphid as antidotes, and aid elimination by large quantities of diluents and potassium iodid. In *lead colic* atropine is of service, and in *lead palsies* electricity (the faradic current when the muscles respond) and strychnine are advantageously employed.

For what medicinal purposes are the lead salts used?

They are used *internally* as *astringents* in *diarrheas* and *dysenteries*, as *hemostatics*, and in the treatment of *internal aneurysm*. Locally, as *astringent injections* in *leukorrhea* and *gonorrhea* and as *sedative* and *astringent lotions* in *inflammations*. The *acetate* is the only lead salt which is administered internally.

What are the preparations of lead and their uses?

Plumbi Oxidum (*lead oxid*), or *litharge*, is occasionally used as a dusting-powder for ulcers, but is chiefly employed to make a *plaster* (*emplastrum plumbi*), which is a basis for medicated plasters; *diachylon ointment* (*unguentum diachylon*) is useful in skin diseases.

PLUMBI ACETAS (*lead acetate* or *sugar of lead*) is used *internally* as an *astringent* in *diarrhea*, often combined with opium, and is also useful in *dysentery*. To lessen the expectoration in *chronic bronchitis* and to check the *night-sweats of phthisis* it is sometimes given. As a *hemostatic* in yellow fever it does some good, and perhaps also in *hemoptysis*. It has been employed as a *sedative* in the treatment of internal *aneurysm*. *Locally* as a *sedative* and *astringent* lotion it is much used in inflammations (not applicable to ocular therapeutics, as it may cause corneal opacity), and to check morbid discharges. Dose, gr. j–viij (0.06–0.5 gm.) two or three times a day. As an injection in gonorrhea, gr. ss–ij (0.03–0.12 gm.)–f℥j (30 c.c.); as a lotion in inflammation, gr. v–x (0.3–0.6 gm.)–f℥j (30 c.c.).

LIQUOR PLUMBI SUBACETATIS (*solution of lead subacetate; Goulard's extract*) contains about 25 per cent. of lead subacetate in solution, and is used externally and in the preparation of *lead-water* (*liquor plumbi subacetatis dilutum; diluted solution of lead subacetate*), which contains 4 per cent. of the stronger solution, and is used as a soothing lotion, and of *Goulard's cerate* (*ceratum plumbi subacetatis; cerate of lead subacetate*).

PLUMBI IODIDUM (*lead iodid*).—It may be used internally, dose, gr. ij–iij (0.13–0.2 gm.), but is chiefly employed externally in the form of *ointment*.

PLUMBI NITRAS (*lead nitrate*) is used as a disinfectant (*Ledoyen's disinfecting fluid* contains ʒj to ℥j—about 4 to 30 c.c.), astringent, and sedative in wounds, ulcers, cracked nipples, onychia maligna, etc.

ALUMEN (ALUM).

What is alum?

Official *alum* is a double sulphate of aluminum and potassium. There are other varieties in which potassium is replaced by some other base, as ammonium or sodium.

What are its effects and uses?

Alum is a powerful astringent, and in large quantity an irritant, whether used locally or internally. In large doses it is emetic, and in excessive doses has caused death from gastro-intestinal irritation. It is *used* in solution as an *astringent*, by atomization in *bronchorrhea*, by injection in *leukorrhea, gonorrhea*, and *gleet*, as a gargle in *sore throat, relaxed palate*, and *uvula*, as a lotion in *conjunctivitis*, and on cotton as a tampon in *cystocele, rectocele*, and *uterine prolapse*. As a *hemostatic* in *hemoptysis* a saturated solution may be used by atomization; and as a *styptic* (*aqua plagiari* consists of alum, compound tincture of benzoin, and water boiled together) it is employed locally to arrest hemorrhage. As an *emetic* it is used in *croup*, in *capillary bronchitis*, and as an adjuvant to other emetics. It is also efficient in the treatment of *lead colic*. Dose as an *astringent*, gr. x–xxx (0.6–2.0 gm.); as an *emetic*, ʒj–iv (4–15 gm.). In lead-poisoning a teaspoonful (4 gm.) may be given every three or four hours.

Dried alum (*alumen exsiccatum*) is alum deprived of its water of crystallization by heat. In excessive doses it has proved fatal. Dose, gr. v–x (0.3–0.6 gm.). Externally it is applied as a mild escharotic to fungous granulations, and as a stimulant to sluggish ulcers.

ALUMINI SULPHAS (ALUMINUM SULPHATE).

What is aluminum sulphate?

It is a powerful *astringent* and *antiseptic*, and is employed for these purposes *externally* and as an *injection in gonorrhea*. Its solution has been used to preserve cadavers for dissection. A solution of *aluminum acetate* is used as an antiseptic and astringent wet-dressing for infected wounds.

ALUMINI HYDROXIDUM (*aluminum hydroxide*) is a feeble astringent.

CUPRUM (COPPER).

What are the sources and effects of copper?

Copper is obtained from copper pyrites, a double sulphid of iron and copper. *The metal* itself is inert. *The salts* are mild *astringents* and *stimulants* when in weak solution, and when strong, act as *irritants*; in powder they are mild *caustics*. Taken *internally in small doses* they are astringent, and are supposed to act as tonics to the nervous system. In *larger doses* they are local *emetics.* In *excessive amounts* they act as *irritant poisons*, causing gastro-intestinal inflammation, hematuria, sometimes jaundice, convulsions, paralysis, delirium, coma, and death. The *postmortem* reveals fatty degeneration of the liver and decomposition of the blood-corpuscles. When taken continuously for a *very long time*, a condition of chronic poisoning results, with giddiness, occasional diarrhea, cramps, wasting, and sometimes progressive palsies, respiratory failure, and death. A *green line* is sometimes observed on the gums.

The *tests* for the soluble copper salts are *potassium ferrocyanid*, which gives a mahogany-colored precipitate; *ammonia*, which gives a beautiful blue color, and *metallic iron*, on which metallic copper will be deposited from a solution. The treatment of *acute poisoning* is albumin (milk or eggs), opium demulcents, and treating symptoms as they arise. In *chronic poisoning* endeavor to eliminate it as if the poison were lead.

For what purpose is copper used in medicine?

It is used *internally* as an *astringent* in *chronic diarrhea*, especially when ulceration exists, as an *emetic* (the sulphate), especially in narcotic poisoning, and occasionally as a *tonic* in nervous debility and functional nervous diseases. *Locally* it is efficacious as a *stimulant* to ulcers, as an *escharotic* in granular conjunctivitis and flabby granulations, and as an *astringent* injection in gonorrhea.

What are the preparations of copper and their doses?

CUPRI SULPHAS (*copper sulphate*), called also *blue vitriol*, or *blue stone;* dose as an *astringent*, gr. ¼–j (0.015–0.06 gm.), in pill; as an *emetic*, gr. iij–v (0.2–0.3 gm.); as an injection in gonorrhea, gr. ¼–j (0.015–0.06 gm.) to ℥j (30 c.c.).

ZINCUM (ZINC).

What are the sources, action, uses, and preparations of zinc?

Zinc is obtained principally from the native carbonate and sulphid. The *effects* of the *zinc salts* are similar to those of copper but are less powerful. In *excessive doses* they cause an *acute poisoning* very similar to that produced by copper, the *antidotes* being milk and eggs, alkalis, and their carbonates. *Chronic poisoning* is so rare as to be disputed. The *test* for zinc in solution is the addition of *ammonium sulphid*, which preciptates *white* zinc sulphid, the only white sulphid met with.

They are used as *astringents* in diarrheas; as *emetics;* as *nerve tonics* in epilepsy and chorea, and locally as *astringents* in conjunctivitis, gonorrhea, etc.; as *sedatives* and *astringents* in eczema and erysipelas; as *dusting-powders*, and as mild *stimulants* to ulcers.

ZINCI SULPHAS (*zinc sulphate; white vitriol*); dose as a *tonic* or *astringent*, gr. ij–v (0.13–0.3 gm.); as an *emetic* (safer than copper sulphate), gr. x–xx (0.6–1.3 gm.). Locally, as a collyrium or as an injection in gonorrhea, gr. j–ij (0.06–0.13 gm.) to ℥j (30 c.c.).

ZINCI PHENOLSULPHONAS (*sulphocarbolate of zinc*) is employed locally as an astringent and stimulant for sluggish ulcers and catarrhal conditions of mucous membranes.

ZINCI OXIDUM (*zinc oxid*) is used internally in *catarrhal diarrhea, membranous enteritis, epilepsy, chorea*, and occasionally to check *colliquative sweats*. Dose, gr. j–v (0.06–0.3 gm.), in pill. It is used also as a *dusting-powder*.

The *ointment* (*unguentum zinci oxidi*) contains 20 per cent. of the salt and is much employed.

ZINCI STEARAS (*zinc stearate*) is a very fine light powder, used externally as a drying and healing *dusting-powder*, or as an *ointment* (*unguentum zinci stearatis*, 50 per cent.).

ZINCI ACETAS (*zinc acetate*) is used as a *collyrium* (gr. ij—0.13 gm.—to ℥j—30 c.c.), as an injection in the third stage of *gonorrhea* (gr. j–xx—0.06–1.3—to ℥j—30 c.c.), and in *leukorrhea* (ʒj to Oj—about 4 to 480 c.c.).

ZINCI CARBONAS PRÆCIPITATUS (*precipitated zinc carbonate* is used as a *dusting-powder* and as a mild *astringent* ointment (ʒj–℥j—about 4 to 30 c.c.), and in skin lotions. *Calamine* is an impure natural zinc carbonate.

ZINCI CHLORIDUM (*zinc chlorid*) is a powerful *caustic* and *antiseptic*, employed to destroy lupus and indolent granulations. It is used also to preserve cadavers for dissection. *Burnett's disinfecting fluid* contains gr. 200 to ℥j (about 13 to 30 c.c.).

Liquor zinci chloridi (*solution of zinc chlorid*) may be used to disinfect water-closets and sinks.

ZINCI IODIDUM (*zinc iodid*) is a local stimulant and caustic.

ZINCI VALERAS (*zinc valerate*) is employed as a *nerve tonic* in epilepsy and chorea; dose, gr. j–ij (0.06–0.13 gm.), t. i. d.

ZINCI BROMIDUM (*zinc bromid*) is also official.

ARGENTUM (SILVER).

What are the physiologic effects of silver?

Metallic silver is inert. Of its soluble salts, the oxid and nitrate are chiefly employed. Locally applied, *the nitrate* coagulates albumin, and is an astringent and superficial caustic, contracting the cutaneous vessels and producing a white stain on the skin which becomes black on exposure to light. Taken *internally* they are astringent, and after absorption exert a tonic influence upon the nervous system. In *large doses* they are gastro-intestinal irritants, often producing also violent convulsions, disturbed respiration, coma, dilated pupils, paralysis, and death from respiratory failure. If *too long continued*, even in minute doses, *chronic argyria* results, consisting in emaciation, impaired memory, and a peculiar indelible *blue discoloration*, first manifesting itself on the mucous membranes, and extending to the skin and internal organs.

What are the tests for silver, and how should argyria be treated?

The addition of *hydrochloric acid* or *sodium chlorid* to a solution of silver produces a white precipitate of silver chlorid, soluble in ammonia. *Acute argyria* is treated by giving immediately, as an *antidote*, a large amount of common salt, and treating symptoms *p. r. n.* In *chronic argyria* nothing does much good as a rule; potassium iodid may be tried as an eliminative agent. Silver nitrate is incompatible with organic substances or with hydrochloric acid or the chlorids.

What are the medicinal uses of the silver salts?

They are used as *astringents* in *chronic diarrheas* and in *dysenteries* (internally or by enema), especially when ulceration is present, and are very useful in organic dyspepsias, especially in *gastric ulcer* and in *chronic gastritis*. As a *nerve tonic* they are employed in *locomotor ataxia* and other *spinal scleroses*. *Externally* as a *stimulant* and *mild caustic* the nitrate is applied to slowly *granulating surfaces*, to unhealthy *ulcers*, and to *warty* growths. As an *antiphlogistic* and *astringent* it is used in solution in various inflammations of the mucous membranes, as *conjunctivitis*, *pharyngitis*, *laryngitis*, etc., and may be used as an injection in the later stages of gonorrhea (gr. j–ij—0.06–0.13 gm.—to f℥j—30 c.c.) in the male, or in *acute vaginitis* (painting the inflamed vagina with strong solutions). It is employed also in superficial inflammations of the skin, in erysipelas, and to prevent pitting in small-pox.

What are the official silver salts and their doses?

ARGENTI NITRAS (*silver nitrate*), dose, gr. $\frac{1}{8}$–$\frac{1}{4}$ (0.008–0.016 gm.), gradually increased to gr. ss–j (0.03–0.06 gm.). Great care should be taken to prevent staining the skin. For external use solutions are employed varying in strength from gr. j–ʒij (0.06–8.0 gm.) to ℥j (30 c.c.) of distilled water.

Molded silver nitrate or *lunar caustic* (*argenti nitras fusus*) is silver nitrate melted and poured into small molds, for external use.

Mitigated silver nitrate (*argenti nitras mitigatus*) is 30 parts of silver nitrate and 60 parts of potassium nitrate, molded as above.

ARGENTI OXIDUM (*silver oxid*), dose, gr. ss–j (0.03–0.06 gm.), in pill.

ARGENTI CYANIDUM (*silver cyanid*), used for preparing diluted hydrocyanic acid.

Are any other silver compounds used?

Certain organic silver compounds are more penetrating and less irritating than silver nitrate, and are much employed. They are:

Argentamin, ethylene diamin silver phosphate.

Argonin, sodium silver caseinate.

Argyrol, silver vitelline, very soluble and scarcely at all irritating in 25 per cent. solution—a valuable remedy.

Itrol, citrate of silver.

Lactate of silver, or "actol."

Largin, a silver albumin compound soluble in 9 parts of water.

Protargol, a soluble silver albumose employed in solutions of ½ to 20 per cent.

BISMUTHUM (BISMUTH).

What are the actions, uses, and preparations of bismuth?

Metallic bismuth is inert. The *less soluble salts* are not actively toxic when pure, as they are absorbed with difficulty. *Bismuth and ammonium citrate* is much more irritant, and in large doses may cause gastro-enteritis. In medicinal doses they are astringent and sedative to the mucous membranes. A portion is absorbed and is eliminated by the kidneys chiefly, while that which is not absorbed is converted into a sulphid and colors the stools black. *Locally* applied they are antiseptic and sedative.

They are *used* internally as *sedatives* and *astringents* to check nausea and vomiting in *gastric irritation*, and to relieve pain in *gastralgia*, *gastric ulcer*, and *cancer*. In *acute diarrheas* from irritation and in *chronic diarrheas*, especially those occurring in children during the summer months, they are very valuable. *Externally* as mild astringents and antiseptics they are useful in the treatment of *ulcers*, and as an injection (suspended in mucilage) in acute *gonorrhea* and in *vaginitis*. They are also used as dusting-powders in *intertrigo* and as snuff in acute *coryza*.

BISMUTHI SUBNITRAS (*bismuth subnitrate*), called also *pearl white* or *magistery of bismuth*, dose, gr. v–ʒj (0.3–4.0 gm.).

BISMUTHI SUBCARBONAS (*bismuth subcarbonate*), dose, gr. v–xxx (0.3–2.0 gm.).

BISMUTHI SUBGALLAS (*bismuth subgallate*), called also "dermatol"; dose, gr. v–xx (0.3–1.3 gm.).

BISMUTHI SUBSALICYLAS (*bismuth subsalicylate*); dose. gr. v–xx (0.3–1.3 gm.).

Bismuthi Citras (*bismuth citrate*), dose, gr. j–v (0.06–0.3 gm.).

Bismuthi et Ammonii Citras (*bismuth and ammonium citrate*), a soluble salt, dose, gr. j–v (0.06–0.3 gm.).

CERII OXALAS (CERIUM OXALATE).

What is cerium oxalate?

It is supposed to resemble the salts of bismuth in its effects. It is *used* with success in *reflex vomiting*, particularly the *vomiting of pregnancy* and in *diarrhea*. Dose, gr. j–iij (0.06–0.2 gm.) t. i. d. in pill or capsule.

ANTACIDS.

What are antacids?

Antacids are remedies capable of neutralizing acids. The term, however, is here used in a more limited sense, and embraces only those remedies which are used in medicine to correct excessive acidity in the alimentary canal, as manifested by heartburn, acid eructations, gastric uneasiness, and diarrhea of infants with "chopped-spinach stools." Excessive acidity may be due to an excessive secretion of acid by the stomach, and here the antacids may be given after meals to neutralize the acid present, or the same effect may be produced by administering an acid before meals, which will decrease the acid secretion. On the other hand, it may be due to organic acids from a deficient secretion of acid and consequent imperfect digestion and fermentation of the food. In these cases an antacid given before meals is useful by increasing the outward osmosis of acid, or a mixture of pepsin and acid after meals may supply the place of the deficient secretion. In acidity due to the development of the *sarcina ventriculi* sulphurous acid, the sulphites, carbolic acid, or other antizymotics give the best results.

Name the antacids employed for the above purposes.

While all the alkalis, alkaline earths, and their carbonates are really antacids, yet in medical practice magnesia and the sodium and calcium salts are chiefly used. *Solution of potassa* (*q. v.*) is sometimes, but not often, employed. The *spirit* and *aromatic spirit of ammonia* (*q. v.*) are frequently used, especially in sick headache or where a stimulating antacid is required.

SODIUM.

What are the effects and uses of the sodium salts?

Caustic soda and its solution are escharotics. The *sodium salts* taken on an empty stomach increase the secretion of acid gastric juice, but if given after a meal in sufficient quantity, they neutralize the acid present. They diffuse readily into the blood, and act somewhat as do the potassium salts, being, however, less irritant, more feebly diuretic, and possessing little, if any, poisonous influence over the (mammalian) heart, nerves, or muscles.

The medicinal uses of the sodium preparations have been considered in discussing the general uses of the antacids.

What are the preparations of sodium?

LIQUOR SODII HYDROXIDI (*solution of sodium hydroxide*); dose, ♏ij–x (0.12–0.3 c.c.), freely diluted.

SODII CARBONAS MONOHYDRATUS (*monohydrated sodium carbonate*) is much used as an antacid in dyspepsia. In over-doses it is a corrosive poison. The antidotes are the vegetable acids. Dose, gr. x–xxx (0.6–2.0 c.c.). The *monohydrated salt* contains but one molecule of water, whereas *sodium carbonate* (*washing soda*) contains 10 molecules of water and is very efflorescent in dry air. It is sometimes deprived of its water of crystallization and prescribed in pill form as the *dried carbonate* (*sodii carbonas exsiccatus*), in doses of gr. v–xv (0.3–1.0 gm.).

SODII BICARBONAS (*sodium bicarbonate*) is preferred to the carbonate because it is a more permanent salt and is less irritating to the stomach. Dose, gr. x–xxx (0.6–2.0 gm.). It is an ingredient of *seidlitz powders* (*q. v.*) and other preparations. The *troches* (*trochisci sodii bicarbonatis*) each contain gr. iij (0.2 gm.) of the bicarbonate.

The other sodium salts are rarely used as antacids, and most of them have been sufficiently described previously.

SODII CITRAS (*sodium citrate*); dose, gr. x–xxx (0.07–2 gm.).

CALCIUM.

What are the effects, uses, and preparations of calcium?

Unslaked lime is a caustic. The *calcium salts* are antacid, slightly astringent, and sedative to the mucous membranes, and are consequently much used in vomiting and in diarrhea. The vapor arising from slaking lime is inhaled with advantage in membranous croup and in diphtheria. The preparations are LIQUOR CALCIS (*lime-solution; lime-water*), used as an antacid and gastric sedative in nausea and vomiting from irritability of the stomach, and often added to milk to increase its digestibility and render it more readily tolerated by the stomach. As an antacid and astringent it is useful in diarrhea, especially in teething children. Locally it is used as an alkaline wash in various skin affections, and as a dressing to burns, scalds, ulcers, etc., in the form of LINIMENTUM CALCIS, often called *carron oil* (equal parts of lime-water and linseed-oil).

SYRUPUS CALCIS (*syrup of lime*), containing 6.5 per cent. of lime in the form of saccharate, is used as an astringent in diarrheas and as an antidote to poisoning by carbolic acid. Dose, f℥ss–ij (2–8 c.c.), freely diluted.

CALCII CARBONAS PRÆCIPITATUS (*precipitated calcium carbonate*) and CRETA PRÆPARATA (*prepared chalk*), dose, gr. x–xxx (0.6–2.0 gm.), have the same chemic composition, but the precipitated chalk is a fine, heavy powder, and is used externally as a dusting-powder or as a tooth-powder, while the prepared chalk is light and adhesive and is used internally. *Compound chalk-powder* (*pulvis cretæ compositus*) contains 30 per cent. of prepared chalk. *Chalk mixture* (*mistura cretæ*) contains 20 per cent. of the compound powder in water and cinnamon water, and is much used, combined with astringents and opium, in diarrheas, especially those of teething children. Dose, ℥j–iv (4–15 c.c.).

Other preparations of calcium have been previously considered.

TOPICAL MEDICINES.

Antiseptics.

What are antiseptics?

Antiseptics are medicines which prevent fermentation and

decomposition by destroying or preventing the development of the germs on which these processes depend. They are not always *germicides* (remedies which kill the germs of disease), for some of them hinder the growth and prevent the development of fresh germs, without destroying those already present; nor are they always *deodorants* (remedies which destroy disagreeable odors), for the microbes of disease may be destroyed, and foul chemic emanations continue, or the latter may exist without the presence of the former.

Name the chief antiseptics.

Antiseptics may be divided, according to their chemic composition into *the inorganic* or *elementary*, and *the organic antiseptics* (or those belonging to the group of carbon compounds, including antiseptic oils and their camphors). To the first group belong hydrogen dioxid, potassium permanganate, chlorin water, chlorinated lime, Labarraque's solution, mercuric chlorid, bromin, iodin, mercuric iodid, iodoform, iodol, sulphurous acid, sulphites, sulphids, boric acid, borates, and many of the mineral salts previously mentioned, as iron sulphate, lead nitrate, etc. In the second division are included carbolic acid and the carbolates, creosote, benzoic acid and the benzoates, naphtalin, naphtol, formaldehyd, the antipyretics (*q. v.*), the antiseptic oils (*vid. Carminatives*), and thymol.

AQUA HYDROGENII DIOXIDI (SOLUTION OF HYDROGEN DIOXID).

What is solution of hydrogen dioxid?

It is a slightly acid, aqueous solution of hydrogen dioxid (also known as *hydrogen peroxid*), containing, when freshly prepared, about 3 per cent., by weight, of the pure dioxid, corresponding to about 10 volumes of available oxygen. It occurs as a colorless liquid, without odor, but having a slightly acidulous taste.

It parts readily with its oxygen, and thus acts as an *oxidizing disinfectant.*

It is, of course, greatly inferior to mercuric chlorid as a disinfectant, antiseptic, and germicide, but has the advantage of being non-poisonous. When brought in contact with pus, as on a suppurating surface, gas is evolved more or less abundantly, depending on the amount of pus present; a slight superficial coagulation forms on the surface, and the pus-corpuscles are disintegrated.

It has been *used* as an *antiseptic injection* into *abscess cavities* after the evacuation of their contents and into *sinuses;* and also as a local application to *superficial wounds* and *ulcers,* whether of common or specific origin. It is also used as an injection in *gonorrhea.* In *scarlatinal* or *diphtheritic sore throat* and in *tonsillitis* it is often used as a gargle or spray.

It is a good *buccal disinfectant,* and may advantageously be used for this purpose in *typhoid* and *other low fevers,* or in any case where the secretions tend to collect in the mouth and become offensive.

On account of the oxygen evolved, it is an active *bleaching agent,* and is used in solutions of 10 to 15 per cent. strength to bleach hair.

POTASSII PERMANGANAS (POTASSIUM PERMANGANATE).

What is potassium permanganate?

Potassium permanganate has been considered with the preparations of manganese (*vid.* Mineral Tonics). Its disinfectant powers are great, but it is decomposed immediately on contact with organic matter, and hence is chiefly used in solution as a gargle in scarlatina and diphtheria, as a lotion to cancerous and other ulcers, to correct fetor in otorrhea, etc., and as an injection (1 : 1000) in leukorrhea and in gonorrhea. It is given internally as an emmenagogue (*q. v.*).

LIQUOR CHLORI COMPOSITUS (CHLORIN WATER).

What is chlorin water?

It is an aqueous solution, containing at least 0.4 per cent. of *chlorin.* It is a powerful irritant and antiseptic. Albumin is the best *antidote.*

It is chiefly used diluted, as a gargle in *diphtheria,* and as a wash for foul *ulcers* and *wounds.*

CALX CHLORINATA (CHLORINATED LIME).

What is chlorinated lime?

It is composed of calcium hypochlorite and chlorid, and

when exposed to the air is decomposed, yielding about 30 per cent. of chlorin. It is an antiseptic, and is used to disinfect the air of sick-rooms, urine, sputum, and fecal discharges and privies.

LIQUOR SODÆ CHLORINATÆ (SOLUTION OF CHLORINATED SODA).

What is this substance?

Solution of chlorinated soda, or *Labarraque's solution*, contains at least 2.4 per cent., by weight, of available chlorin, and may be used for the same purposes as the foregoing preparations.

HYDRARGYRI CHLORIDUM CORROSIVUM (MERCURIC CHLORID).

What is mercuric chlorid?

This preparation has been considered with the mercurial salts (*vid.* Alteratives). It is a valuable germicide, and is used in aqueous solutions of various strength (1 : 1000 to 1 : 16,000) in all manner of surgical operations and affections where an antiseptic is required and can be employed. As several cases of poisoning have been reported, especially from its use in gynecologic and obstetric practice, it should be employed with some caution. It is very irritating to the tissues, and may produce a superficial slough. It attacks steel instruments.

BROMUM (BROMIN); IODUM (IODIN).

Are these substances antiseptic?

Bromin (*vid.* Escharotics) and *iodin* are powerful antiseptics, but are rarely used for this purpose, as their management requires great care and experience.

HYDRARGYRI IODIDUM RUBRUM (MERCURIC IODID).

Is mercuric iodid antiseptic?

Mercuric iodid is a powerful germicide, and has been employed as a substitute for corrosive sublimate, but, so far, has not superseded the latter.

IODOFORMUM (IODOFORM).

What is iodoform?

Iodoform is formyl teriodid, and occurs in minute yellowish crystals with a disagreeable odor. It is insoluble in water, but freely soluble in ether and alcohol.

What are its effects and uses?

The action of iodoform is not well understood. Some of it is absorbed unchanged, and some is changed to alkaline iodids and iod-albuminates. Though not germicidal, it acts in wounds as an antiseptic. It may irritate the skin and cause severe dermatitis. Its local use has often been followed by general poisoning. In mild poisoning there may be nausea and vomiting, headache, and the unpleasant taste and odor of the drug. The pulse is slow at first, then rapid, irregular, and there is sleeplessness and depression of spirits. If the poisoning is more severe, there may be very weak pulse, great restlessness, delirium, maniacal excitement or melancholia; or after a brief period of excitement there is general paralysis, with coma and involuntary discharge of urine and feces. Death follows from cardiac or respiratory paralysis. The autopsy shows fatty degeneration of the heart, liver, and kidneys. Iodids appear in saliva and urine.

Should poisoning occur, remove every particle of the dressing if it has been used locally, give opium and stimulants, and treat symptoms. Iodoform has been *used* internally as a *cardiac tonic* in valvular disease with insufficient hypertrophy, and as an *alterative* in syphilitic rheumatism, neuralgias and the early stages of phthisis. In *diabetes mellitus* it has been advantageously given. *Externally*, it is employed as an anesthetic and antiseptic dressing to irritable ulcers of all kinds, burns, and wounds. In *ethereal solution* it has been injected into the cavities of strumous abscesses, after the evacuation of their contents, to destroy the giant-cells of tubercle, and promote healthy granulation. In *suppositories* it is used in inflammation and ulceration of the vagina, uterus, and rectum. *Bougies* containing iodoform are sometimes used in septic affections of the uterus and in gonorrhea.

Dose, gr. ¼–v (0.01–0.3 gm.), in pill or capsule.

The *ointment* (*unguentum iodoformi*) contains 10 per cent. of iodoform.

What other iodin compounds resemble iodoform?

Among the less disagreeable, iodin-containing substitutes for iodoform are:

THYMOLIS IODIDUM (*thymol iodide; aristol*) is official and is a red-brown, very fine, light, nearly odorless powder, which contains 45 per cent. of iodin.

IODOL (*tetra-iodo-pyrrol*), which is tasteless and odorless and contains 88.9 per cent. of iodin, is official. It is much used in nasal, pharyngeal, and laryngeal cases, especially in tuberculous laryngitis. Its internal dose is gr. ss–iij (0.03–0.2 gm.).

Europhen, isobutyl orthocresol iodid, which contains 25 per cent. of iodin.

Losophan, tri-iodo-metacresol, which is odorless and contains 78.4 per cent. of iodin.

Nosophen, tetra-iodo-phenolphthalein, containing 60 per cent. of iodin.

ACIDUM SULPHUROSUM (SULPHUROUS ACID).

What is sulphurous acid?

Sulphurous acid is an aqueous solution of about 6 per cent. by weight of sulphurous acid gas.

What are its effects and uses?

It is a powerful deoxydizing agent and deodorant. When sufficiently concentrated, the gas is probably a germicide. When inhaled it is irritant, and, if in sufficient amount, causes inflammation and even acts as a caustic from the formation of sulphuric acid. It is eliminated by the urine and feces as sulphates. It is *used internally* (diluted) in *flatulency* depending on fermentation of the food, and *locally* as a wash in various parasitic skin diseases. In the form of burning sulphur it is employed to disinfect rooms. Dose, ♏v–ʒj (0.3–4.0 c.c.), freely diluted. It takes four pounds of sulphur, burnt in the presence of moisture, to disinfect a room containing 1000 cubic feet.

THE SULPHITES AND SULPHIDS.[1]

What are the effects and uses of these salts?

The *effects* of the *sulphites* depend upon the sulphurous acid which they contain, and which is readily evolved on the addition of almost any acid. On exposure to the air they are converted into sulphates. Taken internally they are decomposed by the acid of the gastric juice, evolve sulphurous acid, are finally converted into sulphates, and thus absorbed and eliminated. They are *used* to fulfil the indications for sulphurous acid. The dose of *sodium sulphite* (*sodii sulphis*) is gr. v–xxx (0.3–2.0 gm.), t. i. d.; *sodium bisulphite* (*sodii bisulphis*), gr. v–xx (0.3–1.3 gm.); *sodium thiosulphate* or *hyposulphite* (*sodii thiosulphas*), gr. v–xx (0.3–1.3 gm.).

The *sulphids* are said to stimulate the glands of the skin, and to possess the power of arresting the formation of pus in threatened boils and abscesses. They are used internally for this purpose in acne and furunculosis.

Calx sulphurata (*sulphurated lime*) consists of a mixture containing at least 60 per cent. of calcium monosulphid, together with unchanged calcium sulphate and carbonate, in varying proportions, and is given in doses of gr. $\frac{1}{10}$–$\frac{1}{2}$ (0.006–0.03 gm.), repeated every one-half to one hour.

ACIDUM BORICUM (BORIC ACID); SODII BORAS (BORAX).

What are the effects and uses of boric acid and borax?

Locally, boric acid is antiseptic and deodorant. *Internally* it is somewhat diuretic, and retards the decomposition of the urine. Fatal cases from the injection of large quantities into the pleural sac, the cavity of a large lumbar abscess, and the stomach have been reported, death being due to collapse and cardiac failure.

Boric acid is used as an antiseptic in powder or solution in many external inflammations and wounds, and in inflammations and aphthous or diphtheritic ulcerations of the mouth and fauces, the acid or borax is of undoubted value.

[1] See footnote, p. 72.

In solution it has also been used to wash out *abscess cavities* and as an injection in *gonorrhea.* As a *disinfectant* and *deodorant* in ophthalmic and aural practice it is very useful. Boric acid is recommended internally in *cystitis* depending on ammoniacal decomposition of the urine, and as an injection into the bladder in the cystitis of spinal diseases. Dose of the *acid,* gr. v.–x (0.3–0.6 gm.), t. i. d.; of borax, gr. xx–ʒj (1.2–4.0 gm.).

LIQUOR ANTISEPTICUS (*antiseptic solution*) contains 2 per cent. of boric acid, with benzoic acid, thymol, eucalyptol, the oils of peppermint, gaultheria and thyme, alcohol, and water.

Glyceritum boroglycerini (*glycerite of boroglycerin; glycerite of glyceryl borate; solution of boroglycerite*) is made by dissolving 31 per cent. of boric acid in glycerin by means of heat, and is used as an external application for the disinfection of unhealthy ulcers or suppurating surfaces generally.

It is a useful appplication to burns, and has been applied with advantage to inflamed mucous membranes, as the pharynx, nasal passages, or conjunctiva. It is also used on vaginal tampons in uterine inflammation.

Unguentum acidi borici (*boric acid ointment*) contains 10 per cent. of boric acid, and is employed in various skin diseases, especially those of children.

PHENOL (CARBOLIC ACID).

What is phenol?

Phenol, carbolic acid, or *phenic acid,* is a crystalline solid which readily deliquesces, and can be kept in solution by the addition of 8 per cent. of water or glycerin. It is soluble in 15 parts of water and has a faintly acid reaction. It is derived from coal-tar by fractional distillation.

What are the tests for carbolic acid?

The addition of *ferric sulphate* produces a lilac color; *bromin-water* causes a yellowish precipitate; it coagulates albumin, and precipitates nitrocellulose from collodion.

What are its physiologic actions?

Carbolic acid is a protoplasm poison, capable of destroying the tissues; in full strength it is caustic, producing a white slough of coagulated proteid; in dilute solutions (below 6 per cent.) it is strongly antiseptic and germicidal. Applied to skin or mucous membrane, it is a local anesthetic. Internally it is powerfully irritant and caustic, but if sufficiently diluted, is a gastric sedative and antifermentative.

It first stimulates and then exhausts the vagi (causing slowing, followed by acceleration of the heart's action, which is finally paralyzed), reduces the arterial pressure by paralyzing the vasomotor centers of the cord, increases and then depresses the respiratory movements, from its influence on the vagi and respiratory center, and in large doses lowers the temperature. In poisonous doses it causes vertigo, tremors, contracted pupils, stupor, coma, impaired motion, sensation and reflex action, and in the lower animals convulsions of spinal origin. A large quantity may be followed by immediate unconsciousness. It is eliminated chiefly by the kidneys and lungs, imparting a smoky color to the urine when the dose is excessive.

Carbolic burns are best treated with alcohol or acetic acid, bland oils, or if internal, by whisky or vinegar. The systemic effects are best counteracted by the administration of the alkaline sulphates by mouth, by rectum, and by hypodermoclysis. Atropin, caffein, and camphor should be given to stimulate the central nervous system.

What are its medicinal uses?

In 2 to 5 per cent. solution it is used externally as an antiseptic dressing and lotion in various surgical affections and operations. It has also been used as a local anesthetic previous to minor surgical operations, as the opening of small abscesses and felons, and in dilute solution to allay pruritus. It has been injected into the cavities of chronic abscesses and of the tunica vaginalis, after the withdrawal of the contained fluid, to cause obliteration of their sacs by irritation.

Owing to the combination of an anesthetic effect with its power to destroy tissues, the application of dilute solutions of carbolic acid as a wet dressing has, in many instances, resulted in gangrene.

Internally carbolic acid has been much used as a *gastric sedative* to check *vomiting;* as an *astringent* in *diarrhea;* as an *antifermentative;* as a *germicide* in *sarcina ventriculi;* and as an *antizymotic* in *typhoid fever, small-pox, scarlatina,* and *diphtheria.* It is also used by inhalation in *nasal catarrh, hay-fever, bronchorrhea, pertussis,* and *pulmonary gangrene,* and is a frequent constituent of gargles.

What are its preparations and doses?

PHENOL (*phenol; carbolic acid*), dose, gr. j–ij (0.6–0.13 gm.).

PHENOL LIQUEFACTUM (*liquefied carbolic acid*) is a mixture of 1 part by weight of water and 9 parts of phenol. It is a stable solution, containing not less than 86.4 per cent. by weight of absolute phenol.

GLYCERITUM PHENOLIS (*glycerite of phenol*) contains 20 per cent. of the acid dissolved in glycerin; dose, ♏ij–v (0.12–0.3 c.c.).

UNGUENTUM PHENOLIS (*ointment of phenol*) contains 3 per cent. of phenol in white vaseline.

SODII PHENOLSULPHONAS.

What is sodium phenolsulphonate?

Sodii phenolsulphonas (*sodium sulphocarbolate* or *sodium paraphenolsulphonate*) is used *internally* to fulfil the indications of carbolic acid, and as an antifermentative in flatulency from fermentation of the food and in various bowel complaints. It is also used *locally* as a sedative application to inflamed mucous membranes. Dose, gr. x–xv (0.6–1.0 gm.), t. i. d.

CRESOL.

Cresol is a mixture of the three isomeric cresols obtained from coal-tar, freed from phenol, hydrocarbons, and water. It has a phenol-like odor, is soluble in 60 parts of water, and is freely miscible with alcohol, ether, and glycerin. It is a powerful antiseptic, sometimes spoken of as "coal-tar creosote." Its 50 per cent. solution in linseed oil soap is official under the name of *Liquor Cresolis Compositus,* a substitute for the proprietary "lysol."

CREOSOTUM (CREOSOTE).

What is creosote?

Creosote is obtained from wood-tar by distillation. It is

chiefly made up of guaiacol and creosol and is entirely different from "coal-tar creosote." It does not coagulate albumin or collodion. It has a very disagreeable taste and odor. It is used in respiratory diseases, especially in tuberculosis, producing diminution of cough, night-sweats, and diarrhea (see Guaiacol). The dose of pure creosote is ♏j–iij (0.06–0.2 c.c.), given in milk or with tincture of gentian.

Aqua creosoti (*creosote water*) is a 1 per cent. solution of creosote.

ACIDUM BENZOICUM (BENZOIC ACID).

What is benzoic acid?

Benzoic acid is obtained from benzoin by sublimation, or from hippuric acid or toluol by synthetic processes, and is an ingredient of many of the substances (*the balsams*) previously considered. *Locally* it is an irritant, antiseptic, and germicide. *Internally* it increases the secretions generally, and is eliminated chiefly by the urine, increasing the acidity of that fluid, hence its value in the phosphatic diathesis. Benzoic acid or its salts are of great value in the treatment of *cystitis* from alkaline urine, *phosphatic deposits* in the urine, etc., for by acidulating the urine it renders the phosphates more soluble. They are also used internally as *antiseptics* in *diphtheria, erysipelas,* etc. Benzoic acid is added to unguents, to prevent rancidity, and is an ingredient of the *Liquor Antisepticus* (see *Acidum Boricum*). The dose is gr. v–xx (0.3–1.2 gm.); but for internal administration the salts are generally preferred.

Sodii benzoas (*sodium benzoate*) has been used as an *antipyretic* in *rheumatism,* and as an *antiseptic* in *pertussis, diphtheria,* and *the exanthemata.* Dose, ʒj–ij (4–8 c.c.).

Ammonii benzoas (*ammonium benzoate*) is the best remedy for *incontinence* due to vesical irritation from alkaline decomposition of the urine. Dose, gr. v–xx (0.3–1.2 gm.).

NAPHTHALENUM (NAPHTHALENE).

What is naphthalene?

Naphthalene, also called *naphthalin,* is a hydrocarbon obtained from coal-tar, occurring in colorless, transparent plates, and having a strong, peculiar odor and a burning, somewhat

17

aromatic taste. It is soluble in alcohol but insoluble in water.

Naphthalene is *antiseptic* and *antiparasitic. Locally* it is stimulant to granulations. Given internally in large doses or for a length of time it causes gastric irritation. Very little is absorbed, the greater part being eliminated by the feces and acting as an *intestinal antiseptic.* Some little, however, passes into the system and is eliminated by the kidneys and by the lungs. It is said that its continued administration to animals has resulted in cataract.

It is chiefly *used* as an *intestinal antiseptic* in typhoid fever, diarrheas, and dysentery. It is also used as an *anthelmintic,* given internally for the removal of lumbrici, or used as an injection (gr. x–xx—0.6–1.2 gm.) in sweet oil (f℥iij—90 c.c.) to destroy the oxyuris. It has also been given in *pyelitis, cystitis,* etc., for its antiseptic effect on the urine, and has been employed in the treatment of *bronchorrhea* and *fetid bronchitis.* It has been used as a dressing for *wounds, ulcers,* and *chronic abscesses.* Dose, gr. ij–x (0.12–0.6 gm.), administered in capsules.

BETANAPHTHOL.

What is betanaphthol?

Betanaphthol is a hydrocarbon prepared from naphthalene. It occurs as a white or yellowish-white powder, or in crystalline plates, with a faint, phenol-like odor and a pungent taste. It is freely soluble in alcohol, but only slightly so in water.

In its action it resembles closely naphthalene. In animals large doses cause death by respiratory paralysis. No toxic symptoms have been reported in the human subject from its use.

Its *uses* are similar to those of naphthalene. It is a good *intestinal antiseptic,* preventing fermentation and consequent flatulence, and is used in gastric or intestinal fermentation, in dilated stomach, and in diarrheas and dysentery. Dose, gr. ij–v (0.12–0.32 gm.), although much larger doses have been given without deleterious effect. It is usually administered in capsules, which may be keratin-coated when used as an intestinal antiseptic. It is often advantageously combined with bismuth subnitrate and sodium bicarbonate.

LIQUOR FORMALDEHYDI.

What is this substance?

Liquor Formaldehydi (*solution of formaldehyd*; *formalin*; *formal*) is an aqueous solution, containing not less than 37 per cent. by weight of absolute formaldehyd, an oxidation product of methyl-alcohol. Its vapor is very irritant to the eyes and respiratory organs; taken internally, its solution irritates the stomach, retards digestion, and weakens pulse and respiration. Collapse and death have followed the ingestion of 2 ounces of 4 per cent. solution. The best antidote is ammonia (internally, the aromatic spirit).

As a disinfectant and deodorizer formaldehyd is extensively employed. It is generated in rooms by heating the solution, by passing methyl-alcohol over hot tin or copper strainers, or from the solid cakes of paraformaldehyd. In very weak solution it is added to sprays and mouth-washes, and has been used to irrigate vagina and urethra. It is used also to sterilize and harden catgut, and for the surgeon's hands and instruments. It has been much added to milk and other foods as a preservative.

It requires the vapor of about ℥vj (180 c.c.) of formalin to disinfect a room containing 1000 cubic feet.

THE ANTIPYRETICS AND ANTISEPTIC OILS.

Are these substances used as antiseptics?

The *antipyretics* (*q. v.*) have been sufficiently considered.

The antiseptic properties of the *volatile oils* classed with the Carminatives (*q. v.*) have been alluded to under that head. Those of importance not hitherto mentioned are:

THYMOL.

What is thymol?

Thymol, a *phenol* occurring in the volatile oil of Thymus vulgaris, and in some other volatile oils, is a crystalline substance. *Locally* it is a powerful antiseptic and local anesthetic. Given internally it lowers febrile temperature to some extent, and causes diaphoresis. In excessive amount it causes tinnitus aurium, deafness, diarrhea, and sometimes delirium and collapse. It is used as an *antiseptic* and stimulating *gargle* and *mouth-wash* in aphthous and diphtheritic ulcers of the mouth and fauces, and internally as a *gastric sedative* to allay vomiting. As an *antifermentative*, in flatulency from fermentation of the food, and in intestinal indigestion, it is very useful. Dose, gr. ss–ij (0.03–0.13 gm.). As much as gr. xx–xxx (1.2–2.0 gm.) have been given in twenty-four hours. In dose of gr. xv (1 gm.) it is given as a remedy for hookworm. (See *Anthelmintics*.) It is administered in solution in glycerin, alcohol, and water, and is an ingredient of *liquor antisepticus*.

Thymolis Iodidum (*thymol iodidi*) is an iodin-containing antiseptic. It is a substitute for iodoform, and is a light, brown-colored powder of mild, not unpleasant odor. Its proprietary name is "aristol."

IRRITANTS.

What are irritants?

Irritants are medicines which are used locally to produce counter-irritation or inflammation of the parts to which they are applied. They are divided, according to the violence of their action, into rubefacients, vesicants, suppurants, and escharotics or caustics.

Rubefacients.

What are rubefacients?

Rubefacients are medicines which are employed to produce a powerful but temporary irritation and congestion of the surface. They are useful in arousing the system in shock; in stimulating the circulation of a part in case of frost-bite; to aid in bringing on reaction in the cold stage of a congestive chill; in all cases of congestion and in the formative stages of inflammations. The application of rubefacients for the relief of neuralgic and muscular pains is often followed by improvement which may even be permanent.

Mention the principal rubefacients.

Mustard, capsicum, oil of turpentine, and ammonia.

SINAPIS ALBA (WHITE MUSTARD); SINAPIS NIGRA (BLACK MUSTARD).

What is mustard?

Mustard is the seed of *Sinapis alba*, or white mustard, and *Brassica nigra*, or black mustard (*Fam.* Cruciferæ).

What chemic principles do they contain.

Mustard seed contains a *fixed oil.* Black mustard seed yields on maceration with water a volatile oil (allyl sulpho-cyanid) which does not preëxist in the seed, but is formed by the action of a ferment, *myrosin*, on *sinigrin* or *potassium myronate* in the presence of water. The white seed yields an *acrid fixed principle* which is formed by the action of a ferment on *sinalbin.*

What are the effects and uses of mustard?

Locally, it is an irritant, rapidly causing redness and a sensation of heat; if the application is long continued, inflammation and even gangrene may result. Internally it is a stomachic in small doses, an emetic in larger amounts, and a severe gastro-intestinal irritant if an excessive quantity be taken.

Mustard is *used* as a *rubefacient* in the form of a mustard plaster (made of the powdered seed known as mustard flour), whenever a mild counterirritant effect is desired. The mustard should not be allowed to come in contact with the skin, but should be separated from it by a piece of gauze or a fold of muslin or newspaper. When a prolonged but gentle effect is desirable, the mustard may be added to a flax-seed poultice or diluted with flour. *Internally*, mustard flour is used as an *emetic*, and is especially valuable when torpor of the stomach is present.

What are the preparations of mustard and their doses?

The dose of powdered mustard as an emetic is ʒj–iv (4–15 gm.).

The official preparations are *mustard papers* (*charta sinapis*), a convenient form for external use. Each square inch of paper contains about gr. vj of black mustard deprived of its fixed oil. They should be dipped in warm water before applying. The *volatile oil* (*oleum sinapis volatile*) is very irritant.

CAPSICUM. OIL OF TURPENTINE. AMMONIA.

Are these substances used as rubefacients?

The uses of these substances as rubefacients will be found in detail under the respective drugs.

Linimentum ammoniæ (*liniment of ammonia*) contains 35 per cent. of ammonia water in cotton-seed oil and alcohol.

Vesicants.

What are vesicants?

Vesicants are remedies which, when applied to the skin, cause sufficient inflammation to produce an effusion of serum under the cuticle, or, in other words, to raise a blister. They are also called *epispastics*, or *blisters*. They are occasionally used in inflammations of the serous membranes, especially when accompanied by an outpouring of serum; to deplete the vessels in inflammations of the brain and its membranes; in chronic joint affections; in neuritis, and for the relief of various neuralgic pains; and are sometimes used in inflammations of the parenchymatous viscera. They are contraindicated in the very young or very old, where there is great depression of the vital powers, or where there is very high arterial tension.

Name the principle vesicants.

Spanish fly, potato fly, and stronger water of ammonia.

CANTHARIS (CANTHARIDES).

What is cantharides?

Cantharis vesicatoria, or Spanish fly (*Class*, Insecta; *Order*, Coleoptera), is a beetle found in the temperate parts of Europe, but especially in Spain and Italy. When dried, they contain a *volatile oil* and a neutral crystalline principle, *cantharidin*, the vesicating principle.

What are its effects and uses?

Locally, cantharides is an intense irritant to any surface with which it comes in contact; thus, applied to the skin it causes inflammation of sufficient intensity to result in a serous effusion under the cuticle, and if the application be too long continued, gangrene may result. Constitutional effect may be caused from the local application of cantharides. *Internally, in small doses,* it is diuretic; in *larger amounts* it is an irritant, causing pain on urination, priapism, strangury, and even bloody urine. Sexual desire does not usually occur. In *excessive doses* it is a gastro-enteric irritant, causing vomiting and purging, and even death, often preceded by dilated pupils, delirium, convulsions, and collapse. On *postmortem examination* severe inflammation of the alimentary canal, kidneys, and bladder is found. The *treatment* consists in removing the application or evacuating the contents of the stomach; the free use of diluents; opium (especially by the rectum); and avoiding all oily substances, as these aid the absorption of the poison.

What are its medicinal uses?

The internal uses of cantharides have previously been noticed (*vid.* Emmenagogues and Diuretics). Externally it is used as a blistering agent, almost to the exclusion of other remedies. It must be remembered that poisoning may result from its local application.

What are its preparations and their doses?

The *cerate* (*ceratum cantharidis*) is used locally as a blistering agent, and is often known as *blistering cerate*. *Cantharidal collodion* (*collodium cantharidatum*) is applied with a brush, and is a convenient way of applying a blister to an irregular surface. The *tincture* (*tinctura cantharidis*) is used internally; dose, ♏v–x (0.3–0.6 c.c.).

CANTHARIS VITTATA (POTATO FLY).

What is this substance?

The potato fly (not official) is an indigenous insect which contains *cantharidin*, and may be used as a substitute for the Spanish fly.

AQUA AMMONIÆ FORTIOR (STRONGER WATER OF AMMONIA).

Is this ever used as a blistering agent?

Stronger ammonia water is a rapid but painful vesicant sometimes employed for blistering inflamed gums.

Suppurants.

What are suppurants?

Suppurants are remedies which cause such powerful irritation of the surface to which they are applied as to produce a crop of pustules. They are seldom employed at present except as an *external* application to the throat and chest in *chronic laryngeal* or *bronchial affections*, or to the surface of a joint when *chronic inflammation* is present. The only medicines belonging to this order are *croton oil* and the unofficial *antimonial ointment.* Antimonial ointment is the more painful and its effects are more lasting.

Escharotics.

What are escharotics?

Escharotics are medicines which are applied locally to destroy the structure and vitality of the tissues. The dead tissue excites inflammation, and is thrown off by ulcerative action. It is called the *slough*, or *eschar.* Escharotics are *used* to destroy *morbid growths*, as lupus, epithelium, condylomata, warts, fungous granulations, etc.; to *destroy the virus* of malignant pustule, hospital gangrene, the bites of rabid animals or poisonous reptiles, the virus of chancre, etc.; to substitute a healthy for diseased action, and to stimulate indolent ulcers, sinuses, etc.

Mention the principal medicines used for these purposes.

Caustic potash; caustic soda; arsenous acid; bromin; zinc chlorid; acid nitrate of mercury; corrosive sublimate; potassium dichromate; the mineral acids; silver nitrate; chromium trioxide; glacial acetic acid; trichloracetic acid; copper sulphate; and burnt alum.

POTASSII HYDROXIDUM.

What is potassium hydroxide?

Potassium hydroxide (*potassa*) is formed by the rapid evaporation of the solution of potassa, and is molded into thin, cylindric sticks.

What are its effects and uses?

It is an exceedingly powerful caustic, destroying the surrounding tissues and penetrating to some depth below the surface. It is used when a powerful effect is desired, and it is well to protect the adjoining structures from its action by applying adhesive plaster with a hole cut in its center, through which the caustic is applied.

Potassa cum calce (*potassa with lime*) consists of equal parts of potassa and quicklime, and is a powerful caustic. It is sometimes called *Vienna paste*, and is not official.

SODII HYDROXIDUM.

What is sodium hydroxidum?

Sodium hydroxide (*caustic soda*) is made by the rapid evaporation of the solution of soda, and is a very powerful caustic, resembling potassa in its effects and uses. *London paste* is made by rubbing up equal parts of soda and lime.

ARSENI TRIOXIDUM (ARSENOUS ACID).

Is arsenous acid used as a caustic?

The uses of this substance as a caustic will be found under the article Arsenic (*vid.* Alteratives).

BROMUM (BROMIN).

What is bromin?

Bromin is a halogen element, and is a very powerful caustic. It is a volatile liquid, and has very great affinity for hydrogen. *Locally* it is a powerful deodorant and disinfectant, and a severe and deeply penetrating caustic. When *inhaled*, it is an intense irritant, producing laryngitis, bronchitis, and even pneumonia. *Internally*, if not sufficiently diluted, it is a corrosive poison. It is *used* as a *caustic* in *hospital gangrene* after the removal of the slough. As it is heavier than water, it may be kept in a wide-mouthed bottle half-filled with water, which will prevent it from giving off irritating fumes. From this it may be sucked up with a syringe and injected into the wound which it is desired to cauterize. The fumes are sometimes cautiously inhaled for the cure of *acute coryza, chronic nasal catarrh, ozena, hay asthma,* etc. For purposes of inhalation a solution of ʒss (2 c.c.) in ℥iv (120 c.c.) of alcohol may be used. A weak aqueous solution is also used as a gargle.

ZINCI CHLORIDUM (ZINC CHLORID), LIQUOR HYDRARGYRI NITRATIS (SOLUTION OF MERCURIC NITRATE), HYDRARGYRI CHLORIDUM CORROSIVUM (MERCURIC CHLORID).

Are these medicines escharotics?

The uses of these substances as caustics will be found under Zinc (*vid.* Astringents) and Mercury (*vid.* Alteratives).

POTASSII DICHROMAS (POTASSIUM DICHROMATE).

What is potassium dichromate?

It is an irritant *internally,* and in overdoses a corrosive poison. *Externally* it is a *caustic,* used to destroy syphilitic condylomata, warts, etc. *Internally* it is used as an *alterative* in doses of gr. $\frac{1}{6}$ (0.013 gm.), t. i. d.

CHROMII TRIOXIDUM (CHROMIC ACID).

What is chromium trioxide?

Chromium trioxide, or *chromic acid,* occurs in dark purplish-red deliquescent crystals. It is applied directly to hypertrophied tissues in the nose and throat or to small growths in the ear. Mixed with alcohol or other organic substance it may explode or take fire.

Are the mineral acids used as caustics?

The mineral acids are powerful caustics, and are often employed to remove warts or other excrescences, to cauterize chancres, indolent sinuses, and ulcers. Nitric acid is preferred as an escharotic.

The organic acids, *glacial acetic* and *trichloracetic,* are used for the removal of warts and venereal condylomata.

SILVER NITRATE, COPPER SULPHATE, and ALUM have all been previously spoken of as caustics under their appropriate heads.

DEMULCENTS.

What are demulcents?

Demulcents are bland remedies which, when applied to inflamed or irritated surfaces, exert a soothing influence upon them and are employed internally for this purpose. They are *used* in acute inflammations of the alimentary canal; in pharyngeal, laryngeal, and bronchial irritation; in renal, cystic, and urinary affections generally; and to suspend medicinal substances which are insoluble in water. They are also used as light articles of diet.

Describe the demulcents.

AQUA (*water*) is used in medicine in its purest attainable state—*i. e.*, rain or melted snow. For pharmaceutic purposes it should be used only in the form of *distilled water* (*aqua destillata*). A certain amount of water is necessary for the proper performance of the functions of the body. It is an *active diuretic*, increasing not only the watery, but also the solid, ingredients of the urine. It is *eliminated* by the kidneys, skin, lungs, and bowels. It is *used* as a *diuretic* in acute renal diseases, and is also often serviceable in chronic Bright's disease. To dilute a highly concentrated urine in *ardor urinæ*, especially when there is a tendency to the formation of gravel or calculi, it is invaluable.

It is useful in fevers, as it aids the elimination of the waste-products. *Externally*, it is used in the form of baths, either hot or cold, not only for the purposes of cleanliness, but also as a therapeutic agent. Impregnated with carbonic-acid gas under pressure it makes an agreeable drink known as *soda-water*, which is often useful in allaying nausea and vomiting.

ACACIA, or *gum arabic*, is a *gummy exudation* from *Acacia Senegal* and other species of *acacia* (*Fam.* Leguminosæ), a tree of Africa. It contains *calcium* in combination with *arabic acid*, and is much *used* in solution as a demulcent in various forms of *sore throat*. It is also used in making emulsions and pills.

Its preparations are: a *mucilage* (*mucilago acaciæ*) and a *syrup* (*syrupus acaciæ*). *Emulsion of almonds* (*emulsum amygdalæ*) and *chalk mixture* (*mistura cretæ*) also contain it.

TRAGACANTHA (*tragacanth*) is a *gummy exudation* from *Astragalus gummifer* and other species of *Astragalus* (*Fam.* Leguminosæ), and contains *bassorin* and *tragacanthin.* It is *used* internally as an agent to suspend heavy powders, to give consistence to lozenges, or in making emulsions. A *mucilage* (*mucilago tragacanthæ*) is official.

ULMUS (*elm*) is the *inner bark* of the *Ulmus fulva*, or slippery elm (*Fam.* Ulmaceæ), and contains a large amount of mucilaginous matter, and though more often used *externally* as an emollient poultice, is sometimes employed as a *demulcent* in inflammations of the bowels and in laryngitis. A *mucilage* (*mucilago ulmi*) is official.

ALTHÆA, the *peeled* root of *A. officinalis*, or marshmallow (*Fam.* Malvaceæ), is a pleasant demulcent. There are no official preparations.

LINUM (*flaxseed; linseed*), is the *ripe seed* of *Linum usitatissimum*, or flax (*Fam.* Linaceæ), and contains *fixed oil, mucilaginous matters, vegetable albumin*, etc. The *oil* (*oleum lini*) is a laxative, but is chiefly used externally in emollient liniments. The seed may be used internally as an infusion, flavored with lemon and sugar (*flaxseed tea*), in bronchial catarrhs, enteric inflammations, dysentery, and renal, vesical, or urethral irritations. The ground seeds are much used to make emollient poultices. *Linimentum calcis* consists of equal parts of linseed oil and lime-water.

SASSAFRAS MEDULLA (*sassafras pith*) is the pith of *S. variifolium* (*Fam.* Lauraceæ). The *mucilage* (*mucilago sassafras medullæ*) may be *used* internally as a demulcent, but is chiefly employed locally in inflammations of the eye.

GLYCYRRHIZA, commonly called *licorice-root*, is the rhizome and root of *G. glabra* and of *G. glandulifera* (*Fam.* Leguminosæ). It contains a *glucosid* (*glycyrrhizin*), *asparagin, resin*, etc., and is incompatible with acids. It is chiefly used as a demulcent in catarrhal affections of the respiratory organs and to disguise the taste of quinin, of the ammonium salts, and of other disagreeable medicines; occasionally, also, in kidney and bowel complaints. The preparations are an *extract* (*extractum glycyrrhizæ*), often called *licorice; refined extract* (*extractum glycyrrhizæ purum*); *fluid extract* (*fluidextractum glycyrrhizæ*), used as an addendum to cough medicines and an ingredient of *elixir adjuvans; ammoniated glycyrrhizin* (*glycyrrhizinum ammoniatum*), dose, gr. v–x (0.3–0.6 gm.); *compound glycyrrhiza mixture* (*mistura glycyrrhizæ composita; brown mixture*), contains the refined extract, mucilage of acacia, syrup, paregoric (12 per cent.), antimonial wine (6 per cent.), sweet spirits of niter and water; dose, f℥ss (15 c.c.). *Compound licorice powder* (containing sulphur and senna—used as a laxative) has been previously mentioned.

Chondrus.—*Chondrus crispus*, Irish moss, or carrageen (*Fam.* Gigartinaceæ), is a sea-weed found on the coast of Ireland and New England. It contains *carrageenin*, etc., and is used as a nutritive (in the form of a blanc-mange), as a demulcent, as an emollient poultice, and in making emulsions.

Amylum (*starch*) is the starch grains obtained from the *fruit* of *Zea mays* (*Fam.* Gramineæ). With iodin its solution forms a rich blue iodid. It is converted into glucose in the alimentary canal, and thus absorbed. It is used as an article of diet, and locally as a dusting-powder. Its solution is employed as a vehicle for laudanum enemata.

Glyceritum amyli (*glycerite of starch* or *plasmine*) is used as a vehicle for astringent applications to the eye, and as an unguent in scarlatina and small-pox.

Kaolinum (*kaolin*) is a native aluminum silicate; the *cataplasma kaolini*, a clay-like poultice of kaolin, boric acid, methyl salicylate, glycerin, thymol, and oil of peppermint, is official.

Talcum (*talc*), a native hydrous magnesium silicate, and Talcum Purificatum (*purified talc*), talc treated with hydrochloric acid, are employed as dusting-powders, and in the manufacture of medicated waters.

Lycopodium, the *sporules* of *L. clavatum*, or club-moss, and other species of lycopodium (*Fam.* Lycopodiaceæ), is used as a dusting-powder for intertrigo, and is very useful in the excoriated nates of children.

EMOLLIENTS.

What are emollients?

Emollients are bland, fatty substances used externally to soften the skin and render it more pliable, or to serve as a vehicle for other medicaments.

Describe the emollients.

Adeps (*lard*), the prepared internal fat of the abdomen of *Sus scrofa*, var. *domesticus* (the hog), consists of olein and stearin and is used in the preparation of unguents. *Adeps benzoinatus* (*benzoinated lard*) contains 2 per cent. of benzoin to prevent rancidity. *Ointment* (*unguentum*) consists of benzoinated lard (80 per cent.) melted with white wax. *Cerate* (*ceratum*) contains 50 per cent. of benzoinated lard.

Adeps Lanæ (*wool-fat*) is the purified fat of the wool of sheep (*Ovis aries*), and Adeps Lanæ Hydrosus (*hydrous wool-fat; lanolin*) is the purified fat of the wool of sheep, mixed with not more than 30 per cent. of water. Wool-fat is capable of taking up more than half its weight of watery solutions, and is rapidly absorbed by the skin.

Sevum Præparatum (*prepared suet*), the internal fat of the abdomen of *Ovis aries* (the sheep), consists, when purified, almost entirely of stearin.

Cetaceum (*spermaceti*), a peculiar, concrete, fatty substance obtained from the head of *Physeter macrocephalus*, or sperm-whale. It enters into the preparation of *cold cream.*

Cera Flava (*yellow*) and Cera Alba (*white wax*). The former is a solid substance, prepared from the honeycomb of the bee, *Apis mellifera.* The latter is the former which has been bleached. They are used in making cerates, plasters, and ointments.

ACIDUM OLEICUM (*oleic acid*), used chiefly in preparing the oleates.

GLYCERINUM (*glycerin*) is the hydroxid of glyceryl and exists in animal oils combined with fatty acids. Internally it is nutrient, demulcent, and, in large doses, laxative. Administered by the bowel it is laxative even in small amounts, for which purpose the *suppositories* (*suppositoria glycerini*) are much used. Locally, it is much used as an emollient. *Glycerite of starch* (*vid.* Amylum) is used externally; the *glycerite of the phosphates of iron, quinine and strychnine, of phenol, of tannic acid, of boroglycerin,* and *of hydrastis* are also official.

GELATINUM GLYCERINATUM (*glycerinated gelatin*) is a mixture of equal parts of glycerin and gelatin, solid when cold, but easily melted by gentle heat. It is employed as a basis for suppositories.

OLEUM THEOBROMATIS (*oil of theobroma*), or cacao butter, is the *fixed oil expressed* from the roasted *seed* of *Theobroma Cacao* (*Fam.* Sterculiaceæ), and is used as an unguent and to give form and consistence to suppositories. It is solid at ordinary temperature.

OLEUM GOSSYPII SEMINIS (*cotton-seed oil*), *a fixed oil expressed* from the *seed* of *Gossypium herbaceum* (*q. v.*), is used as a substitute for almond or olive oil, and enters into the composition of numerous liniments.

PETROLATUM (*petrolatum*) is a mixture of hydrocarbons, chiefly of the marsh-gas series, obtained by distilling off the lighter and more volatile portions from petroleum and purifying the residue.

It differs from *petrolatum liquidum* (*liquid petrolatum*) chiefly in its consistence, in its melting-point, and in its specific gravity. Under the names of vaselin and cosmolin, the heavier petroleum oils are much used externally as emollients and as a basis for ointments, and internally to allay irritation of the mucous membranes. They are not readily absorbed by the skin, but have the advantage of not becoming rancid.

PETROLATUM ALBUM (*white petrolatum; white vaselin; solid albolene*) is of the same nature and consistence as *petrolatum*, but white and less sticky.

Many of the Demulcents also are employed in the form of poultices as emollients.

PROTECTIVES.

What are protectives?

Protectives are substances used to exclude light or air from the surface to which they are applied, or otherwise to protect it from injurious influences. Many *surgical appliances* are thus "protectives," but do not belong to the domain of Materia Medica. The *plasters* and *unguents*, when simply used to protect the surface, come under this class. The following agents have not been previously considered: plaster-of-Paris, collodion, solution of gutta-percha, and solution of sodium silicate.

What are these substances?

CALCII SULPHAS EXSICCATUS (*dried gypsum; dried calcium sulphate, or plaster-of-Paris*) is a powder containing about 95 per cent., by weight, of calcium sulphate.

It is used as a permanent dressing in the treatment of fractures, caries of the vertebræ, etc., where it is necssary to give continual support to the parts for some time. For this purpose it is moistened and thoroughly rubbed into successive layers of previously moistened roller bandage. It *sets* very rapidly, forming with the bandage a stiff, board-like support.

COLLODIUM (*collodion*) is a solution of *pyroxylin* or soluble gun-cotton (*pyroxylinum*) (4 per cent.), in stronger ether and alcohol. When applied to the skin, the solvents rapidly evaporate, leaving a colorless, transparent, flexible, and strongly contractile film, closely adherent, difficult to detach, and impervious alike to air and water. It has been used in surgery as an antiphlogistic in inflammation, on account of its contractile power, and also applied on gauze, as a substitute for adhesive plaster in the treatment of wounds. Its contractile power is an objection to its use as a simple protective, for which purpose it is better to employ *flexible collodion* (*collodium flexile*), which contains Canada turpentine (5 per cent.) and castor oil (3 per cent.), and is more pliable and elastic. *Styptic collodion* (*collodium stypticum*) contains, in addition to collodion, tannic acid (20 per cent.), ether (25 per cent.), and alcohol (5 per cent.).

ELASTICA (*India rubber or caoutchouc*) is the prepared *milk-juice* of various species of Hevea (*Fam.* Euphorbiaceæ), known in commerce as Para rubber. It is used in making plasters, bougies, etc., and has been used dissolved in chloroform as a protective to small abrasions, chaps, threatened bedsores, etc. It forms 2 per cent. of the *emplastrum adhæsivum* (adhesive plaster).

COLORING AGENTS.

What are coloring agents?

They are employed almost exclusively to give their particular color to tinctures, spirits, and ointments, and are—

COCCUS (*cochineal*), the *dried female insect, Pseudococcus cacti*, a native of Mexico and Central America, containing *carminic acid*, to which it owes its pecu'iar red color. It has been used also as an *antispasmodic;* dose, gr. $\frac{1}{3}$ (0.02 gm.), t. i. d.

SANTALUM RUBRUM (*red saunders*), the *heart-wood* of *Pterocarpus santalinus* (*Fam.* Leguminosæ), contains *santalic acid* and *pterocarpin*, and is used to give a red color to pharmaceutic preparations.

SWEETENING AGENT.

BENZOSULPHINIDUM (SACCHARIN).

What is saccharin?

Saccharin is a sweetening agent to replace sugar in the food of diabetics. It is about 200 times as sweet as cane sugar, and is soluble in 250 parts of water and 25 of alcohol. It is more soluble in water in the presence of an alkali, and is frequently dispensed in one-half or one-grain tablets made with an equal quantity of sodium bicarbonate.

SERUM THERAPY.

What is serum therapy?

Serum therapy is the treatment of disease by the employment of a serum which is antagonistic either to the poisons produced in the disease or to the development of the bacteria of the disease. The only official serum is—

SERUM ANTIDIPHTHERICUM (*diphtheria antitoxin*), "a fluid separated from the coagulated blood of a horse immunized through the inoculation of diphtheric serum." It gradually deteriorates on keeping; dose, 2000 to 20,000 units for the treatment of diphtheria, or 500 to 1000 units for immunizing, injected beneath the skin. A *unit* is as much serum as will protect a 250-gm. guinea-pig from 100 fatal doses of diphtheria toxin.

ORGANO-THERAPY.

Certain organs of the body, the thyroid gland, the suprarenals, ovaries, testicles, spleen, pituitary body, etc., have been found to have a decided influence when administered as medicine. The only official ones are *suprarenal* (see page 155) and *thyroid.*

GLANDULÆ THYROIDEÆ SICCÆ (*desiccated thyroid glands*) are the cleaned, dried, and powdered thyroid glands of the sheep, freed from fat. They are employed in *myxedema* to replace the normal thyroid secretion, and have been used in numerous other diseases of metabolism, such as diabetes, Addison's disease, eclampsia, obesity, etc., with varying success; dose, gr. j–v (0.06–0.3 gm.). In overdose *thyroid* causes flushing and sweating of the skin, rapid feeble heart, and great nervousness, with a tremor of the hands.

INDEX

ABSINTHE, 40
Absinthin, 40
Absinthium, 39, 40, 41
  oil, 40
Absinthol, 40
Absolute alcohol, 148
Acacia, 267
  syrup, 267
Aceta, 23
Acetanilid, 80
  powder compound, 81
Acetanilidum, 80
Acetic acid, 167, 168
    glacial, 168, 266
Acetphenetidin, 81
Acetum opii, 91
  scillæ, 210
Acetylpara-amidophenol salicylate, 85
Acid, acetic, 167, 168
    glacial, 168, 266
  anthemic, 40
  arsenous, 69, 265
    solution, 69
  benzoic, 228, 257
  boric, 253
  calumbic, 37
  cambogic, 199
  camphoric, 131
  carbolic, 254, 256
  carminic, 273
  cathartic, 191
  chromic, 266
  chrysophanic, 192, 194
  cinchotannic, 43
  citric, 167, 169
  cocatannic, 113
  crotonic, 200
  crotonoleic, 200
  cubebic, 218
  digallic, 331
  digitallic, 153
Acid, ergotinic, 171
  euonic, 195
  filicic, 202
  gallic, 233
  gallotannic, 231
  gelseminic, 139
  gentisic, 37
  guaiacic, 75
  guaiaconic, 75
  guaiacresinic, 75
  hydriodic, 67
  hydrobromic, diluted, 99
  hydrochloric, 56, 58
  hydrocyanic, 140, 142
  hypophosphorous, 58
  igasuric, 132
  ipecacuanhic, 179
  kinic, 43
  kinotannic, 232, 234
  kinovic, 43
  kombic, 159
  kramerotannic, 234
  lactic, 47, 59
  lobelic, 145
  lupamaric, 105
  mineral, 47, 56
  muriatic, 56, 58
  nitric, 56, 58
  nitrohydrochloric, 56, 58
  nitromuriatic, 56, 58
  oleic, 271
  ophelic, 37
  phenic, 254, 256
  phosphoric, 56, 58
  polygalic, 226
  prussic, 140
  pyroligneous, 229
  quercitannic, 234
  rheotannic, 192
  rheumic, 192
  salicylic, 82, 84
  santalic, 273

Acid, sphacelic, 171
sulphuric, 56, 57
sulphurous, 252
tannic, 158, 231
tartaric, 167, 169
trichloracetic, 168, 266
urochloralic, 97
valerianic, 128, 175
vegetable, 167
Acidum. See *Acid.*
Aconin, 163
Aconite, 163
fluid extract, 165
tincture, 126, 165
Aconitin, 163, 165
Aconitina, 163, 165
Aconitum, 163
Actol, 244
Adeps, 270
benzoinatus, 229, 270
hydrosus, 270
lanæ, 270
Adhesive plaster, 273
Adjuvant of inscription, 27
Administration of medicines, 32
Adonidin, 158
Adrenalin, 155
chlorid solution, 156
Æther, 116, 119, 149
fortior (U. S. P. 1880), 119
Æthylis carbamas, 103
chloridum, 123, 125
Age, dosage and, 31
Albolene, solid, 272
Alcohol, 147, 149
absolutum, 148
dilutum, 149
narcosis, 148
Alimentary canal, medicines affecting, 178
Allium, 227
Allspice, 186
oil, 186
Allyl sulphocyanid, 261
Almond, bitter, essence, 142
oil, 142
spirit, 142
water, 142
emulsion, 142, 267
milk, 142
syrup, 142
Alœ purificata, 193
Aloes, 193
and iron pills, 194
and mastiche pills, 193
Aloes and myrrh pills, 194
tincture, 194
extract, 194
pills, 193
tincture, 194
Aloin, 194
pills, 135
Aloinum, 194
Alpha-eucain, 126
Alteratives, 59
Althæa, 268
Alum, 182, 238
ammonioferric, 51
dried, 239
Alumen, 182, 238
exsiccatum, 239
Alumini hydroxidum, 239
sulphas, 239
Aluminum acetate, 239
hydroxid, 239
sulphate, 239
Amidophenacetin, 81
Aminoform, 219
Ammonia, 262
gas, 150
liniment, 262
spirit, 152
aromatic, 152
water, 151
stronger, 151, 263
Ammoniac, 228
Ammoniacum, 228
Ammoniated mercury, 63
ointment, 63
tincture, 22
Ammonii benzoas, 257
bromidum, 98
carbonas, 152
chloridum, 73, 225
iodidum, 67
salicylas, 152
valeras, 128
Ammonioferric alum, 51
Ammonium, 50
acetate, 152
and iron solution, 50
solution, 221
and bismuth citrate, 245
and iron citrate, 51
tartrate, 51
benzoate, 257
bromid, 98
carbonate, 152
chlorid, 73, 225
troches, 225

Ammonium citrate, 244
iodid, 67
muriate, 225
nitrate, 152
salicylate, 84, 152
valerate, 128
Amygdalin, 142
Amyl nitrate, 137, 138
Amylis nitris, 137, 138
Amylum, 269
Anaphrodisiacs, 170
Anesthetics, 116
local, 124
Anise, 188
oil, 188
spirit, 188
water, 188
Anisum, 188
Anodynes, 89
Hoffmann's, 131
mydriatic, 106
Antacids, 245
Anthelmintics, 201
Anthemic acid, 40
Anthemis, 39, 41
Antifebrin, 80
Antimonial ointment, 264
Antimonii et potassii tartras, 162, 182
Antimonium, 161
and potassium tartrate, 162, 182
Antimony, 161
tartrated, 162
wine, 163
Antipyretics, 77, 259
Antipyrin, 78
Antiseptic oils, 259
solution, 254
Antiseptics, 247
Antispasmodics, 126
Aphrodisiacs, 169
Apiol, 177
Apocynein, 211
Apocynin, 211
Apocynum, 211
fluid extract, 211
Apomorphin hydrochlorid, 180
Apomorphinæ hydrochloridum, 180
Aporetin, 192
Apothecaries' measure, 24
weight, 24
metric system and, relation, 25
Aqua, 22, 267
ammoniæ, 151
fortior, 151, 263
Aqua, amygdale amaræ, 142
anisi, 188
aurantii florum, 189
fortior, 189
camphoræ, 130
chloroformi, 122
cinnamomi, 185
creosoti, 257
destillata, 267
fœniculi, 188
hamamelidis, 235
hydrogenii dioxidi, 248
menthæ piperitæ, 188
viridis, 188
regia, 58
rosæ, 235
fortior, 235
Arbutin, 214
Argentamin, 243
Argenti cyanidum, 142, 243
nitras, 243
fusus, 242
mitigatus, 243
oxidum, 243
Argentum, 242
Argonin, 243
Argyria, 242
Argyrol, 241
Aristol, 252, 260
Aristolochin, 40
Arnica, 167
tincture, 167
Arnicin, 167
Aromatic bitters, 39
elixir, 189
fluid extract, 187
powder, 185, 186
Arseni iodidum, 70
trioxidum, 69, 265
Arsenic, 67
and mercuric iodid solution, 70
iodid, 70
poisoning, 68
trioxid, 69, 265
white, 69, 265
Arsenous acid, 69, 265
solution, 69
Arsenum, 67
Arthralgia, lead, 236
Asafetida, 128
emulsion, 129
pills, 129
tincture, 129
Ascarides, remedies for, 203
Aspidium, 202

Aspidium oleoresin, 202
Aspidosperma, 226
Aspidospermatin, 226
Aspidospermin, 226
Astringents, 231
mineral, 235
vegetable, 231
Atropamin, 107
Atropin, 152
Atropinæ, 107, 110, 111, 113, 152, 222
oleatum, 110
sulphas, 110
Aurantii amari cortex, 188
dulcis cortex, 188
Auri et sodii chloridum, 65
Aurum, 64

Balsam, Canada, 216
gauge, 229
of fir, 216
of peru, 229
of tolu, 229
Balsamum peruvianum, 229
tolutanum, 229
Basham's mixture, 50
Basis of inscription, 27
Bassorin, 268
Belladonna, 107
leaves, extract, 110
tincture, 110
liniment, 110
ointment, 110
pills, 135, 198
plaster, 110
root, fluid extract, 110
Belladonnin, 107
Benzoic acid, 228, 257
aldehyd, 142
Benzoin, 228
tincture, 229
compound, 229
Benzoinated lard, 229
Benzoinum, 228
Benzosol, 86
Benzosulphinidum, 273
Benzoylecgonin, 113
Berberin, 37, 38, 46
Berberis, 37
fluid extract, 39
Beta-eucain, 125
Beta-naphthol, 258
Betula oil, 84
Bichlorid of gold, 65
Birch, sweet, oil, 84
Bismuth, 244
Bismuth and ammonium citrate, 245
citrate, 244, 245
magistery of, 244
subcarbonate, 244
subgallate, 244
subnitrate, 244
subsalicylate, 84, 244
Bismuthi citras, 245
et ammonii citras, 245
subcarbonas, 244
subgallas, 244
subnitras, 244
subsalicylas, 244
Bismuthum, 244
Bitter almond essence, 142
oil, 142
spirit, 142
water, 142
orange-peel, 188
fluid extract, 189
tincture, 189
wine of iron, 51
Bitters, aromatic, 39
peculiar, 42
simple, 37
Black draft, 194
drop, 94
Blaud's pills, 49
Blistering cerate, 263
Blisters, 262
Blue mass, 62, 195
ointment, 62
stones, 240
vitriol, 240
Borax, 253
Boric acid, 253
ointment, 254
Boroglycerin glycerite, 254, 271
Boroglycerite solution, 254
Bozoic acid, 228, 257
Brandy, 149
Brayera, 203
Bromids, 97
Bromin, 71, 250, 265
Bromism, 98
Bromoform, 123
Bromoformum, 123
Bromum, 71, 250, 265
Brown mixture, 269
Brucin, 132
Brunton's rule for dosage in children, 31
Bryonia, 198
Bryonin, 198

Bryony, 198
  tincture, 198
Buchu, 213
  fluid extract, 213
Burnett's disinfecting fluid, 241
Burns, carbolic acid, 255
Butyl-chloral hydrate, 96
Buxin, 213

CACAO butter, 271
Cade oil, 230
Caffein, 156, 158, 210
  citrated, 158
  effervescent, 158
Caffeina, 156, 158, 210
  citrata, 158
  effervescens, 158
Cajuput oil, 187
Calabar bean, 135
Calabarin, 135
Calamin, 241
Calamus, 187
  fluid extract, 187
Calcii bromidum, 99
  carbonas præcipitatus, 247
  chloridum, 73
  hypophosphis, 73
  phosphas præcipitatus, 72
  sulphas exsiccatus, 272
Calcined magnesia, 195
Calcium, 247
  bromid, 99
  carbonate, precipitated, 247
  chlorid, 73
  hypophosphite, 73
  lactophosphate syrup, 73
  phosphate, 72
  sulphate, dried, 272
Calendula, 76
  tincture, 76
Calendulin, 76
Calomel, 62, 64, 195, 203, 212
Calumba, 37
  fluid extract, 38
  tincture, 38
Calumbic acid, 37
Calumbin, 37
Calx chlorinata, 249
  sulphurata, 253
Cambogia, 199
Cambogic acid, 199
Campeachy wood, 234
Camphor, 129, 130
  cerate, 130
  liniment, 130
Camphor mixture, Hope's, 130
  monobromated, 130
  parsley-, 177
  spirit, 130
  tobacco-, 145
  water, 130
Camphora, 129, 130
  monobromata, 130
Camphorated oil, 130
Camphoric acid, 131
Canada balsam, 216
  turpentine, 216
Canadian hemp, 211
Cannabin, 104
Cannabis Indica, 104
    extract, 105
      fluid, 105
    tinctura, 105
Cantharidal collodion, 263
Cantharides, 178, 219, 262
  cerate, 263
  tincture, 219, 263
Cantharidin, 262, 263
Cantharis, 219, 262
  vesicatoria, 262
  vittata, 263
Caoutchouc, 273
Capsicum, 184, 262
  fluid extract, 184
  oleoresin, 184
  pills, 198
  plaster, 184
  tincture, 184
Capsules, 23
Caraway, 188
  oil, 188
Carbolic acid, 251, 256
Cardamom, 186
  tincture, 186
    compound, 186
Cardamomum, 186
Cardiac sedatives, 161
  stimulants, 146
Carminatives, 183
Carminic acid, 273
Carrageen, 269
Carrageenin, 269
Carron oil, 247
Carum, 188
Caryophyllin, 186
Caryophyllus, 185
Cascara sagrada, 191
Cascarilla, 39, 41
Cascarillin, 40
Cassia fistula, 190

Castor oil, 191
Cataplasm, 21
 kaolini, 269
Cataplasma, 21
 kaolini, 269
Catechol, 86
Catechu, 234
Cathartic acid, 194
 enemata, 201
 pills, compound, 200
  vegetable, 200
Cathartics, 189
 drastic, 197
 mercurial, 195
 saline, 195
Caustic soda, 246, 265
Centimeter, 25
Cephaelin, 179
Cera alba, 270
 flava, 270
Cerata, 21
Cerates, 21
Ceratum camphoræ, 130
 cantharidis, 263
 plumbi subacetatis, 238
Cerii oxalas, 245
Cerium oxalate, 245
Cetaceum, 270
Cevadillin, 167
Cevadin, 167
Ceylon cinnamon, 185
Chalk mixture, 247, 267
 prepared, 247
Chalk-powder, compound, 247
Chamomile tea, 41
Charta, 21
 potassii nitratis, 21
 sinapis, 21, 261
Chenopodium, 202
Chimaphila, 214
 fluid extract, 214
Chimaphilin, 214
Chinolin, 88
Chirata, 37
 fluid extract, 39
Chiratin, 37
Chittem bark, 191
Chloral, 95
 anhydrous, 95
 habit, 95
 hydrate, official, 95
Chloralamid, 97
Chloralformamidum, 97
Chloralism, 95
Chloralum hydratum, 95
Chlorin, 71
 water, 249
Chlorinated lime, 249
 soda solution, 250
Chloroform, 120, 122
 and ether, comparison of effects, 121
 emulsion, 122
 liniment, 122
 spirit, 122
 water, 122
Chloroformum, 120, 122
Cholin, 105, 155
Chondrus, 269
 crispus, 269
Chromic acid, 266
Chromii trioxidum, 266
Chromium trioxid, 265
Chrysophan, 192
Chrysophanic acid, 192, 194
Chrysotoxin, 171
Cimicifuga, 160
 fluid extract, 160
 tincture, 160
Cinchona, 42
 bark, 42
 fluid extract, 45
 tincture, 45
  compound, 41, 45
Cinchonicin, 43
Cinchonidin, 43
 sulphate, 46
Cinchonidinæ sulphas, 46
Cinchonin, 43
 sulphate, 46
Cinchoninæ sulphas, 46
Cinchonism, 44
Cinchotannic acid, 43
Cinnaldehydum, 185
Cinnamic aldehyd, 185
Cinnamomum Saigonicum, 185
 Zeylonicum, 185
Cinnamon, Ceylon, 185
 oil, 185
 Saigon, 185
 spirit, 185
 tincture, 185
 water, 185
Circulatory organs, medicines affecting, 146
Citric acid, 167, 169
 syrup, 169
Citrin ointment, 63
Classifications of medicines, 33
Cloves, 185

Cloves, oil, 186
Coca, 113
wine, 116
Cocain, 113, 116, 125
hydrochlorid, 116
oleate, 116
Cocaina, 113, 116
Cocainæ hydrochloridum, 116
Cocatannic acid, 113
Coccus, 273
Cochineal, 273
Codein, 92, 94
phosphate, 94
sulphate, 94
Codeina, 94
Codeinæ phosphas, 94
sulphas, 94
Cod-liver oil, 71
emulsion, 71
with hypophosphites, 72
Colchicein, 74
Colchicin, 74, 75
Colchicina, 74, 75
Colchicum, 74
corns, extract, 74
seed, fluid extract, 74
tincture, 74
wine, 75
Cold as anesthetic, 124
cream, 235
Colic, lead, 236, 237
Collodion, 272
flexible, 273
styptic, 273
tannic acid, 233
Collodium, 272
cantharidatum, 263
flexile, 273
stypticum, 233, 273
Colocynth, 199
extract, 199
Colocynthin, 199
Colocynthis, 199
Colocynthitin, 199
Coloring agents, 273
Confectio rosæ, 235
sennæ, 191
Confection, 20
Coniin, 113
Conium, 113
fluid extract, 144
Conserves, 20
Convallamarin, 160
Convallaria, 160
fluid extract, 160
Convallarin, 160
Conydrin, 144
Copaiba, 218
oil, 218
Copper, 239
sulphate, 182, 240
Copperas, 50
Coriander, 188
Coriandri oil, 188
Coriandrum, 188
Corn-silk, 215
Cornutin, 171
Corrective of inscription, 27
Corrosive sublimate, 63, 64, 213
poisoning, 61
Cosmolin, 271
Cotarnin hydrochlorid, 174
Cotton-root bark, 174
Cotton-seed oil, 271
Cough lozenges, Wistar's, 93
Cowling's rules for dosage for children, 31
Coxe's hive syrup, 163, 210
Cream of tartar, 197, 207
Cremor tartar, 197, 207
Creosote, 256
water, 257
Creosotum, 256
Cresol, 256
Creta præparata, 247
Croton oil, 200, 264
Croton-chloral hydrate, 96
Crotonic acid, 200
Crotonoleic acid, 200
Cubeb, 218
fluid extract, 219
oil, 218
oleoresin, 218
tincture, 219
troches, 219
Cubeba, 218
Cubebic acid, 218
Cubebin, 218
Cupri sulphas, 182, 240
Cuprum, 239
Curare, 145
Curarin, 145
Cusso, 203
Cyanids, 142
Cymol, 40
Cypripedium, 131
fluid extract, 131
Cystogen, 219

DAPHNIN, 76
Decimal system of weights, 24
apothecaries' weights and, relations, 24, 25
Decocta, 22
dosage, 30
Decoctions, 22
dosage, 30
Demulcents, 267
Deodorants, 248
Depressomotors, 135
Dermatol, 241
Diachylon ointment, 237
Diaphoretics, 220
nauseating, 220
saline, 221
sedative, 220
special, 222
Diastase, 35
Diethylsulphon-diethylmethane, 103
Diethylsulphon-dimethylmethane, 100, 103
Diethylsulphon-methylethylmethane, 102, 103
Digallic acid, 231
Digestants, 34
Digitaleic acid, 153
Digitalein, 153
Digitalin, 152, 155
Digitalis, 152, 210
extract, 155
fluid, 155
pills, 154
tincture, 155
Digitonin, 153
Digitophyllin, 153
Digitoxin, 152
Dimethylxanthin, 211
Dipentene, 230
Diphtheria antitoxin, 274
Dispensatory, definition, 19
Diuretics, 204
alkaline, 204
alterative, 213
hydragogue, 209
Diuretin, 211
Donovan's solution, 70
Dosage, age and, 31
conditions modifying effect, 30
for children, 31
general rules for, 30
Dose, calculating, 29
Dover's powder, 93, 220
Drops, 26
EFFERVESCENT salt, granular, 21
Effervescing draft, 206
powder, compound, 197
Elastica, 273
Elaterin, 200
trituration, 200
Elaterinum, 200
Elixir aromaticum, 189
ferri, quinine et strychninæ phosphatum, 51, 73
of phosphorus, 55
of vitriol, 57
Ellis' magnesia, 196
Elm, 268
Emetics, 178
local, 178
systemic, 178
Emetin, 179
Emmenagogues, 176
stimulating, 176
Emodin, 191
Emollients, 270
Emplastrum, 21
adhæsivum, 273
belladonnæ, 110
capsici, 84
hydrargyri, 62
opii, 93
plumbi, 237
Emulsi, 23
Emulsin, 40, 142
Emulsions, 23
Emulsum amygdalæ, 142, 267
asafœtidæ, 129
chloroformi, 122
olei morrhuæ, 71
cum hypophosphitibus, 72
Encephalopathy, lead, 236
Endermic administration of medicines, 32
Enemata, 23, 201
Enepidermic administration of medicines, 32
Epidermic administration of medicines, 32
Epispastics, 262
Epsom salt, 196
Ergochrysin, 171
Ergot, 171
extract, 173
fluid, 173
wine, 173
Ergota, 171
Ergotinic acid, 171
Ergotisin, 172

Ericolin, 214
Erigeron oil, 215
Eriodictyon, 227
fluid extract, 227
Erythrol tetranitrate, 137, 139
Erythroretin, 192
Erythroxylon, 113
fluid extract, 116
Eschar, 264
Escharotics, 264
Eserin, 135
Ether, 116, 119, 149
and chloroform, comparison of effects, 121
hydrochloric, 125
nitrous, spirit, 212, 221
spirit, 119
compound, 119, 131
Ethereal oil, 131
Ethyl bromid, 123
carbamate, 103
chlorid, 123, 125
hydroxid, 147
oxid, 116
Ethylene-diamin silver phosphate, 243
Eucain, alpha-, 126
beta-, 125
Eucalyptol, 40, 41
Eucalyptus, 39, 40
fluid extract, 41
oil, 40, 41
Eugenol, 186
Euonic acid, 195
Euonymin, 195
Euonymus, 194, 195
extract, 195
fluid, 195
Eupatorin, 40
Eupatorium, 39
fluid extract, 41
Europhen, 252
Excitomotors, 132
Expectorants, 223
sedative, 224
stimulating, 224
Extracts, 20
fluid. See *Fluidextractum.*
Extractum aloes, 194
belladonnæ foliorum, 110
cannabis indicæ, 105
cimicifugæ, 160
colchici cormi, 74
colocynthidis, 199
compositum, 199
Extractum digitalis, 155
ergotæ, 173
euonymi, 195
gentianæ, 38
glycyrrhizæ, 269
purum, 269
hæmatoxyli, 234
hyoscyami, 112
iridis, 199
juglandis, 193
krameriæ, 234
leptandræ, 195
malti, 35, 36
nucis vomicæ, 134
opii, 93
physostigmatis, 136
quassiæ, 38
rhamni purshianæ, 191
rhei, 193
scopolæ, 113
stramonii, 111
sumbul, 127
taraxaci, 212

FENNEL, 188
oil, 188
water, 188
Ferri carbonas saccharatus, 49
chloridum, 50
citras, 51
et ammonii sulphas, 51
citras, 51
tartras, 51
et potassii tartras, 51
et quininæ citras, 51
solubilis, 51
et strychninæ citras, 51
hydroxid with magnesium oxid, 49
hydroxidum, 49
cum magnesii oxido, 49
hypophosphis, 51
phosphas solubilis, 51
pyrophosphas solubilis, 51
sulphas, 50
exsiccatus, 50
granulatus, 50
Ferric ammonium sulphate, 51
chlorid, 50
solution, 50
tincture, 50
citrate, 51
hydroxid, 49
hypophosphite, 51
phosphate, soluble, 51

Ferric pyrophosphate, soluble, 51
  subsulphate solution, 50
  sulphate solution, 50
Ferrous carbonate mass, 49
    pills, 49
    saccharated, 49
  iodid pills, 50
    syrup, 50
  sulphate, 49, 50
    dried, 50
    granulated, 50
Ferrum, 47, 48
  reductum, 49
Filicic acid, 202
Flaxseed, 268
  tea, 268
Flowers of sulphur, 192
Fluid extracts. See *Fluidextractum.*
Fluidextractum, 22
  aconiti, 165
  apocyni, 211
  aromaticum, 187
  aspidospermæ, 227
  aurantii amari, 189
  belladonnæ radicis, 110
  berberidis, 39
  buchu, 213
  calami, 187
  calumbæ, 38
  cannabis indicæ, 105
  capsici, 184
  chimaphilæ, 214
  chiratæ, 39
  cimicifugæ, 160
  cinchonæ, 45
  cocæ, 116
  colchici seminis, 74
  conii, 144
  convallariæ, 160
  cubebæ, 219
  cypri pedii, 131
  digitalis, 155
  dosage of, 30
  ergotæ, 173
  eriodictyi, 227
  eucalypti, 41
  euonymi, 195
  eupatorii, 41
  frangulæ, 191
  gelsemii, 140
  gentianæ, 38
  geranii, 235
  glycyrrhizæ, 269
  granati, 203
  grindeliæ, 224
Fluidextractum guaranæ, 158
  hamamelidis, 235
  hydrastis, 47
  hyoscyami, 112
  ipecacuanhæ, 180
  iridis, 199
  krameriæ, 234
  lappæ, 77
  leptandræ, 195
  lobeliæ, 143
  lupulini, 106
  matico, 219
  mezerei, 76
  nucis vomicæ, 134
  pareiræ, 213
  pilocarpi, 223
  podophylli, 198
  pruni virginianæ, 41
  quassiæ, 38
  quercus, 235
  quillajæ, 226
  rhamni purshianæ, 191
      aromaticum, 191
  rhei, 193
  rhoïs glabræ, 235
  rosæ, 235
  sabinæ, 177
  sanguinariæ, 228
  sarsaparillæ, 75
    compositum, 75
  scillæ, 210
  scoparii, 212
  scopolæ, 113
  scutellariæ, 131
  senegæ, 226
  sennæ, 194
  serpentariæ, 41
  spigeliæ, 202
  stillingiæ, 77
  stramonii, 111
  sumbul, 127
  taraxaci, 212
  tritici, 214
  uvæ ursi, 214
  valerianæ, 128
  veratri, 166
  viburni opuli, 176
    prunifolii, 175
  zingiberis, 186
Fœniculum, 188
Fomentations, 23
Forced enemata, 201
Formal, 259
Formaldehyd solution, 259
Formalin, 259

Formulas, extemporized, 26
Formyl terchlorid, 120
 teriodid, 251
Fowler's solution, 69
Frangula, 190
 fluid extract, 191
Frangulin, 190
Fraxin, 190
Freezing as anesthetic, 124

GADUIN, 71
Galla, 233
 ointment, 233
 tincture, 233
Gallic acid, 233
Gallotannic acid, 231
Gambir, 234
 tincture, compound, 234
 troches, 234
Gamboge, 199
Gargles, 23
Garlic, 227
 syrup, 227
Gastric sedatives, 182
Gaultheria oil, 81, 187
 spirit, 187
Gelatin, glycerinated, 271
Gelatinum glycerinatum, 271
Gelsemin, 139
Gelseminic acid, 139
Gelseminin, 139
Gelsemium, 139, 167
 fluid extract, 140
 tincture, 140
Gentian, 37
 extract, 38
  fluid, 38
 tincture, compound, 38
Gentiana, 37
Gentianin, 37
Gentiopicrin, 37
Gentisic acid, 37
Gentisin, 37
Geranium, 235
 fluid extract, 235
Germicides, 248
Ginger, 186
 fluid extract, 186
 oleoresin, 186
 syrup, 186
 tincture, 186
Glacial acetic acid, 266
Glandulæ suprarenales siccæ, 155, 156
 thyroideæ siccæ, 274
Glauber's salt, 196
Glonoin, 137
Glycerin, 271
 suppositories, 271
Glycerinum, 271
Glycerita, 23
Glycerites, 23
Glyceritum acidi tannici, 233
 amyli, 269
 boroglycerini, 254
 ferri, quininæ, et strychninæ phosphatum, 51, 73
 hydrastis, 47
 phenolis, 256
Glyceryl borate glycerite, 254
 hydroxid, 271
 trinitrate, 137
  spirit, 138
Glycyrrhiza, 268
 and opium troches, 93
 mixture, compound, 269
 powder, compound, 194
Glycyrrhizin, 268
 ammoniated, 269
Glycyrrhizinum ammoniatum, 269
Gold, 64
 and sodium chlorid, 65
 bichlorid, 65
Gossypii cortex, 174
Goulard's cerate, 238
 extract, 238
Grains, metric value, 25
Gram, 24
Granatum, 202
Granular effervescent salt, 21
Granules, 23
Gray powder, 62
Green vitriol, 50
Griffith's antihectic mixture, 50
Grindelia, 224
 fluid extract, 224
Guaiac, 75, 178
 beta-resin, 75
 tincture, 76
Guaiacic acid, 75
Guaiacin, 75
Guaiacol, 86, 126
 benzoate, 86
 carbonate, 86
 phosphate, 86
 valerianate, 86
Guaiacolis carbonas, 86
Guaiaconic acid, 75
Guaiacresinic acid, 75
Guaiacum, 75

Guarana, 157, 158
fluid extract, 158
Gum arabic, 267
Gun-cotton, soluble, 272
Gypsum, dried, 272

HÆMATOXYLON, 234
extract, 234
Hamamelis, 235
fluid extract, 235
water, 235
Heart sedatives, 161
stimulants, 146
Heavy magnesia, 195
Hedeoma, 188
oil, 188
Hellebore, 165
Hematinics, 47
Hemp, Canadian, 211
Henry's magnesia, 196
Hexamethylenamina, 219
Hexamethylene, 219
Hive syrup, Coxe's, 163, 210
Hoffmann's anodyne, 119, 131
Homatropin hydrobromid, 110
Homatropinæ hydrobromidum, 110
Honey, 23
of red rose, 235
Hope's camphor mixture, 130
Hop-pillows, 106
Hops, 105
Horehound, 188
Hot lotions, 24
Humulus, 105
Husband's magnesia, 196
Huxham's tincture of cinchona, 45
Hydragogues, 197
Hydrargyri ammoniatum, 63
chloridum corrosivum, 63, 250
mite, 62, 195, 203, 212
iodidum flavum, 63
rubrum, 63, 250
oxidum flavum, 62
rubrum, 62
subsulphas flavus, 64, 182
Hydrargyrum, 60
cum creta, 62
Hydrastin, 46, 47
Hydrastinin hydrochlorid, 47, 173
Hydrastininæ hydrochloridum, 47, 173
Hydrastis, 42, 46, 173
fluid extract, 47
glycerite, 47, 271
tincture, 47
Hydriodic acid, diluted, 67
syrup, 67
Hydrobromic acid, diluted, 99
Hydrochloric acid, 56, 58
ether, 125
Hydrocyanic acid, 142
diluted, 140, 142
Hydrogen dioxid solution, 248
peroxid, 248
Hydroquinon, 88
Hyoscin, 111
hydrobromid, 99, 113
Hyoscinæ hydrobromidum, 99, 113
Hyoscyamin, 107, 111
hydrobromid, 113
sulphate, 113
Hyoscyaminæ hydrobromidum, 113
sulphas, 113
Hyoscyamus, 111
extract, 112
fluid, 112
tincture, 112
Hypnotics, 89
Hypodermic administration of medicine, 32
Hypophosphites, 72
syrup, 73
compound, 73
Hypophosphorous acid, 58
Hypoquebrachin, 226

IGASURIC acid, 132
India rubber, 273
Indian cannabis, 104
Incin, 159
Infusa, 22
dosage, 30
Infusions, 22
dosage, 30
Infusum digitalis, 155
pruni virginianæ, 41
sennæ compositum, 194
Ingluvin, 34, 35, 36
Inhalations, 23
Injections, 23
intravenous, 33
Inscription of prescription, 27
Intestinal worms, medicines for, 201
Intravenous injections, 33
Inulin, 212
Iodids, 65
Iodin, 65, 71, 250
ointment, 66
solution, compound, 66, 67
tincture, 66

Iodism, 65
Iodoform, 251
 ointment, 252
Iodoformum, 251
Iodol, 252
Iodum, 65, 71, 250
Ipecac, 179, 220
 and opium powder, 93
  tincture, 91
 fluid extract, 180
 pills, 135
 powder, 180
 syrup, 180
 wine, 180
Ipecacuanha, 179
Ipecacuanhic acid, 179
Iris, 199
 extract, 199
  fluid, 199
Irish moss, 269
Iron, 47, 48
 and aloes pills, 194
 and ammonium acetate solution, 50
  citrate, 51
  tartrate, 51
 and potassium tartrate, 51
 and quinin citrate, 51
 and strychnin citrate, 51
 carbonate pills, 49
 chlorids, 48
 hydrated oxid of, 49
 mixture, compound, 50
 nitrate, 48
 phosphate glycerite, 271
 potassiotartrate, 51
 Quevenne's, 49
 quinin and strychnin phosphates,
   elixir of, 51, 73
   glycerite, 51, 73
   syrup, 51, 73
 reduced, 49
 sulphate, 48
 wine, 51
  bitter, 51
Irritants, 260
Isaconitin, 163
Isobutyl orthocresol iodid, 252
Isorottlerin, 203
Itrol, 244

JABORANDI, 222
Jaborandin, 222
Jaborin, 222
Jalap, 197
Jalap powder, compound, 198
Jalapa, 197
Jecorin, 155
Jervin, 165
Juglans, 193
 extract, 193
Juniper oil, 214
 spirit, 215
  compound, 215

KAIRIN, 88
Kamala, 203
Kaolin, 269
Kaolinum, 269
Keeley cure, 65
Kinic acid, 43
Kino, 234
 tincture, 234
Kinoïn, 234
Kinotannic acid, 232, 234
Kinovic acid, 43
Knock-out drops, 96
Kombic acid, 159
Kosotoxin, 203
Kousso, 203
Krameria, 231
 extract, 234
  fluid, 234
 syrup, 234
 tincture, 234
 troches, 234
Kramerotannic acid, 234

LABARRAQUE'S solution, 250
Lac asafœtidæ, 129
Lactic acid, 47, 59
Lactucarium, 106
 syrup, 106
 tincture, 106
Lactucin, 106
Lady Webster's dinner pill, 194
Lanolin, 270
Lappa, 77
 fluid extract, 77
Lard, 270
 benzoinated, 270
 cerate, 270
 ointment, 270
Largin, 244
Latin, medical, 27, 28
Laudanum, 93
Lavender flower oil, 187
 spirit, 187
 tincture, compound, 187
Laxative pills, compound, 135

Laxatives, 190
Lead, 236
  acetate, 238
  arthralgia, 236
  colic, 236, 237
  encephalopathy, 236
  iodid, 238
  nitrate, 238
  oxid, 237
  paralysis, 236, 237
  plaster, 237
  subacetate, cerate of, 238
    solution, 238
  sugar, 238
Lecithin, 155
Ledoyen's disinfecting fluid, 238
Lemon-juice, 169
  oil, 169
Lemon-peel tincture, 169
Leptandra, 194
  extract, 195
    fluid, 195
Leptandrin, 194
Licorice, 269
  powder, compound, 194, 269
  root, 268
    extract, 269
      fluid, 269
      refined, 269
Lime, chlorinated, 249
  potassa with, 265
  solution, 247
  sulphurated, 253
  syrup, 247
  unslaked, 247
Lime water, 247
Limonis succus, 169
Linimenta, 23
Liniments, 23
Linimentum ammoniæ, 262
  belladonnæ, 110
  calcis, 247, 268
  camphoræ, 130
  chloroformi, 122
  saponis, 130
  terebinthinæ, 217
Linseed, 268
Linum, 268
  oil, 268
Liquids, 20, 22
Liquor acidi arsenosi, 69
  ammonii acetatis, 221
  antisepticus, 254
  arseni et hydrargyri iodidi, 70
  calcis, 247
Liquor chlori compositus, 249
  cresolis compositus, 256
  ferri chloridi, 50
    et ammonii acetatis, 50
    subsulphatis, 50
    tersulphatis, 50
  formaldehydi, 259
  hydrargyri nitratis, 64
  iodi compositus, 66, 67
  plumbi subacetatis, 238
  potassii arsenitas, 69
    citratis, 206
    hydroxidi, 206
  sodæ chlorinatæ, 250
  sodii arsenatis, 70
    hydroxidi, 246
    phosphatis compositus, 196
  zinci chloridi, 241
Liquores, 20, 22
Litharge, 237
Lithii benzoas, 209
  carbonas, 208
  citras, 208
    effervescens, 208
  salicylas, 84
Lithium, 208
  benzoate, 209
  carbonate, 208
  citrate, 208
    effervescent, 208
  salicylate, 84
Lobelia, 143
  fluid extract, 143
  tincture, 143
Lobelic acid, 143
Lobelin, 143
Local anesthetics, 124
Logwood, 234
London paste, 265
Losophan, 252
Lotions, 23
  hot, 24
Lozenges, 20
Lugol's solution, 66, 67
Lunar caustic, 243
Lupamaric acid, 105
Lupulin, 105, 106
  fluid extract, 106
  oleoresin, 106
Lupulinum, 105, 106
Lycopodium, 270

Mace, 185
Macis, 185
Magendie's solution, 94

Magistery of bismuth, 244
Magnesia, 195
  alba, 196
Magnesii carbonas, 196
  oxidum, 195
    ponderosum, 195
  sulphas, 196
    effervescens, 196
Magnesium carbonate, 196
  citrate solution, 196
  oxid, ferric hydroxid with, 49
  sulphate, 196
Malt extract, 35, 36
Manganese, 47, 52
  dioxid, 52
    precipitated, 53
  hypophosphite, 53
  sulphate, 53, 197
Mangani dioxidum præcipitatum, 53
  hypophosphis, 53
  sulphas, 53, 197
Manganum, 47, 52
Manna, 190
Mannit, 190
Marrubium, 188
Marshmallow, 268
Mass, 20
Massa, 20
  ferri carbonatis, 49
  hydrargyri, 62, 195
Mastiche and aloes pills, 193
Materia medica, definition, 17
Matico, 219
  fluid extract, 219
Matricaria, 39, 41
Measures, 24
  approximate, 26
Medical Latin, 27, 28
Medicines, administration, 32
  affecting alimentary canal, 178
    circulatory organs, 116
    excretions, 204
    secretions, 204
    sexual organs, 169
  classification, 33
  conditions influencing effects, 31, 32
  systemic, 33, 34
  topical, 34, 247
Mel rosæ, 235
Mellita, 23
Mentha piperita, 187
  viridis, 187
Menthol, 126
Mercurial cathartics, 195
  nitrate ointment, 63
  ointment, 62
  oleate, 62
  plaster, 62
  subsulphate, yellow, 182
Mercurials, 212
Mercuric and arsenic iodid solution, 70
  chlorid, 63, 64, 213, 250
  iodid, 63, 250
  nitrate solution, 64
  oxid, red, 62
      ointment, 62
    yellow, 62
      ointment, 62
Mercurous chlorid, 62, 195, 203, 212
  iodid, 63
Mercury, 60
  ammoniated, 63
    ointment, 63
  mass, 62
  metallic, 60
  with chalk, 62
Metallic mercury, 60
Methyl salicylate, 84
  chlorid, 120
Methylconiin, 144
Methylene bichlorid, 123
  blue, 219
Methylis salicylas, 84
Methylpyrocatechin, 86
Methylthionin hydrochlorid, 219
Methylthioninæ hydrochloridum, 219
Metric system of weights, 24
    apothecaries' weight and, relations, 25
Mezereum, 76
  fluid extract, 76
Milk-weed, 211
Mindererus spirit, 221
Mineral acids, 47, 56
  tonics, 47
Minims, metric value, 25
Mistura, 22
  cretæ, 247, 267
  ferri compositæ, 50
  glycyrrhizæ composita, 269
  rhei et sodæ, 193
Mixtures, 22
Monsel's solution, 49, 50
Morphin, 92
  acetate, 94
  hydrochlorid, 94

Morphinæ acetas, 94
hydrochloridum, 94
sulphas, 94
Morphine powder, compound, 94
sulphate, 94
Moschus, 127
Mucilage, 267
Mucilago acaciæ, 267
sassafras medullæ, 268
tragacanthæ, 268
ulmi, 268
Mucous tracts, medication through, 33
Muriatic acid, 56, 58
Musk, 127
tincture, 127
vegetable, 127
extract, 127
fluid, 127
Mustard, 181
black, 261
oil, volatile, 261
papers, 261
powder, 261
white, 261
Mydriatic anodynes, 106
Myristica, 185
Myrosin, 261
Myrrh and aloes pills, 194
tincture, 194

NAPHTHALENE, 257
Naphthalenum, 257
Naphthalin, 257
Narcosis, alcohol-, 148
Narcotics, 89
Nervous system, medicines acting on, 89
Neurin, 155
Neutral mixture as diuretic, 206
Nicotianin, 145
Nicotin, 145
Niter, 207
sweet spirit, 212, 221
Nitric acid, 56, 58
Nitrites, 137
Nitrogen monoxid, 122
Nitroglycerin, 137
spirit, 138
triturates, 138
Nitrohydrochloric acid, 56, 58
Nitromuriatic acid, 56, 58
Nitrosyl chlorid, 58
Nitrous ether spirit, 212, 221
oxid, 122
Nosophen, 252
Nutgall, 233
Nutmeg, 185
oil, 185
Nutritive enemata, 201
Nux vomica, extract, 134
fluid, 134
tincture, 134

OFFICIAL preparations, classification, 19
definition, 19
Oil. See also *Oleum*.
of vitriol, 56, 57
of wine, 131
Oils, volatile, dosage, 30
Ointment, 21. See also *Unguentum*.
Oleata, 21
Oleates, 21
Oleatum atropinæ, 110
cocainæ, 116
hydrargyri, 62
quininæ, 46
veratrinæ, 167
Oleic acid, 271
Oleoresina, 23
aspidii, 202
capsici, 184
cubebæ, 218
lupulini, 106
piperis, 185
zingiberis, 186
Oleoresins, 23
Oleum æthereum, 131
amygdale amaræ, 142
anisi, 188
aurantii corticis, 189
betulæ, 84
cadinum, 230
cajuputi, 187
cari, 188
caryophylli, 186
cinnamomi, 185
copaibæ, 218
coriandri, 188
cubebæ, 218
erigerontis, 215
eucalypti, 40, 41
fœniculi, 188
gaultheriæ, 84, 187
gossypii seminis, 271
hedeomæ, 188
juniperi, 214
lavandulæ florum, 187
limonis, 169

Oleum lini, 268
  menthæ piperitæ, 187
    viridis, 187
  morrhuæ, 71
  myristicæ, 185
  picis liquidæ, 230
  pimentæ, 186
  ricini, 191
  rosmarini, 188
  sabinæ, 177
  santali, 215
  sassafras, 77
  sinapis volatile, 261
  terebinthinæ, 203, 216
    rectificatum, 217
  theobromatis, 271
  thymi, 188
  tiglii, 200
Ophelic acid, 37
Opii pulvis, 93
Opium, 89
  and glycyrrhiza troches, 93
  and ipecac powder, 93
    tincture, 94
  deodoratum, 93
  deodorized, 93
  extract, 93
  granulated, 93
  granulatum, 93
  habit, 93
  pills, 93
  plaster, 93
  powdered, 93
  tincture, 93
    camphorated, 93
    deodorized, 93
  vinegar, 94
  wine, 94
Orange peel, bitter, 188
    fluid extract, 189
  oil, 189
  sweet, 188
  syrup, 189
  tinctures, 189
  spirit, compound, 189
Orange-flower syrup, 189
  waters, 189
Organotherapy, 274
Orthoanisidin, 86
Oxyatropin, 107
Oxytocics, 170

PAINTERS' colic, 236, 237
Palmetto, saw, 170
Pancreatin, 34, 35, 36
Pancreatinum, 34, 35, 36
Papain, 35, 36
Papers, 21
  mustard, 261
Paraldehyd, 100
Paraldehydum, 100
Paralysis, lead, 236, 237
Paregoric, 93
Pareira, 213
  fluid extract, 213
Parsley-camphor, 177
Parvules, 23
Pearl white, 241
Peculiar bitters, 42
Pelletierin, 202
  tannate, 203
Pennyroyal, 188
Pepper, 184
  oleoresin, 185
  red, 184
Peppermint, 187
  oil, 187
  spirit, 188
  troches, 188
  water, 188
Pepo, 203
Pepsin, 34, 35, 36
Pepsinum, 34, 35, 36
Petrolatum, 271
  album, 272
  liquidum, 271
Phaeoretin, 192
Pharmacology, definition, 17
Pharmacopeia, definition, 19
Pharmacy, definition, 17
Phenacetin, 81
Phenic acid, 254, 256
Phenocoll, 81
Phenol, 254, 256
  glycerite, 256, 271
  liquefactum, 256
  ointment, 256
Phenyl salicylate, 84, 85
Phenyldimethyl pyrazolon, 78
Phosphates, 72
Phosphids, 72
Phosphites, 72
Phosphorated oil, 55
Phosphoric acid, 56, 58
Phosphorus, 47, 53
  elixir, 55
  pills, 55
  poisoning, 54
Physostigma, 135
  extract, 136

Physostigma, tincture, 136
Physostigmin, 135
  salicylate, 84, 137
  sulphate, 136
Physostigminæ salicylas, 84, 137
  sulphas, 136
Picraconitin, 163
Pills. See also *Pilulæ*.
Pilocarpidin, 222
  hydrochlorid, 223
  nitrate, 223
Pilocarpinæ hydrochloridum, 223
  nitras, 223
Pilocarpus, 222
  fluid extract, 223
Pilulæ, 20
  aloes, 193
    et ferri, 194
    et mastiches, 193
    et myrrhæ, 194
  asafœtidæ, 129
  belladonnæ, 198
  capsici, 198
  catharticæ compositæ, 200
    vegetabiles, 200
  ferri iodidi, 50
  Lady Webster's dinner, 194
  laxativæ compositæ, 194
  opii, 93
  phosphori, 55
  podophylli, 198
  rhei compositæ, 193
  Rufus', 194
Pimenta, 186
Pinkroot, 201
Piper, 184
Piperin, 184, 185
Piperinum, 185
Pix liquida, 229
Plasmin, 269
Plaster, 21. See also *Emplastrum*.
Plaster-of-Paris, 272
Plumbi acetas, 238
  iodidum, 238
  nitras, 238
  oxidum, 237
Plumbum, 236
Podophyllotoxin, 198
Podophyllum, 198
  fluid extract, 198
  pills, 198
Poisoning, aconite, 164
  ammonia, 150
  antimony, 161, 162
  antipyrin, 78
Poisoning, arsenic, 68
  atropin, 108
  bromid, 98
  calabar bean, 136
  colchicum, 74
  chloral, 95
  chloralamid, 97
  cocain, 114
  conium, 144
  copper, 240
  corrosive sublimate, 61
  digitalis, 153, 154
  ergot, 171, 172
  hydrocyanic acid, 141
  iodin, 66
  iodoform, 251
  lead, 236, 237
  lobelia, 143
  mercuric chlorid, 61
  mercury, 60
  mineral acid, 56
  nicotin, 146
  opium, 90
  phosphorus, 54
  physostigma, 136
  potassium nitrate, 207
  prussic acid, 141
  salicin, 84
  salicylic acid, 84
  saturnin, 236, 237
  silver, 242
  squill, 210
  strychnin, 133
  sulphonal, 101
  trional, 102
  turpentine oil, 217
  veratrum, 165
  woorara, 145
  zinc, 240
Polygalic acid, 226
Pomegranate, 202
  fluid extract, 203
Potassa, 264
  cum calce, 265
Potassii acetas, 206
  bicarbonas, 205, 206
  bitartras, 197, 207
  bromidum, 97, 98
  carbonas, 206
  chloras, 207
  citras, 206
    effervescens, 206
  cyanidum, 142
  dichromas, 266
  et sodii tartras, 197

Potassii hydroxidum, 264
  hypophosphis, 73
  iodidum, 67
  nitras, 207
  nitris, 137, 138
  permanganas, 53, 249
  sulphas, 197
Potassium, 205
  acetate, 206
  and antimonium tartrate, 162, 182
  and iron tartrate, 51
  and sodium tartrate, 197
  arsenite solution, 69
  bicarbonate, 205, 206
  bitartrate, 197, 207
  bromid, 97, 98
  carbonate, 206
  chlorate, 207
    troches, 208
  citrate, 206
    effervescent, 206
  cyanid, 142
  dichromate, 266
  hydroxid, 264
    solution, 206
  hypophosphite, 73
  iodid, 67
    ointment, 67
  myronate, 261
  natural mixture, 206
  nitrate, 207
    papers, 207
  nitrite, 137, 138
  permanganate, 53, 249
  sulphate, 197
Potato fly, 263
Poultices, 23
Powder, 20. See also *Pulvis*.
  dosage, 30
Preparations, official, 19
Prepared chalk, 247
    classification, 19
Prescription, doses, 29
  parts, 27
  writing, method, 28
    precautions, 26
Protectives, 272
Proto-iodid, 63
Prunus Virginiana, 39, 40, 41
    fluid extract, 41
    infusion, 41
    oil, 40
    syrup, 41
Prussic acid, 140
Pseudoconydrine, 144
Pseudojervine, 165
Psychotrin, 179
Pterocarpin, 273
Pulveres, 20
  dosage, 30
Pulvis acetanilidi compositus, 81
  aromaticus, 185, 186
  cretæ compositus, 247
  effervescens compositus, 197
  glycyrrhizæ compositus, 194
  ipecacuanhæ et opii, 93
  jalapæ compositus, 198
  morphinæ compositus, 94
  rhei compositus, 193
Pumpkin-seed, 203
Purgatives, simple, 192
Pyrocatechin, 88, 155, 234
Pyroligneous acid, 229
Pyroxylin, 272
Pyroxylinum, 272

QUASSIA, 37
  extract, 38
    fluid, 38
  tincture, 38
Quassin, 37, 38
Quebrachamin, 226
Quebrachin, 226
Quebracho, 226
Quercitannic acid, 234
Quercus, 234
  fluid extract, 235
Quevenne's iron, 49
Quicksilver, 60
Quillaja, 226
  fluid extract, 226
  tincture, 226
Quinicin, 43
Quinidin, 43
Quinin, 42, 44, 45, 82, 174
  and iron citrate, 51
      soluble, 51
  bisulphate, 45
  hydrobromid, 45
  hydrochlorid, 45
  iron, and strychnin phosphates,
        elixir, 51, 73
      glycerite, 51, 73
      syrup, 51, 73
  oleate, 46
  phosphate glycerite, 271
  salicylate, 45, 84
  sulphate, 45
Quinina, 45, 174

Quininæ bisulphas, 45
hydrobromidum, 45
hydrochloridum, 45
salicylas, 45

RECTAL suppository, 21
Red mercuric oxid, 62
ointment, 62
pepper, 184
precipitate ointment, 62
rose, 235
saunders, 273
wine, 149
Remedies, classification, 18
combination, 26
definition, 18
dietetic, 18
hygienic, 19
mechanical, 18
pharmaceutic, 19
physical, 18
Resina jalapæ, 198
scammonii, 199
Resorcin, 88
Resorcinol, 88
Rhamnus purshiana, 191
extract, 191
fluid, 191
Rheotannic acid, 192
Rheum, 192
Rheumic acid, 192
Rhigolene, 124
Rhubarb, 192
and soda mixture, 193
extract, 193
fluid, 193
pills, compound, 193
powder, compound, 193
syrup, 193
tincture, 193
Rhus glabra, 235
Rochelle salt, 197
Rosa gallica, 235
Rose ointment, 235
red, 235
confection, 235
fluid extract, 235
honey, 235
syrup, 235
water, 235
Rosemary oil, 188
Rottlerin, 203
Rubefacients, 260
Rubijervine, 165
Rufus' pills, 194

SABADIX, 167
Sabadinin, 167
Sabal, 170
Sabina, 177
Saccharin, 273
Sage, 188
Saigon cinnamon, 185
Sal ammoniac, 225
granulatus effervescens, 21
Saleratus, 206
Salicin, 82, 83
Salicinum, 82, 83
Salicylates, 82
Salicylic acid, 82, 84
Saline cathartics, 195
Salol, 85
Salophen, 85
Salt, granular effervescent, 21
Saltpeter, 207
Salvia, 188
Sandal-wood oil, 215
Sanguinaria, 227
fluid extract, 228
tincture, 228
Sanguinarin, 227, 228
Santal oil, 215
Santalic acid, 273
Santalum rubrum, 273
Santonica, 202
Santonin, 202
troches, 202
Santoninum, 202
Saponin, 226
Sarsaparilla, 75
fluid extract, 75
compound, 75
syrup, compound, 75
Sassafras, 77
medulla, 268
oil, 77
pith, 268
Saturnin poisoning, 236, 237
Savin, 177
fluid extract, 177
oil, 177
Saw palmetto, 170
Scammonin, 199
Scammonium, 199
Scammony, 199
Scilla, 209
Scillin, 209, 210
Scillipicrin, 209, 210
Scillitoxin, 209, 210
Scoparin, 212
Scoparius, 211

Scoparius, fluid extract, 212
Scopola, 113
 extract, 113
  fluid, 113
Scopolamin, 113
 hydrobromid, 99, 113
Scopolaminæ hydrobromidum, 99, 113
Scutellaria, 131
 fluid extract, 131
Sedatives, cardiac, 161
 gastric, 182
 uterine, 175
Seidlitz powder, 197
Semisolids, 19, 20
Senega, 226
 fluid extract, 226
 syrup, 226
Senegin, 226
Senna, 194
 confection, 194
 fluid extract, 194
 infusion, compound, 194
 syrup, 194
Sennacrol, 194
Sennit, 194
Serpentaria, 39, 40
 fluid extract, 41
 tincture, 41
Serum antidiphthericum, 274
 therapy, 274
Sevum præparatum, 270
Sex, action of drugs and, 31
Sexual organs, medicines affecting, 169
Signature of prescription, 27
Silver, 242
 albumose, soluble, 244
 caseinate, sodium, 243
 citrate, 244
 cyanid, 142, 243
 lactate, 244
 nitrate, 243
  mitigated, 243
  molded, 243
 oxid, 243
 phosphate, ethylene diamin, 243
 vitelline, 244
Simple bitters, 37
 syrup, 23
Sinalbin, 261
Sinapis, 181
 alba, 261
 nigra, 261
Sinigrin, 261
Skin, medication through, 32
Slippery elm, 268
Slough, 264
Soap liniment, 130
Soda and rhubarb mixture, 193
Soda-water, 267
Sodii acetas, 209
 arsenas, 70
  exsiccatus, 70
 benzoas, 257
 bicarbonas, 246
 bisulphis, 253
 boras, 253
 bromidum, 98
 carbonas exsiccatus, 246
  monohydratus, 246
 citras, 246
 hydroxidum, 265
 hypophosphis, 73
 iodidum, 67
 nitris, 137, 138
 phenolsulphonas, 256
 phosphas, 196
  effervescens, 196
  exsiccatus, 196
 pyrophosphas, 197
 salicylas, 84
 sulphas, 196, 253
 thiosulphas, 253
Sodiotheobromin salicylate, 211
Sodium, 246
 acetate, 209
 and gold chlorid, 65
 and potassium tartrate, 197
 arsenate, 70
  dried, 70
  solution, 70
 benzoate, 257
 bicarbonate, 246
  troches, 246
 bisulphid, 253
 bromid, 98
 carbonate, 246
  dried, 246
  monohydrated, 246
 citrate, 246
 hydroxide, 265
  solution, 246
 hypophosphite, 73
 hyposulphite, 253
 iodid, 67
 nitrite, 137, 138
 paraphenolsulphonate, 256
 phenolsulphonate, 256
 phosphate, 196

Sodium phosphate, dried, 196
effervescent, 196
solution, compound, 197
pyrophosphate, 197
salicylate, 84
silver caseinate, 243
sulphate, 196
sulphite, 253
sulphocarbolate, 256
thiosulphate, 253
Solids, 19, 20
Solutions, 22
Spanish flies, 262
Sparteine, 159, 212
sulphate, 159, 212
Sparteinæ sulphas, 159, 212
Spearmint, 187
oil, 187
spirit, 188
water, 188
Spermaceti, 270
Sphacelic acid, 171
Sphacelotoxin, 171
Spigelia, 201
fluid extract, 202
Spiriti, 22
Spirits, 22
Spiritus ætheris, 119
compositus, 119, 131
nitrosi, 212, 221
ammoniæ, 152
aromaticus, 152
amygdalæ amaræ, 142
anisi, 188
aurantii compositus, 189
camphoræ, 130
chloroformi, 122
cinnamomi, 185
frumenti, 149
gaultheriæ, 187
glycerylis nitratis, 138
juniperi, 215
compositus, 215
lavandulæ, 187
menthæ piperitæ, 188
viridis, 188
mindereri, 221
vini gallici, 149
Squill, 209
fluid extract, 210
syrup, 210
compound, 163, 210
tincture, 210
vinegar, 210
Starch, 269
Starch glycerite, 269, 271
Stillingia, 77
fluid extract, 77
Stimulants, cardiac, 146
Stramonium, 111
extract, 111
fluid, 111
ointment, 111
tincture, 111
Strontii bromidum, 99
iodidum, 67
salicylas, 84
Strontium bromid, 99
iodid, 67
lactate, 209
salicylate, 84
Strophanthin, 159
Strophanthinum, 159
Strophanthus, 159
tincture, 159
Strychnin, 132, 134
and iron citrate, 51
iron, and quinin phosphates
elixir, 51, 73
glycerite, 51, 73
syrup, 51, 73
nitrate, 134
phosphate glycerite, 271
pills, 135
sulphate, 134
Strychnina, 132, 134
Strychninæ nitras, 134
sulphas, 134
Stypticin, 174
Sublimed sulphur, 192
Subscription of prescription, 27
Suet, prepared, 270
Sugar of lead, 238
Sulphids, 253
Sulphites, 253
Sulphonal, 100, 103
Sulphonethylmethane, 102, 103
Sulphonmethanum, 100, 103
Sulphur, 191
flowers, 192
iodid, 67
lotum, 192
ointment, 192
præcipitatum, 192
sublimatum, 192
washed, 192
Sulphurated lime 253
Sulphuric acid, 56, 57
Sulphuris iodidum, 67
Sulphurous acid, 252

Sumach, 235
  fluid extract, 235
Sumbul, 127
  extract, 127
    fluid, 127
Superscription of prescription, 27
Suppositoria glycerini, 271
Suppositories, 271
Suppositorium, 21
Suppository, 21
Suppurants, 264
Suprarenal extract, 156
  glands, 155, 156, 274
Sweet birch oil, 84
  orange peel, 188
    tincture, 189
  spirit of niter, 212, 221
Sweetening agents, 273
Sydenham's laudanum, 94
Syrupi, 23
  dosage, 30
Syrups, 23
  dosage, 30
Syrupus acaciæ, 267
  acidi citrici, 169
    hydriodici, 67
  allii, 227
  amygdalæ, 142
  aurantii, 189
    florum, 189
  calcii lactophosphatis, 73
  calcis, 247
  ferri iodidi, 50
    quininæ et strychninæ phosphatum, 51, 73
  hypophosphitum, 73
    compositus, 73
  ipecacuanhæ, 180
  krameriæ, 234
  lactucarii, 106
  picis liquidæ, 230
  pruni Virginianæ, 41
  rhei, 193
    aromaticus, 193
  rosæ, 235
  sarsaparillæ compositus, 75
  scillæ, 210
    compositus, 163, 210
  senegæ, 226
  sennæ, 194
  tolutanus, 229
  zingiberis, 186
Systemic medicines, 33, 34

TABÁCUM, 145
Tablespoonful, 26
Talc, 269
  purified, 269
Talcum, 269
  purificatum, 269
Tamarind, 190
Tamarindus, 190
Tanacetin, 177
Tannic acid, 158, 231
    collodion, 233
    glycerite, 233, 271
    ointment, 233
    troches, 232
Tansy, 177
Tar, 229
  oil, 230
  ointment, 230
  syrup, 230
Taraxacerin, 212
Taraxacin, 212
Taraxacum, 212
  extract, 212
    fluid, 212
Tartar emetic, 162, 182
  salts, 206
Tartaric acid, 167, 169
Tar-water, 230
Tea, chamomile, 41
Teaspoonful, 26
Terebene, 230
Terebenum, 230
Terebinthina, 216
  canadensis, 216
Terpin hydrate, 230
Terpini hydras, 230
Tetra-iodo-phenolphthalein, 252
Tetra-iodo-pyrrol, 252
Tetronal, 103
Thallin, 88
Thein, 156, 158
Theobroma oil, 271
Theobromin, 158, 210, 211
Theocin, 158
Theophyllin, 158, 210
Therapeutics, definition, 18
  empirical, 18
  rational, 18
Thyme oil, 188
Thymol, 188, 203, 259
  iodid, 252
  iodidi, 260
Thymolis iodidum, 252, 260
Thyroid glands, desiccated, 274
Tinctura, 22

Tinctura aconiti, 126, 165
aloes, 194
et myrrhæ, 194
arnicæ, 167
asafœtidæ, 129
aurantii amari, 189
dulcis, 189
belladonnæ foliorum, 110
benzoini, 229
composita, 229
bryoniæ, 198
calendulæ, 76
cannabis indicæ, 105
cantharidis, 219, 263
capsici, 184
cardamomi, 186
composita, 186
cimicifugæ, 160
cinchonæ, 45
composita, 41, 45
cinnamomi, 185
colchici seminis, 74
columbæ, 38
cubebæ, 219
digitalis, 155
dosage, 30
ferri chloridi, 50
gallæ, 233
gambir composita, 234
gelsemii, 140
gentianæ composita, 38
guaiaci, 76
ammoniata, 76
hydrastis, 47
hyoscyami, 112
iodi, 66
ipecacuanhæ et opii, 94
kino, 234
krameriæ, 234
lactucarii, 106
lavandulæ composita, 187
limonis corticis, 169
lobeliæ, 143
moschi, 127
nucis vomicæ, 134
opii, 93
camphorata, 93
deodorati, 93
physostigmatis, 136
quassiæ, 38
quillajæ, 226
rhei 193
aromaticus, 193
sanguinariæ, 228
scillæ, 210
Tinctura serpentariæ, 41
stramonii, 111
strophanthi, 159
tolutana, 229
valerianæ, 128
ammoniata, 128
vanillæ, 189
veratri, 166
zingiberis, 186
Tinctures, 22. (See also *Tinctura.*)
Tobacco, 145
Tobacco-camphor, 145
Tolene, 229
Tonics, 36
mineral, 47
vegetable, 37
Topical medicines, 34, 247
Tragacanth, 268
Tragacantha, 268
Tragacanthin, 268
Trapp's test for veratrin, 166
Trichloracetic acid, 168, 266
Trichloraldehyd, 95
Tri-iodo-metacresol, 252
Trimethylxanthin, 211
Trinitroglycerin, 137
Trinitrin, 137
Trional, 102, 103
Triticin, 214
Triticum, 214
fluid extract, 214
Trituratio elaterini, 200
Triturationes, 20
Triturations, 20
Troches, 20
Trochisci, 20
acidi tannici, 232
ammonii chloridi, 225
cubebæ, 219
gambir, 234
glycyrrhizæ et opii, 93
krameriæ, 234
potassii chloratis, 208
santonini, 202
sodii bicarbonatis, 246
Trypsin, 35
Tully's powder, 94
Turpentine, 216
Canada, 216
liniment, 217
oil, 189, 203, 216, 262
rectified, 217
white, 216
Turpeth mineral, 64, 182

ULMUS, 268
Unguenta, 21
Unguentum acidi borici, 254
    tannici, 233
  aquæ rosæ, 235
  belladonnæ, 110
  diachylon, 237
  gallæ, 233
  hydrargyri, 62
    ammoniati, 63
    dilutum, 62
    nitratis. 63
    oxidi flavi, 62
      rubri, 62
  iodi, 66
  iodoformi, 252
  phenolis, 256
  picis liquidæ, 230
  potassii iodidi, 67
  stramonii, 111
  sulphuris, 192
  veratrinæ, 167
  zinci oxidi, 241
    stearatis, 241
Urethan, 103
Urethral suppository, 22
Urochloralic acid, 97
Urotropin, 219
Uterine sedatives, 175
Uva ursi, 214
    fluid extract, 214

VAGINAL suppository, 21
Valerian, 127
  fluid extract, 128
  tincture, 128
    ammoniated, 128
Valeriana, 128
Valerianic acid, 128, 175
Vanilla, 189
  tincture, 189
Vanillin, 189
Vanillinum, 189
Vaselin, 271
  white, 272
Vegetable acids, 167
  tonics, 37
Vehicle of inscription, 27
Veratridin, 167
Veratrine, 165, 166
  ointment, 167
  oleate, 167
Veratrina, 166
Veratrum, 165
  fluid extract, 166
Veratrum, tincture, 166
Vermicides, 201
Vermifuges, 201
Vesicants, 262
Viburnin, 175
  opulus, 176
    fluid extract, 176
  prunifolium, 175
    fluid extract, 175
Vienna paste, 265
Vina, 22
Vinegars, 23
Vinum album, 149
  antimonii, 163
  cocæ, 116
  colchici seminis, 75
  ergotæ, 173
  ferri, 51
    amarum, 51
  ipecacuanhæ, 180
  opii, 94
  rubrum, 149
Virginia snakeroot, 39, 40
Vitriol blue, 240
  elixir, 57
  green, 50
  oil, 56, 57
  white, 241
Volatile oils, dosage, 30

WAHOO, 195
Washes, 23
Washing soda, 246
Water, 22, 267. (See also *Aqua*.)
Wax, white, 270
  yellow, 270
Weights, 24
Whisky, 149
White arsenic, 69
  precipitate, 63
  turpentine, 216
  vitriol, 241
  wine, 149
Wild cherry bark, 39, 41
Wine. (See *Vinum*.)
  measure, 24
  oil, 131
Wineglassful, 26
Wintergreen oil, 187
    artificial, 84
Wistar's cough lozenges, 93
Witch-hazel, 235
  extract, 235
Wool-fat, 270
  hydrous, 270

Woorali, 145
Woorara, 145
Wormseed, 202

YELLOW mercurial subsulphate, 182
  mercuric oxid, 62
    ointment, 62
Yerba santa, 227
Young's rule for dosage for children, 31

ZEA, 215
Zinc, 240
  acetate, 241
  bromid, 99, 242
  carbonate, precipitated, 241
  chlorid, 241
    solution, 241
  iodid, 242
  oxid, 241
Zinc oxid ointment, 241
  phosphid, 47, 55
  stearate, 241
    ointment, 241
  sulphate, 182, 241
  sulphocarbolate, 241
  valerate, 128, 242
Zinci acetas, 241
  bromidum, 99, 242
  carbonas præcipitatus, 241
  chloridum, 241
  iodidum, 242
  oxidum, 241
  phenolsulphonas, 241
  phosphidum, 55
  stearas, 241
  sulphas, 182, 241
  valeras, 242
Zincum, 240
Zingiber, 186

Peterson *and* Haines' Legal Medicine & Toxicology

A Text-Book of Legal Medicine and Toxicology. Edited by FREDERICK PETERSON, M. D., Clinical Professor of Psychiatry, Columbia University (College of Physicians and Surgeons), New York; and WALTER S. HAINES, M. D., Professor of Chemistry, Pharmacy, and Toxicology, Rush Medical College, in affiliation with the University of Chicago. Two imperial octavo volumes of about 750 pages each, fully illustrated. Per volume: Cloth, $5.00 net; Sheep or Half Morocco, $6.00 net. *Sold by Subscription.*

BOTH VOLUMES NOW READY

The object of the present work is to give to the medical and legal professions a comprehensive survey of forensic medicine and toxicology in moderate compass. An interesting and important chapter is that on "The Destruction and Attempted Destruction of the Human Body by Fire and Chemicals." A chapter not usually found in works on legal medicine is that on "The Medicolegal Relations of the X-Rays." This section will be found of unusual importance. The responsibility of pharmacists in the compounding of prescriptions, in the selling of poisons, in substituting drugs other than those prescribed, etc., furnishes a chapter of the greatest interest. Also included in the work is the enumeration of the laws of the various states relating to the commitment and retention of the insane.

OPINIONS OF THE MEDICAL PRESS

Medical News, New York

"It not only fills a need from the standpoint of timeliness, but it also sets a standard of what a text-book on Legal Medicine and Toxicology should be."

Columbia Law Review

"For practitioners in criminal law and for those in medicine who are called upon to give court testimony in any of its various forms . . . it is extremely valuable."

Pennsylvania Medical Journal

"If the excellence of this volume is equaled by the second, the work will easily take rank as the standing text-book on Legal Medicine and Toxicology."

Frühwald *and* Westcott's Diseases of Children

Diseases of Children. A Practical Reference Book for Students and Practitioners. By PROFESSOR DR. FERDINAND FRÜHWALD, of Vienna. Edited, with additions, by THOMPSON S. WESTCOTT, M. D., Associate in Diseases of Children, University of Pennsylvania. Octavo volume of 533 pages, containing 176 illustrations. Cloth, $4.50 net.

JUST READY

This work represents the author's twenty years' experience, and is intended as a practical reference work for the student and practitioner. With this reference feature in view, the individual diseases have been arranged alphabetically. The prophylactic, therapeutic, and dietetic treatments are elaborately discussed. Edited by such a distinguished pediatrist as Dr. Westcott, the American edition of this excellent work fully maintains the reputation won by the original German.

Ruhräh's Diseases of Children

A Manual of Diseases of Children. By JOHN RUHRAH, M. D., Clinical Professor of Diseases of Children, College of Physicians and Surgeons, Baltimore. 12mo of 404 pages, fully illustrated. Flexible leather, $2.00 net.

JUST READY

In writing this manual Dr. Ruhrah's aim was to present a work that would be of the greatest value to students. All the important facts are given concisely and explicitly, the therapeutics of infancy and childhood being outlined very carefully and clearly. There are also directions for dosage and prescribing, and a number of useful prescriptions are included. The feeding of infants is given in detail, and the entire work is amply illustrated with practical illustrations.

Brower & Bannister on Insanity

A Practical Manual of Insanity. For the Student and General Practitioner. By DANIEL R. BROWER, A. M., M. D., LL. D., Professor of Nervous and Mental Diseases in Rush Medical College, in affiliation with the University of Chicago; and HENRY M. BANNISTER, A. M., M. D., formerly Senior Assistant Physician, Illinois Eastern Hospital for the Insane. Handsome octavo of 426 pages, with a number of full-page inserts. Cloth, $3.00 net.

This work, intended for the student and general practitioner, is an intelligible, up-to-date exposition of the leading facts of psychiatry, and will be found of invaluable service, especially to the busy practitioner unable to yield the time for a more exhaustive study.

American Medicine

"Commends itself for lucid expression in clear-cut English. . . . Treatment is one of the best features of the book, and for this aspect is especially commended"

Bergey's Hygiene

The Principles of Hygiene: A Practical Manual for Students, Physicians, and Health Officers. By D. H. BERGEY, A. M., M. D., Assistant Professor of Bacteriology, University of Pennsylvania. Octavo of 536 pages, illust. Cloth, $3.00 net.

RECENTLY ISSUED—SECOND REVISED EDITION

This book is intended to meet the needs of students of medicine in the acquirement of a knowledge of those principles upon which modern hygienic practices are based, and to aid physicians and health officers in familiarizing themselves with the advances made in hygiene and sanitation in recent years.

Buffalo Medical Journal

"It will be found of value to the practitioner of medicine and the practical sanitarian; and students of architecture, who need to consider problems of heating, lighting, ventilation, water supply, and sewage disposal, may consult it with profit."

Galbraith's Four Epochs *of* Woman's Life

Second Revised Edition—Recently Issued

The Four Epochs of Woman's Life: A Study in Hygiene. By ANNA M. GALBRAITH, M. D., Fellow of the New York Academy of Medicine, etc. With an Introductory Note by JOHN H. MUSSER, M. D., Professor of Clinical Medicine, University of Pennsylvania. 12mo volume of 247 pages. Cloth, $1.50 net.

In this instructive work are stated, in a modest, pleasing, and conclusive manner, those truths of which every woman should have a thorough knowledge. Written, as it is, for the laity, the subject is discussed in language readily grasped even by those most unfamiliar with medical subjects.

Birmingham Medical Review, England

"We do not as a rule care for medical books written for the instruction of the public. But we must admit that the advice in Dr. Galbraith's work is in the main wise and wholesome."

Pyle's Personal Hygiene

A Manual of Personal Hygiene: Proper Living upon a Physiologic Basis. By Eminent Specialists. Edited by WALTER L. PYLE, A. M., M. D., Assistant Surgeon to Wills Eye Hospital, Philadelphia. Octavo volume of 441 pages, fully illustrated. Cloth, $1.50 net.

NEW (2d) EDITION—RECENTLY ISSUED

In this new second edition there have been added new chapters on Home Gymnastics and Domestic Hygiene, besides an Appendix of Emergency Procedures.

Boston Medical and Surgical Journal

"The work has been excellently done, there is no undue repetition, and the writers have succeeded unusually well in presenting facts of practical significance based on sound knowledge."

Draper's Legal Medicine

A Text-Book of Legal Medicine. By FRANK WINTHROP DRAPER, A. M., M. D., Professor of Legal Medicine in Harvard University, Boston. Handsome octavo of 573 pages, illustrated. Cloth, $4.00 net.

RECENTLY ISSUED

The author of this work has had twenty-six years' experience as Medical Examiner for the city of Boston, his investigations comprising nearly eight thousand deaths under a suspicion of violence.

Hon. Olin Bryan, LL. B.

Professor of Medical Jurisprudence, Baltimore Medical College

"It is comprehensive, thorough, and must, of a necessity, prove a splendid acquisition to the libraries of those who are interested in medical jurisprudence."

Jakob *and* Fisher's Nervous System and its Diseases

Atlas and Epitome of the Nervous System and its Diseases. By PROFESSOR DR. CHR. JAKOB, of Erlangen. *From the Second Revised German Edition.* Edited, with additions, by EDWARD D. FISHER, M. D., Professor of Diseases of the Nervous System, University and Bellevue Hospital Medical College, New York. With 83 plates and copious text. Cloth, $3.50 net. *In Saunders' Hand-Atlas Series.*

The matter is divided into Anatomy, Pathology, and Description of Diseases of the Nervous System. The plates illustrate these divisions most completely; especially is this so in regard to pathology. The exact site and character of the lesion are portrayed in such a way that they cannot fail to impress themselves on the memory of the reader.

Philadelphia Medical Journal

"We know of no one work of anything like equal size which covers this important and complicated field with the clearness and scientific fidelity of this hand-atlas."

American Text-Book of Diseases of Children

American Text-Book of Diseases of Children. Edited by LOUIS STARR, M. D., Consulting Pediatrist to the Maternity Hospital, etc.; assisted by THOMPSON S. WESTCOTT, M. D., Attending Physician to the Dispensary for Diseases of Children, Hospital of tne University of Pennsylvania. Handsome octavo, 1244 pages, profusely illustrated. Cloth, $7.00 net; Sheep or Half Morocco, $8.00 net.

SECOND REVISED EDITION

To keep up with the rapid advances in the field of pediatrics, the whole subject-matter embraced in the first edition has been carefully revised, new articles added, some original papers amended, and a number entirely rewritten and brought up to date.

British Medical Journal

"May be recommended as a thoroughly trustworthy and satisfactory guide to the subject of the diseases of children."

Paul's Fever Nursing

Nursing in the Acute Infectious Fevers. By GEORGE P. PAUL, M.D., Assistant Visiting Physician to the Samaritan Hospital, Troy, N. Y. 12mo of 200 pages. Cloth, $1.00 net.

JUST ISSUED

Dr. Paul has written his book especially for the trained nurse, so that all extraneous matter has been studiously avoided. Great stress has been laid upon care and management in each disease, as this relates directly to the duties of the nurse. The work discusses fever in general, then each acute infectious fever separately, and finally those practical procedures necessary to the proper management of the fevers described.

Friedenwald & Ruhräh's Dietetics for Nurses

Dietetics for Nurses. By JULIUS FRIEDENWALD, M. D., Clinical Professor of Diseases of the Stomach, College of Physicians and Surgeons, Baltimore; and JOHN RUHRAH, M. D., Clinical Professor of Diseases of Children, College of Physicians and Surgeons, Baltimore. 12mo of 363 pages. Cloth, $1.50 net.

JUST ISSUED

This work has been prepared to meet the needs of the nurse, both in the training school and after graduation. An outline is given of the principles involved in the nourishment of patients suffering from the various diseases in which diet plays an important part in treatment. Rectal alimentation and the feeding of operative cases are fully described.

Lewis' Anatomy and Physiology for Nurses

Anatomy and Physiology for Nurses. By LEROY LEWIS, M. D., Surgeon to and Lecturer on Anatomy and Physiology for Nurses at the Lewis Hospital, Bay City, Michigan. 12mo of 317 pages, with 146 illustrations. Cloth, $1.75 net.

JUST ISSUED

The author has based the plan and scope of the work on the methods he has employed in teaching the subjects, and has made the text unusually simple and clear. The object was so to deal with anatomy and physiology that the student might easily grasp the primary principles, at the same time laying a broad foundation for a wider study.

Hofmann and Peterson's Legal Medicine

Atlas of Legal Medicine. By DR. E. VON HOFMANN, of Vienna. Edited by FREDERICK PETERSON, M. D., Clinical Professor of Psychiatry in the College of Physicians and Surgeons, New York. With 120 colored figures on 56 plates, and 193 half-tone illustrations. Cloth $3.50 net. *In Saunders' Hand-Atlas Series.*

By reason of the wealth of illustrations and the fidelity of the colored plates, the book supplements all the text-books on the subject. Moreover, it furnishes to every physician, student, and lawyer a veritable treasure-house of information.

The Practitioner, London

"The illustrations appear to be the best that have ever been published in connection with this department of medicine, and they cannot fail to be useful alike to the medical jurist and to the student of forensic medicine."

Chapman's Medical Jurisprudence

Medical Jurisprudence, Insanity, and Toxicology. By HENRY C. CHAPMAN, M. D., Professor of Institutes of Medicine and Medical Jurisprudence in Jefferson Medical College, Philadelphia. Handsome 12mo of 329 pages, fully illustrated. Cloth, $1.75 net.

RECENTLY ISSUED—THIRD REVISED EDITION, ENLARGED

This third edition has been thoroughly revised and greatly enlarged, so as tc bring it absolutely in accord with the very latest advances in this important branch of medical science.

Medical Record, New York

"The manual is essentially practical, and is a useful guide for the general practitioner, besides possessing literary merit."

Golebiewski and Bailey's Accident Diseases

Atlas and Epitome of Diseases Caused by Accidents. By DR. ED. GOLEBIEWSKI, of Berlin. Edited, with additions, by PEARCE BAILEY, M. D., Consulting Neurologist to St. Luke's Hospital, New York. With 71 colored illustrations on 40 plates, 143 text-illustrations, and 549 pages of text. Cloth, $4.00 net. *In Saunders' Hand-Atlas Series.*

This work contains a full and scientific treatment of the subject of accident injury; the functional disability caused thereby; the medicolegal questions involved, and the amount of indemnity justified in given cases.

The Medical Record, New York

"This volume is upon an important and only recently systematized subject, which is growing in extent all the time. The pictorial part of the book is very satisfactory."

Stoney's Materia Medica for Nurses

Practical Materia Medica for Nurses, with an Appendix containing Poisons and their Antidotes, with Poison-Emergencies; Mineral Waters; Weights and Measures, etc. By EMILY M. A. STONEY, Superintendent of the Training School for Nurses at the Carney Hospital, South Boston, Mass. 12mo, 300 pages. $1.50 net.

RECENTLY ISSUED—SECOND REVISED EDITION

In this work the consideration of the drugs includes their names, their sources and composition, their various preparations, physiologic actions, directions for handling and administering, and the symptoms and treatment of poisoning.

Journal of the American Medical Association

"So far as we can see, it contains everything that a nurse ought to know in regard to drugs. As a reference-book for nurses it will without question be very useful."

Stoney's Nursing

Practical Points in Nursing: for Nurses in Private Practice. By EMILY M. A. STONEY, Superintendent of the Training School for Nurses at the Carney Hospital, South Boston, Mass. 466 pages, fully illustrated. Cloth, $1.75 net.

THIRD REVISED EDITION—RECENTLY ISSUED

In this volume the author explains the entire range of *private* nursing as distinguished from *hospital* nursing, and the nurse is instructed how best to meet the various emergencies of medical and surgical cases when distant from medical or surgical aid or when thrown on her own resources. An especially valuable feature will be found in the direction how to *improvise* everything ordinarily needed in the sick-room.

The Lancet, London

"A very complete exposition of practical nursing in its various branches, including obstetric and gynecologic nursing. The instructions given are full of useful detail."

Stoney's Technic for Nurses

Bacteriology and Surgical Technic for Nurses. By EMILY M. A. STONEY, Superintendent of the Training School, Carney Hospital, South Boston. Revised by FREDERIC R. GRIFFITH, M. D., Surgeon, N. Y. 12mo, 278 pages, illus. $1.50 net.

RECENTLY ISSUED—NEW (2d) EDITION

Spratling on Epilepsy

Epilepsy and Its Treatment. By WILLIAM P. SPRATLING, M. D., Medical Superintendent of the Craig Colony for Epileptics, Sonyea, New York. Octavo of 522 pages, fully illustrated. Cloth, $4.00 net.

American Pocket Dictionary **4th Ed.—Recently Issued**

AMERICAN POCKET MEDICAL DICTIONARY. Edited by W. A. NEWMAN DORLAND, M. D., Assistant Obstetrician to the Hospital of the University of Pennsylvania. Containing the pronunciation and definition of the principal words used in medicine and kindred sciences, with 64 extensive tables. Handsomely bound in flexible leather, with gold edges, $1.00 net; with patent thumb index, $1.25 net.

"I can recommend it to our students without reserve."—J. H. HOLLAND, M. D., *Dean of the Jefferson Medical College*, Philadelphia.

Warwick and Tunstall's First Aid

FIRST AID TO THE INJURED AND SICK. By F. J. WARWICK, B. A., M. B. Contab., Associate of King's College, London; and A. C. TUNSTALL, M. D., F. R. C. S. Edin., Surgeon-Captain Commanding the East London Volunteer Brigade Bearer Company. 16mo of 232 pages and nearly 200 illustrations. Cloth, $1.00 net.

Starr's Diets for Infants and Children

DIETS FOR INFANTS AND CHILDREN IN HEALTH AND IN DISEASE. By LOUIS STARR, M. D., Consulting Pediatrist to the Maternity Hospital, Philadelphia. 230 blanks (pocket-book size). Bound in flexible Morocco, $1.25 net.

Grafstrom's Mechano-Therapy **Recently Issued 2d Revised Edition**

A TEXT-BOOK OF MECHANO-THERAPY (Massage and Medical Gymnastics). By AXEL V. GRAFSTROM, B. Sc., M.D., Attending Physician to the Gustavus Adolphus Orphanage, Jamestown, New York. 12mo, 200 pages, illustrated. Cloth, $1.25 net.

Shaw on Nervous Diseases and Insanity

Recently Issued—Fourth Edition, Revised

ESSENTIALS OF NERVOUS DISEASES AND INSANITY: their Symptoms and Treatment. A Manual for Students and Practitioners. By the late JOHN C. SHAW, M. D., Clinical Professor of Diseases of the Mind and Nervous System, Long Island College Hospital, New York. 12mo of 204 pages, illustrated. Cloth, $1.00 net. *In Saunders' Question-Compend Series.*

Powell's Diseases of Children **3d Edition, Revised**

ESSENTIALS OF THE DISEASES OF CHILDREN. By WILLIAM M. POWELL, M. D. Revised by ALFRED HAND, JR., A. B., M. D., Dispensary Physician and Pathologist to the Children's Hospital, Philadelphia. 12mo volume of 259 pages. Cloth, $1.00 net. *In Saunders' Question-Compend Series.*

Published by

Facsimile Publisher
Ashok Vihar, Delhi-110052 (India)
Website: www.facsimilepublisher.com

Distributed by

Gyan Books Pvt. Ltd.
5, Ansari Road, Daryaganj, New Delhi-110002 (India)
E-mail: books@gyanbooks.com, Website: www.gyanbooks.com

2 222000 000424